S0-CLU-874

Family Planning Operations Research

Family Planning Operations Research

A Book of Readings

JAMES R. FOREIT
TOMAS FREJKA

EDITORS

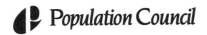 Population Council

◖▌ Population Council

The Population Council is an international, nonprofit, nongovernmental institution that seeks to improve the wellbeing and reproductive health of current and future generations around the world and to help achieve a humane, equitable, and sustainable balance between people and resources. The Council conducts biomedical, social science, and public health research and helps build research capacities in developing countries. Established in 1952, the Council is governed by an international board of trustees. Its New York headquarters supports a global network of regional and country offices.

Population Council
One Dag Hammarskjold Plaza
New York, NY 10017 USA

© 1998 by The Population Council, Inc. All rights reserved.

Library of Congress Cataloging-in-Publication Data

Family planning operations research : a book of readings / James R. Foreit,
    Tomas Frejka, editors.
       p.   cm.
    Includes bibliographical references.
    ISBN 0-87834-092-0 (pbk. : alk. paper)
    1. Birth control—Research. 2. Birth control clinics—Management—Research.
    3. Operations research. I. Foreit, James R. II. Frejka, Tomas.
    HQ763.5.F34 1998
    363.9'6'072–dc21   98-40823
                                                CIP

Spanish edition, *Investigación operativa en planificación familiar: lecturas selectas*, with a preface by Jorge Balán, forthcoming 1998.

French edition, *La recherche opérationnelle en planification familiale: un recueil d'articles*, forthcoming 1999.

Printed in the United States of America

This book is dedicated to the memory of
Bernard Berelson
whose thoughtfulness and leadership
put an indelible mark on the development
of family planning research.

CONTENTS

RESOURCES

QUALITY OF CARE

CONDUCT

FOREWORD

This book assembles some of the best family planning operations research literature to emerge over a 35-year period. It draws examples from all three developing continents and across a remarkable range of subjects. It covers methods as well as results, and it shows the diversity of institutions studied.

Some 40 years have elapsed since the first operations research projects were carried out. Even some of the top professionals in the field today are not familiar with such projects as the Singur, India, experiment that, starting in late 1957, increased contraceptive use and reduced fertility, with careful measurement of results in both control and experimental villages. The famous Taichung experiment of the 1960s used a 12-cell design and found gradients of response that tracked intensity of effort, all compared to cost. In Thailand, the Photaram experiment established in 1964, helped to set the stage for a national program, as did trials in other countries. The news of such activities spread internationally, and by 1977, some 96 OR projects had been described. Meanwhile family planning surveys had proliferated: By 1969, some 400 had been catalogued; most of these were local, but more than 300 national surveys in 98 countries were to follow.

The ensuing decades saw literally thousands of pilot projects and quasi-experiments conducted throughout the developing world. These continue today; the editors note that 75–100 projects are running at any one time—far too many for any one person to follow. The full literature now exceeds anyone's grasp. Fortunately, there are index services and rare volumes like this one, to winnow out what is relevant and best.

OR personnel have faced extremely diverse working conditions in three respects: in the problems posed to them, in the program settings involved, and in the data at hand or collectable. They have been forced to invent new methods and adapt old ones, thus enriching the battery of research techniques now available. A notable example is that of situation analysis. After its demonstration on 99 Kenyan service points, the technique spread rapidly to be used in countries in all three developing continents. Focus groups and other qualitative methods have also come to the fore and done much to inform quantitative survey approaches.

During its long history, OR has found its place in the "middle ground" of management concerns. Trivial matters are to be avoided, and issues of grand strategy are uncommon. In between is a wealth of pressing problems, as well as key opportunities, to be examined. Illustrative cases fall under the book's five section headings of impact, access, resources, quality of care, and conduct. Each of the five has its own importance. For resources, for example, it is the dual squeeze of growth in both numbers and proportions who will use contraceptives, matched with increased demands resulting from the International Conference on Population and Development of 1994. OR is responding to these challenges from a strong base, as it is firmly entrenched as part of the family planning and reproductive health establishment. It commands sizable shares of donor funding, organizational resources, research talent, and publication exposure. Therefore, it is fair to ask how far its findings are applied in practice, and the editors address such questions as the generalizability of OR results. Many studies are, in fact, limited to a particular program; this limiting fits the results to the local setting and makes their adoption more likely. However, some studies produce lessons that are broadly applicable, such as the rise in contraceptive use when several methods, not just one, are offered to the public.

Whether managers pay attention to the findings that researchers offer them depends on several factors; more managers do so when they are brought into the early planning of a study, and more do so when they grasp that OR is meant to serve their particular concerns. The editors stress that, properly understood, OR is distinguished by its orientation to the administration and improvement of action programs. However, managers and researchers tend to speak different languages and respond to different pressures. Managers also have less time to read. Nevertheless, they may listen to people who do read, so key persons located in the interface between the researcher and the manager can play important roles.

Although this book is directed to young people just entering the field, it will also remind older heads of important studies they may have forgotten and save them from needlessly repeating them. Some selections have not been published before, and one, the update on the Taichung study, is an original contribution for this volume. The editors' section introductions are must readings for the perspectives they provide on the individual studies, as is the overview of the field in the general introduction that follows. Operations research, with its long history, methodological depth, and rich geographic and substantive variety, is well represented in this volume.

JOHN A. ROSS
Senior Fellow
The Futures Group International

ACKNOWLEDGMENTS

The editors wish to express special thanks to Rodolfo Bulatao, Karen Foreit, Sarah Harbison, and Nancy Sloan for their helpful comments on earlier drafts of this book. We also wish to acknowledge the contribution, written especially for this volume, of Ronald Freedman, distinguished scholar of family planning at the University of Michigan. We are most grateful to Guille Herrera for her dedicated work in producing the Spanish version. We also wish to thank Silvia Llaguno for her valuable contribution in coordinating the Spanish translation. Last but not least, we are grateful to the editorial staff of the New York Office of the Population Council, especially Robert Heidel, Julie Sitney, Y. Christina Tse, and Karen Tweedy-Holmes for their assistance in bringing this book into print. Publication was financed by the United States Agency for International Development, Office of Population, as part of contract AID/CCP-C-00-95-00007-00, "Latin America and the Caribbean Operations Research and Technical Assistance in Family Planning and Reproductive Health."

Introduction

James R. Foreit and Tomas Frejka

For as long as there have been family planning programs, there has been family planning research. At the theoretical level, researchers examine the effect of fertility on health and socioeconomic development and study the determinants of fertility for individuals and populations. At the policy level, studies explore the role of family planning programs in modifying fertility and health. The development of new contraceptives is accompanied by clinical and preintroductory trials carried out in program settings. Surveys are conducted to measure changes in contraceptive use and fertility, and the results are used to make decisions affecting programs. Finally, programs themselves carry out operations research (OR) to improve service delivery.

The aim of this volume is to provide an overview of how operations research is used by family planning programs. The readings in this book illustrate many of the major issues and topics that have benefitted from operations research, as well as many of the research designs encountered among OR studies. The book also provides information about the problems that programs and researchers encounter in carrying out operations research and the challenges faced in translating research findings into changes in day-to-day program operations.

The first four sections in this book deal with major operations research topic areas including program impact, access, resources, and quality of care. The last section deals with issues in the conduct of OR studies and the use of OR findings. Each section begins with a brief introduction intended to provide the reader with basic information about the topic under consideration, and about the programmatic and research issues dealt with in the readings. Occasionally, section introductions also suggest areas within the section topics requiring further study. Finally, most papers are prefaced by brief remarks by the editors designed to identify the salient aspects and issues raised by each study.

The field of family planning has broadened into reproductive health as other services (for example, treatment for reproductive tract infections) are integrated into previously single-purpose family planning programs or, conversely, as other reproductive health services (for example, postabortion care) have begun to include family planning. So far, reproductive health operations research is still in a formative stage. However, we believe that many of the definitions, principles, and lessons learned in this book will be as applicable to the newer field of reproductive health operations research as to the narrower field of family planning operations research.

What Is Operations Research? When to Do It and How to Do It

In defining the domain of operations research, we distinguish OR from other kinds of technical assistance for decisionmaking and from other kinds of family planning research. What distinguishes OR from other technical assistance activities is the application of systematic research techniques to program improvement (Ross et al., 1987). What distinguishes OR from other types of research is the focus on factors under the control of managers and the inclusion of indicators of program success.

We consider a family planning program to be any organized effort whose purpose is to help individuals regulate their fertility. Family planning programs are directed by managers who function at many different levels, from the individual service-delivery point, as in the case of a family planning clinic administrator, to the national cabinet level, as in the case of a Minister of Health. Some managers have immediate "hands-on" responsibility for seeing that services are delivered in a small area, whereas other managers are high-level policymakers responsible for the general oversight and planning of the program at a national level.

All family planning program managers—whether their programmatic mission is to provide information and services for individuals already motivated to regulate their fertility, to stimulate demand for contraceptive goods and services, or a combination of the two—must make decisions: what goods and services to offer, what kinds of workers to recruit, where to locate facilities, what prices to charge, and what promotional avenues to employ. The goal of operations research is to provide program managers with information they can use to make decisions to improve their programs' operations. Operations Research can help managers decide between alternative courses of action, identify and take advantage of opportunities, and find solutions to service-delivery problems that limit program effectiveness and efficiency.

To phrase these criteria in the language of experimental design, we would say that independent variables in operations research are factors that can be manipulated by managers—type of training, frequency of supervision, prices charged—and that dependent variables are indicators of program success—program outputs (number of clinic visits, contraceptives distributed), outcomes (client knowledge, contraceptive continuation rates, prevalence rates), and individual or population impacts (fulfillment of individual fertility desires, prevention of unwanted pregnancies, fertility rates, maternal morbidity), or cost-effectiveness of program operations (cost per unit of output). Research that does not fulfill both the criteria of managerial control over the independent variables and inclusion of indicators of program success as dependent variables is not OR. Thus, studies that report lack of education, rural residence, or adherence to traditional value systems as barriers to family planning program use are not operations research because none of these is a factor under the control of managers. This definition is not proposed to argue that factors not potentially under the control of managers are unimportant. On the contrary, the program manager's responsibility is to design and test interventions to overcome the barriers posed by these contextual factors. Thus, research that tests strategies for removing barriers to use, such as mobile clinics employed to provide services in rural areas, qualifies as operations research.

Operations research addresses major program concerns including problems related to impact, access, resource allocation and mobilization, quality, and their interrelationships. *Impact* refers to program effects as measured by changes in individuals' lives and well-being, improvements in health, and declines in unwanted fertility. *Access* refers to making services available geographically, economically, administratively, and psychologically. *Resources* refers to the ability of a program manager to make the most efficient use of existing resources and to obtain additional resources, and *quality of care* refers to the appropriateness of the service provided, and the degree of competence with which it is provided. These factors are interrelated, and changes in one will result in changes in the others (Chelminsky, 1993). These changes may be either positive or negative. Throughout this book we draw attention to the inter-relatedness of the themes to encourage researchers and managers to examine the effects of interventions as broadly as possible.

In dealing with these themes, OR focuses on inputs and processes such as planning, financing, evaluation, and monitoring; selection and training of staff; supervision; logistics; and client education, all of which are under the control of managers. Thus, if we wish to improve the quality of a program, we may manipulate processes such as provider training or supervision or information given to the client. If the problem is to improve access, OR may focus on factors such as price, number and location of services, publicity, or logistics.

In common with many other disciplines, the process of operations research follows several steps including (1) problem definition; (2) solution generation; (3) solution testing; (4) analysis of the success of the solutions; and (4) results dissemination (Fisher et al., 1991). The two broad types of operations research are diagnostic studies, which do not include manipulation of an independent variable, and intervention studies, which do include manipulation of an independent variable. We conduct diagnostic studies to determine whether problems exist, to set priorities for their solution, and to generate hypotheses for program improvement. Diagnostic studies are not conducted for their own sakes, but because the information they obtain is potentially useful in the design of intervention studies. The Senegal situation analysis presented in the Quality of Care section and the article on developing a culturally appropriate family planning program in Navrongo, Ghana, which appears in the Conduct section, are examples of diagnostic operations research.

Intervention OR manipulates inputs and processes to improve outputs, outcomes, and impacts. It either compares altered inputs and processes with routine (unchanged) practices, or else compares two or more new alternatives to see which produce the more effective or efficient program. Intervention research includes demonstration projects, experiments, and simulations. The latter often have the advantage of being easier and quicker to conduct than a demonstration or experiment, but the findings of simulations must be validated empirically, reducing their advantages over other types of intervention research. Every section in this book contains examples of intervention studies. The paper on intrauterine device revisit norms in the CEMOPLAF program in Ecuador (Foreit et al., 1998) that appears in the Resources section is an example of an operations research simulation.

Various commentators have asked the question, "What is the right way to do OR?" This question focuses on methodological techniques and the process of OR rather than on its outcome. Family planning operations research is not limited to specific research techniques. Both quantitative and qualitative methods can be used, including observations, demonstrations, experiments, and quasi-experiments, models, surveys, focus groups, in-depth interviews, and mystery clients. Advocates of applied research in family planning and reproductive health programs are sometimes divided into different methodological camps: those who argue that true experimental designs should be used because they provide the most powerful tests of program effects (see Bauman, 1997 and Bauman et al., 1994) and those who argue for nonexperimental designs because of lower cost and ease of implementation (see Reynolds, 1991). We feel that both camps miss an essential point by focusing on design issues rather than on the nature of the program problem and the decision that the manager needs to make. In combination, the nature of the information needed to make the decision, the program setting, the degree of precision required of the information, and the cost of making a wrong decision all determine the appropriate methodological approach. In this book, we present studies demonstrating a variety of approaches to a wide range of problems, and discuss, for each study, why the particular design employed was appropriate for that problem in that setting.

A paradox of operations research is that testing a successful program interven-tion does not equal successful operations research. The success criterion for OR is the amount of program change that results from the research. The implication of this criterion is that the operations research process must include steps that maxi-mize the potential for using the results, and that the operations researcher be-comes an advocate for the research. She or he must have access to decision-makers and be able to communicate with them effectively and concisely. Expe-rience suggests that findings are more likely to be used if researchers, managers, and other stakeholders are involved in the research process from the very begin-ning and if the research is conducted in the context of a long-term commitment between researchers and policymakers (Davis and Howden-Chapman, 1996). In the Conduct section of this book, the Stevens and Stevens (1992) paper about the in-troduction of small cash incentives to promote child spacing in an Indian family planning program details the many steps and activities involved in moving interven-tions from the research to the routine program level.

Origins and Scope of Family Planning Operations Research

Family planning OR has origins different from operations research programs in military, health, and industrial settings, which rely heavily on techniques devel-oped by mathematicians, engineers, and experimental psychologists (Austin and Boxerman, 1995). Operations research that draws on these disciplines is often referred to as operations analysis and is defined by a set of methodologies. Un-like operations analysis, family planning OR is not methodologically defined, and it has been influenced by many social science disciplines including anthropology, demography, economics, social psychology, marketing, and sociology (Freedman, 1965 and 1967). The term operations research as applied to family planning did not come into general use until the 1970s. The term was probably first used by the United States Agency for International Development (USAID) in a contract when it established a program of applied research in Asia in 1981 that was car-ried out by the Population Council.

Operations research has also been heavily influenced by international po-litical developments. The first OR grew out of the need to counter political oppo-sition and indifference to family planning programs, and OR's continuing devel-opment has been heavily influenced by changes in local and international family planning program environments. Thus, the emphasis of early operations research was on demonstrating that family planning programs could have an effect on reproductive health and well-being, and many early operations research studies were embedded in broader programs of policy research (Freedman, 1998, in this volume). The need to measure fertility impacts also led to the involvement of demographers in OR and contributed to the emphasis on counting users that characterizes many program output and outcome indicators.

Once family planning programs were accepted as a way to reduce fertility and improve health, researchers began to experiment with new service-delivery strategies to improve access to and the impact of programs. Beginning in the 1960s, OR was used to test community-based distribution (CBD) of contraceptives, mobile clinics, postpartum family planning programs, and a variety of family planning promotional strategies. Later, the fear of reductions in international donor funding stimulated interest in resource allocation and mobilization. Most recently, the emergence of an international women's movement often critical of family planning programs has provided the impetus for study of quality of care.

Studies entirely devoted to problems of quality of services began to appear in the OR literature in the 1990s, and after the International Conference on Population and Development (ICPD), held in Cairo in 1994, endorsed a program for achieving universal reproductive health and reproductive rights, OR began to focus on the problems of integrating family planning and other reproductive health services.

The first family planning operations research studies in developing countries were conducted in the 1950s in India, Puerto Rico, and Sri Lanka (Cuca and Pierce, 1977), and in the early 1960s in Korea (Keeny, 1966), Taiwan (Chow et al., 1966; Hsu et al., 1966), Thailand, Bangladesh and Pakistan (Cuca and Pierce, 1977). Technical assistance was provided to many of these projects by the Ford Foundation, Harvard University, the Population Council, and the University of Michigan. The national family planning programs in many Asian countries rapidly built up their research capacities and had institutionalized programs of applied research by the early 1970s. Operations research began in Latin America in the 1960s and in sub-Saharan Africa in the 1970s.

Cuca and Pierce (1977) identified 96 family planning program "experiments" conducted in developing countries between 1961 and 1972. In 1965, the United States began to provide support to family planning programs in developing countries, and since that date, USAID has been the major international family planning operations research donor. USAID supports applied research in Africa, Asia, and Latin America. The combined annual budget of these projects is now approximately $15 million and about 75–100 research projects are under way at any given time. Other operations research donors (Ross et al., 1987) include the United Nations Population Fund (UNFPA) and the World Health Organization (WHO).

The applicability of operations research to a variety of health programs other than family planning has been recognized by donors and programs alike. OR components are now included in AIDS, child-survival, breastfeeding-promotion, and primary health-care initiatives. The existence of applied programmatic research in these fields owes a great deal to the ground-breaking field of family planning operations research.

A Note on the Readings Selected for This Book

We have selected papers that illustrate the variety of family planning program settings where OR has been used, the specific questions addressed, and the methodological approaches employed. General inclusion criteria included the subject matter, quality, and conciseness of the study. Most of the papers were previously published in peer-reviewed journals. The volume also contains some previously unpublished papers that represent newer research themes, especially quality of care. One of the unpublished papers was written at the request of the editors by Ronald Freedman of the University of Michigan. Students should also find the readings in this book useful companions to the *Handbook for Family Planning Operations Research Design* (Fisher et al., 1991) and other treatises on field research, and on quasi-experimental and experimental design.

Readers interested in learning more about family planning operations research will find the book, *Operations Research: Helping Family Planning Programs Work Better* (Seidman and Horn, 1991) a useful guide to issues related to the substance and conduct of operations research. The monographs, *Operations Research: Lessons for Policy and Programs* (Gallen and Rinehart, 1986), *Findings From Two Decades of Family Planning Research* (Ross and Frankenberg, 1993), and *How Operations Research Is Improving Reproductive Health Services* (Shane and Chalkley, 1998) summarize many important operations research studies not included in this reader. The article "Perspectives on Operations Research" (Ross et al., 1987) contains many valuable insights into the role of operations research in family planning programs. Finally, those seeking reports and articles on specific OR projects, or simply wishing to remain current on operations research activities, should consult the POPLINE database, keyword "operations research," available online from Johns Hopkins University at http://www.jhuccp.org/popwel.stm.

References

Austin, Charles J. and Stuart B. Boxerman. 1995. *Quantitative Analysis for Health Services Administration.* Ann Arbor, MI: AUPHA Press/Health Administration Press.

Bauman, Karl. 1997. "The effectiveness of family planning programs evaluated with true experimental designs." *American Journal of Public Health* 7,4: 666–669.

Bauman, Karl et al. 1994. "Use of experimental designs for family planning program evaluation: Merits, problems and solutions." *International Family Planning Perspectives*, 20: 108–113.

Chelminsky, E. 1993. "The political debate about health care: Are we losing sight of quality?" *Science* 262: 525–528.

Chow, L.P. et al. 1966. "Taiwan: Experimental Series." *Studies in Family Planning* no. 13: 1–5.

Cuca, Roberto and Catherine S. Pierce. 1977. *Experiments in Family Planning, Lessons from the Developing World*. Baltimore and London: The Johns Hopkins University Press.

Davis, Peter and Philippa Howden-Chapman. 1996. "Translating research findings into health policy." *Social Science Medicine* 43,5: 865–872.

Fisher, Andrew et al. 1991. *Handbook for Family Planning Operations Research Design*. New York: The Population Council.

Freedman, Ronald. 1965. "Family planning programs today: Major themes of the Geneva conference." *Studies in Family Planning* no. 8 (supplement).

———. 1967. "The behavioral sciences and family planning programs: Report on a conference." *Studies in Family Planning* no. 23: 1–12.

Gallen, M. and W. ,-Rinehart. 1986. "Operations research: Lessons for policy and programs." *Population Reports*, Series J, no. 31. Baltimore, MD: The Johns Hopkins University Press.

Hsu, S.C. et al. 1966. "Cost analysis of the Taichung experiment." *Studies in Family Planning* no. 10: 6–15.

Keeny, S.M. 1966. "Korea and Taiwan: The 1965 story." *Studies in Family Planning* no. 10: 1–6.

Reynolds, Jack. 1991. "A reconsideration of operations research experimental design." In Myrna Seidman and Marjorie C. Horn, op. cit. Pp. 377–394.

Ross, John A. et al. 1987. "Perspectives on operations research." *International Family Planning Perspectives* 13,4: 128–135.

Ross, John and Elizabeth Frankenberg. 1993. *Findings From Two Decades of Family Planning Research*. New York: The Population Council.

Seidman, Myrna and Marjorie C. Horn. 1991. *Operations Research: Helping Family Planning Programs Work Better. Progress in Clinical and Biological Research* vol. 371. New York: Wiley-Liss.

Shane, Barbara and Kate Chalkley. 1998. *How Operations Research is Improving Reproductive Health Services*. Washington, DC: Population Reference Bureau.

IMPACT

Introduction

Tomas Frejka

Operations research projects described in the papers presented in this section were designed to demonstrate that family planning programs can have an impact on fertility, fertility regulation, and health. Historically, these were the first operations research projects, even though the term was not used before the 1970s. Impact studies were considered necessary to convince policymakers of the utility of family planning programs for social and economic progress in their respective countries. Critics of family planning programs argued that no demand for contraceptives existed, or that once demand for fertility regulation appeared, fertility would decline as rapidly without a program as with one (Davis, 1967). The need to demonstrate the effectiveness of family planning programs is illustrated in papers included in this section, in particular by Faúndes-Latham et al. and by Berelson and Freedman, and is discussed in detail by Freedman.

Program impact is measured by:

- declines in fertility;
- changes in the prevalence and composition of means of fertility regulation; and
- improvements in health.

From the beginning, programs aimed to lower fertility, because high fertility was regarded as a barrier to economic and social progress, and because rapid population growth incurs high social costs, mainly in education, health, employment, and housing (Coale and Hoover, 1958; Robinson, 1975). Fertility declines are brought about by increased fertility regulation, although regulation is not the only proximate cause of this decline. Changes in patterns of cohabitation have been the other significant factor in fertility decline. Almost universally, in those developing countries where the fertility transition is well under way, marriages are being postponed with the result that proportions of married women are declining, bringing about a meaningful fertility-depressing impact. In other words, the historical fertility decline of the past several decades in the developing countries has been achieved by a combination of increased fertility regulation and changes in cohabitation patterns.

Changes in the prevalence and composition of means of fertility regulation involve increases in the use of contraceptives, primarily of effective modern contraceptives, such as the IUD, hormonal methods, and voluntary sterilization. Moreover, an expanding body of experience indicates that a widening choice of contraceptives tends to increase their attractiveness to clients and leads to increased use (Potter, 1971; Jain, 1989).

High fertility also implies poor reproductive health status. The improvements in health that early family planning programs strived for were declines in maternal, perinatal, and infant morbidity and mortality. From the time when the first family planning programs were organized, pregnancies of very young and of older women, short intervals between births, unwanted pregnancies, and unsafe induced abortions were understood to be potential health hazards for women and the children they were bearing. Thus, family planning programs were designed and organized to ameliorate these hazards (see also *International Encyclopedia of Population*, 1982).

A simultaneous objective for some programs was to lower the incidence of unsafe abortions, which are widespread throughout the developing world. In Latin America, the prevention of abortion was among the objectives of the earliest organized family planning programs, for example of BEMFAM in Brazil and of PROFAMILIA in Colombia. In countries where induced abortion is legal, family planning programs included the procedure as a program method, for example, in South Korea (Hong and Watson, 1976). To date there appear to be no operations research projects in the published literature dealing with aspects of induced abortion, probably because of the subject's political sensitivity.

During the 1960s, 1970s, and 1980s, other threats to maternal and child health surfaced. These included considerable declines in the duration of breastfeeding in numerous developing countries and the spread of sexually transmitted diseases (STDs), including HIV/AIDS. The realization that prolonged breastfeeding strengthens infant health and extends the period of postpartum infertility stimulated the inclusion of breastfeeding promotion as part of postpartum family planning programs. The prevention of STDs, especially HIV/AIDS, began to be integrated into family planning programs in the 1980s, a decade that saw the revitalization of condom promotion because the condom serves the double purpose of fertility regulation and STD prevention.

The International Conference on Population and Development (ICPD) in 1994 further expanded the concern for reproductive health to many new areas such as maternal nutrition, adolescent fertility, female genital mutilation and other violence against women.

In the early days of family planning, operations research often accompanied the implementation of a new program (see, for example, Faúndes-Latham et al., in this volume). Thus, researchers studied the program per se as the intervention, and used fertility or contraceptive behavior as the dependent variable. Currently, in already existing programs, OR is usually designed to improve specific aspects, namely access, resource allocation and mobilization, or quality. As a result, the program is expected to increase contraceptive use, thereby producing impacts on health and fertility. In these studies, indicators of increased access or quality are the interventions and contraceptive use or fertility is the dependent variable. A number of papers in other sections of this volume are of this nature (for example, León and Cuesta; K. Foreit et al.; and the two articles by J. Foreit et al.).

The opposite is also true. Studies designed to demonstrate a program impact, whether on health, fertility regulation, or fertility, will often improve access, enhance resource allocation and mobilization, or refine the quality of services. All of the projects discussed in this section have improved access to family planning, demonstrating that program impact and access tend to be closely related. The Thai project, in which auxiliary midwives were trained to prescribe oral contraceptives, could just as well have been included in the Access section of the reader. In this project, Rosenfield and Limcharoen (reprinted here) considered the significant impact of the respective activities as being the result of "bringing services closer to the people."

Many impact projects also enhance the quality of the services being provided. For instance, the Bangladesh project (Phillips et al., in this volume) demonstrated that a user-oriented program with a wide choice of methods that incorporates skilled counseling, the treatment of side effects, and ancillary health services will be substantially more effective than a program based on one or two methods distributed by unskilled workers.

Impact projects frequently incorporate explicit concerns for the allocation of resources, because programs almost always face a scarcity of funds. An objective of the Taiwan project (Berelson and Freedman) was to determine how much family planning could be achieved at what cost (money, personnel, and time). Important findings included the information that visiting both husbands and wives compared with visiting wives alone was not worth the additional cost and that one-time methods, such as the IUD, were the most cost-effective in reducing fertility.

A number of the issues dealt with in the Conduct section are also present in the papers of this section. Prominent among them is the concern for scaling up. The majority of impact projects are designed and implemented with the objective of applying the experience gained on a larger scale, be it national or international, as happened in Taiwan (Berelson and Freedman; Freedman).

So far, most research has focused on measuring program impact in terms of changes in fertility and contraceptive use as a result of widespread interest in lowering fertility in order to achieve slower population growth. Few OR projects measure improved health—not because health is a low priority, but because changes in health status are difficult to measure. As stated earlier, high fertility implies poor maternal and child health, and researchers used fertility as a proxy for maternal and child morbidity and mortality. The new ICPD agenda goes beyond maternal and child health and requires a broader focus. Future impact research must deal explicitly with health outcomes. For example, OR should attempt to determine how effective integrated programs are in reducing STD infections and in producing other desirable reproductive health outcomes.

In reviewing the projects described in the selected papers, all achieved a clear impact on fertility regulation by increasing contraceptive prevalence and by providing a wider choice of methods. An impact on lowering the prevalence of induced abortion is implied only in the Chilean project. However, the project did not devise appropriate and simple methods to measure a decline in induced abortion, presumably because of the inherent difficulty of measuring impact on a behavior that is often illegal and socially censured. Moreover, trends in induced abortion are influenced by a number of factors other than contraceptive use and method choice. Analogous problems occurred in documenting impact on maternal or child health in the other studies, although making an impact on health was likely to have been an objective in all of the studies.

The papers selected for this section all played an important role in establishing the value of family planning programs. The paper by Berelson and Freedman is arguably the first of its kind. It illustrates how many different and complex issues need to be addressed to plan and evaluate a family planning program that functions well. At the same time, it shows that a number of hypotheses can be dealt with and tested in a single project. The paper also illustrates the importance of conducting experiments that provide valuable experience on how to implement and expand programs as well as what to avoid. Experiments can also provide strong evidence for influencing high-level decisions on the implementation, expansion, and continuation of programs.

Freedman's contribution is valuable for several reasons. It summarizes the experience with operations and other research of one of the foremost social scientists in the field of family planning who has followed developments throughout the history of these programs for the past four decades. It gives examples of the relationship between operations research and other social science research in this field. Finally, it closes the circle. Among all the papers selected for the reader, the *Scientific American* paper by Berelson and Freedman, discussing the Taichung study in Taiwan, was published first, and Freedman, which deals with the same study as well as with the Taiwanese historical experience, was the last to be written.

The paper by Faúndes-Latham et al. is a good example of how to provide evidence of the extent of impact a family planning program has had on fertility. At the time it was published, the paper was important because it provided evidence that family planning programs were taking hold in Latin America. The decisive rationale in that region for introducing family planning programs was to improve reproductive health in general, and to curb unsafe abortions, in particular.

Rosenfield and Limcharoen was one of the first studies to legitimize the use of paraprofessionals for tasks that were hitherto performed only by physicians. This paper proved that one way of remedying the shortage of family planning physicians in developing countries is by training nonphysicians such as auxiliary midwives to provide services. It also shows that nonphysicians can significantly broaden access for the population to some family planning methods and thereby increase contraceptive prevalence and lower fertility.

That family planning programs can make a considerable difference in increasing contraceptive prevalence and lowering fertility in a poor rural population is an important contribution of the project described by Phillips et al. This project demonstrated that almost invariably, a demand for fertility regulation exists among poor rural populations, which, if appropriately approached, can be satisfied.

References

Coale, Ansley J. and Edgar M. Hoover. 1958. *Population Growth and Economic Development in Low-Income Countries: A Case Study of India's Prospects.* Princeton: Princeton University Press.

Davis, Kingsley. 1967. "Population policy: Will current programs succeed?" *Science* 153: 730–739.

Hong, Sung Bon and Walter Watson. 1976. *The Increasing Utilization of Induced Abortion in Korea.* Seoul: Korea University Press.

International Encyclopedia of Population, vol. 1. 1982. New York: The Free Press. Pp. 205–215, 341.

Jain, Anrudh. 1989. "Fertility reduction and the quality of family planning services." *Studies in Family Planning* 20,1: 1–16.

Potter, Robert G. 1971. "Inadequacy of a one-method family planning program." *Studies in Family Planning* 20,1: 1–6.

Robinson, Warren C. (ed.) 1975. *Population and Development Planning.* New York: The Population Council.

A Study in Fertility Control

Bernard Berelson and Ronald Freedman

Programmatic issue: *In Taiwan in 1962 preliminary findings indicated that many women/couples desired to have fewer children than they were having and that they were attempting to limit their family size largely by ineffective means. The desire for fewer children was widespread and evident because fertility had started its decline in 1959 and was declining in cities, towns, and rural areas. The general issue was to explore whether an organized family planning program could assist couples to realize their desires for reduced childbearing.*

Programmatic processes/components: *The program was the process being tested to determine if it would reduce fertility. A special focus was placed on promotional activities to determine the costs and effectiveness of home visits, mailings, and the involvement of husbands.*

Research design: *The city of Taichung with 300,000 inhabitants of which 36,000 were married women aged 20–39 was selected. 1. Public health nurses conducted a baseline and a follow-up survey with more than 2,400 of these women; 2. An experimental family planning program, which covered all 36,000 households, was designed and implemented. Posters were used and meetings with community leaders were held throughout the city. Four types of "treatments" were applied selectively in 2,400 neighborhoods (lin's), each with 20–30 families: (a) home visits with wives and husbands; (b) home visits with wives only; (c) mailing of information to newlyweds and to couples with two or more children; and (d) no effort in addition to the posters and meetings. To test the diffusion effect, the four treatments were applied in different concentrations in three different parts of the city. A concentration or density was defined by the proportion of home visits. These were administered to half the lin's in the high-density sector; to a third of the lin's in the medium sector; and to a fifth in the light sector.*

Findings: *1. The baseline survey found that couples were having more children than they wanted; they wanted a moderate number (an average of four); they approved of family limitation; they were trying to limit the number of offspring; they were poorly informed about family planning* *methods and about the physiology of reproduction; and they had a strong interest in learning about and adopting better methods. 2. The paper reported on initial findings regarding program effects. The proportion of pregnant women declined by a fifth, from 14.2 percent of married women aged 20–39 at the end of 1962 (1–2 months before the start of the program) to 11.4 percent at the end of 1963, and the proportion of women practicing contraception increased from 16 percent in February 1963 to 27 percent in March 1964, a 70 percent increase. It was later established that the program accelerated the ongoing fertility decline. Also, the proportions accepting contraception were higher in the lin's where home visits were conducted. However, home visits to husbands and wives were not more effective than home visits to wives alone. The effect of diffusion was meaningful, but family planning does not diffuse evenly. It depends on education, age, and the number of children a woman has borne, that is, it depends on the intensity of motivation.*

Program response to findings: *This project was the first of its kind and was arguably "one of the most extensive and elaborate social science experiments ever carried out in a natural setting." It was the basis for extending the program to the whole island within a few years. It influenced the development of family planning programs in many other developing countries.*

Discussion: *Although the project was complex, its implementation lived up to expectations, because it was well conceptualized, planned, and carried out by appropriately trained personnel. Although the principal aim of the project was general "impact" in modifying fertility, all other aspects of operations research were of concern and were addressed. Rational resource allocation permeated all project activities. As it became clear that people with low education have little knowledge about family planning but desire to limit their number of children, special attention was given to increase their cognitive, but also geographic and economic, access to family planning. A concern for the quality of delivery of services was also an inherent component. The principles of this 1963 program remain principles of a good program in the 1990s: to assist women to achieve their desired family size, provide a choice of contraceptive methods, provide education about the physiology of reproduction, and foster knowledge about contraceptive methods.*

A Study in Fertility Control

Bernard Berelson and Ronald Freedman

It is widely recognized that in many parts of the world there is a "population problem": the high rate of increase in population makes social and economic development difficult if not impossible. Can anything be done about the problem? Practical means of fertility control are available to individual couples, but can the control of fertility actually be implemented on a large scale in the developing areas? This article will describe an experiment designed to find out what can be done in one of the world's most densely populated places: the island of Taiwan off the coast of mainland China.

Large-scale efforts to control fertility are, to be sure, not unknown. A number of governments have assumed the responsibility of providing their people with information and services on family planning, and some countries have organized major national programs. Lowering a birthrate is a novel objective for a government, however, and no country has yet managed to achieve widespread family limitation through a planned social effort. Current programs are therefore handicapped by a lack of information on attitudes toward fertility control and by a lack of experience with programs to implement family planning.

Since any change in birthrate depends on individual decisions by large numbers of husbands and wives, it is essential to know first of all how the people concerned feel about family size and limitation. Do they need to be motivated toward family planning? If they are so motivated, how can they best be helped to accomplish their aim? To investigate these questions the Taiwan study was inaugurated a year and a half ago under the sponsorship of the provincial health department of Taiwan with the support of the Population Council, a U.S. foundation that advances scientific training and study in population matters. The most significant preliminary finding is that the people do not need to be motivated. They want to plan their families, but they need to know how. Teaching them how—implementing a family planning program—has proved to be feasible.

Taiwan has a population of about 12 million in an area of 14,000 square miles, and its population is increasing rapidly [see Fig. 1]. In recent years mortality has fallen almost to Western levels: life expectancy is more than 60 years and

---

Reprinted with the permission of *Scientific American* from *Scientific American* 1964. 21,5: 29–37, © 1964 by Scientific American, Inc. All rights reserved.

Figure 1. Rate of increase in Taiwan's population *(shaded area)* has grown because the birthrate (solid line) has remained high while the death rate *(broken line)* has fallen.

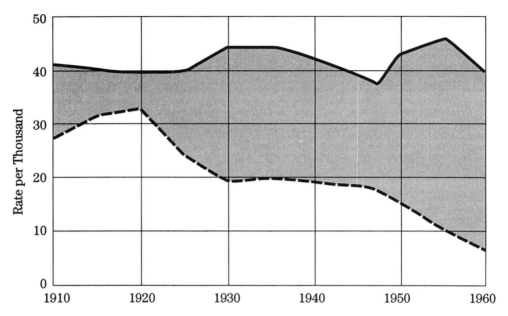

the death rate is less than eight per 1,000 of population per year. The birthrate is about 37 per 1,000, so the rate of increase is almost 3 percent per year, or enough to double the population in 25 years. Nevertheless, compared with other parts of Asia, Taiwan provides a favorable situation for the diffusion of family planning. The island is relatively urbanized and industrialized, the farmers are oriented toward a market economy, literacy and popular education are fairly widespread, there is a good transportation and communication system and a solid network of medical facilities. The standard of living is high for a population of this size in Asia outside of Japan. The society is highly organized. Women are not sharply subordinated and there are few religious or ideological objections to contraception.

The birthrate in Taiwan has been falling slowly since 1958. When fertility rates are analyzed by age group [see Fig. 2], it becomes apparent that they have decreased first and most for the older women of the childbearing population. This is exactly what one would expect if many women wanted to have a moderate number of children, had them with low mortality by the age of 30 and then tried to limit the size of their families in some way. The same pattern was observed earlier in a number of Western countries at the beginning of the declines in fertility that have tended to follow declines in mortality.

Figure 2. Fertility rates, shown here for Taiwan women in seven age groups *(figures at right)*, have fallen since 1958 in the case of the older women, presumably because they are trying to limit their families. The rates are birthrates per 1,000 women of the relevant age groups.

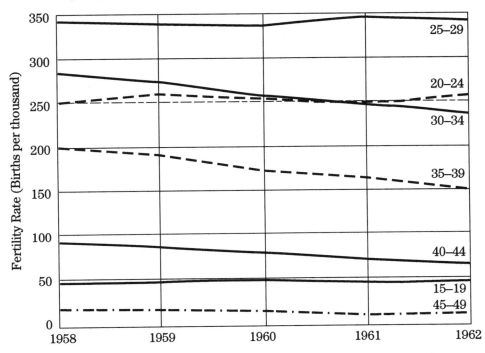

Although the situation in Taiwan was quite favorable for family planning and the birthrate trend had been downward, this was not to say that it would be a simple matter to accelerate the decline in fertility. As a first step in that effort the population studies centers in Taiwan and at the University of Michigan undertook a survey that would serve as a base line and also as a guide for a program of action. Between October, 1962, and January, 1963, public health nurses interviewed nearly 2,500 married women of the city of Taichung in the prime reproductive age group (ages 20 to 39) as to their attitudes toward family planning, their information about it and what they did about it. The survey made it clear that these women as a group wanted to have a moderate number of children, were having more children than they wanted, approved of the idea of family limitation and were trying—ineffectively—to limit the size of their families.

The number of children most of the women wanted was four, and women who had already borne more than that number acknowledged that they would have preferred fewer children [see Fig. 3]. More than 90 percent of Taichung's wives (and their husbands too, according to the wives) were favorably inclined

Figure 3. Family-size preferences are charted for Taichung wives according to the number of children they have. The chart shows the percent of wives in each group who said they would have preferred fewer children (*solid bars*) or more children (*shaded bars*) than they had or were satisfied with the number of children they had (*clear bars*).

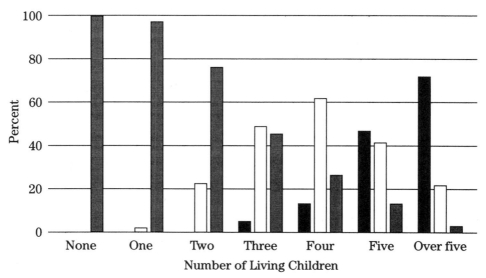

toward limiting family size. They had few objections in principle, they saw the value of such limitation for the economic welfare of their families and they did not believe that the number of children should be left to "fate" or "providence." In this regard (and the same has been found to be true in other countries) their attitudes are more advanced than some officials believe them to be.

The women were in general poorly informed about family planning methods and indeed about the physiology of reproduction. About a fourth of them had employed some means of contraception, but in most cases only after four or five pregnancies and in many cases without success. The women expressed strong interest in learning and adopting better methods. And in their own minds family planning did not conflict with their traditional feelings about the Chinese family or its central role in their lives.

Experience with contraception or other methods of limiting family size was naturally most common in the "modernized" sectors of the population: the best-educated women, the most literate and those with an urban background. The women's actual and desired fertility were also related to these characteristics [see Fig. 4], but we found that on every educational level the average woman between 35 and 39, when childbearing is not yet over, had borne more children than she wanted. This was true even of groups in which substantial numbers of women

Figure 4. Education affects family size and the use of contraceptives. The chart groups women 35 to 39 years old according to the level of schooling they had reached. The bars show the average number of children they said they had wanted *(clear bars)* and the number they had borne *(solid bars)*, and the percent of each group practicing contraception *(shaded bars)*.

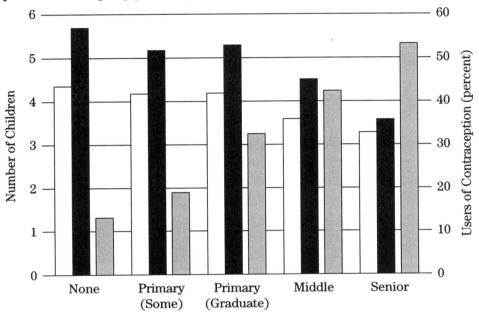

had tried to limit the size of their families: contraception had arrived on the scene too late and was too ineffective to enable such women to attain their goals.

The survey data made it clear that the women had become aware of the decline of infant mortality in their community. This is an important perception, and one that does not follow automatically on the event. (Other surveys have shown that women sometimes perceive a decrease in infant mortality as an increase in births.) Because they recognized that more children were surviving, the women appreciated that, unlike their parents, they did not need to have five to seven children in order to see three or four survive to adulthood.

The salient message of the survey was that in Taichung people have more children than they want. There are indications that the same thing is true in many similar societies. It seems clear that if throughout the world unwanted children were not conceived, a large part of the "population problem" would disappear.

The next task was to facilitate the matching of behavior to attitude—to implement family planning. Several things were required beyond the mere wish to limit the number of children: information and knowledge, supplies and services, public acceptance and social support. To study how best to enable the people of Taiwan to do what they themselves said they wanted to do, the provincial health authorities undertook to develop a program of action to make the practice of family planning more readily available in the city of Taichung. This effort, we think, is one of the most extensive and elaborate social science experiments ever carried out in a natural setting.

Taichung has a population of about 300,000, including about 36,000 married women from 20 to 39 years old, of whom 60 percent have had three or more children. Most of the people live in a central region of shops, offices and residences, but there are also rural areas within the city's administrative limits. A number of government health stations and hospital clinics provide focal points for the action program.

The city as a whole was exposed to only two aspects of the program: a general distribution of posters pointing out the advantages of family planning and a series of meetings with community leaders to inform them about the program, get their advice and enlist their support. That was the extent of the community-wide effort; the remainder of the program was designed as a differentiated experiment involving various kinds and degrees of effort. The objective was to learn how much family planning could be achieved at how much cost in money, personnel and time. To this end the local health authorities and a cooperating team from the U.S. devised four different "treatments," and applied one of them to each of the 2,389 *lin's*, or neighborhoods of 20 to 30 families, into which Taichung is divided. In order of increasing effort, the treatments were designated "Nothing," "Mail," "Everything (wives only)" and "Everything (wives and husbands)."

In the "Nothing" *lin's* there was no activity beyond the distribution of posters and the meetings with leaders. In the "Mail" *lin's* there was a direct-mail campaign addressed to two groups: newlywed couples and parents with two or more children. It was in the "Everything" neighborhoods that the major effort was made to increase family planning. The primary procedure was a personal visit to the home of every married woman from 20 to 39 years old by a specially trained staff of nurse-midwives. The fieldworkers made appointments for people at the health stations, provided contraceptive supplies, answered questions and did whatever else was necessary to satisfy a couple's desire for family planning guidance. In half of the "Everything" *lin's* the visits were made to wives only; in the other half the visits were extended to both husbands and wives, who were seen either separately or together.

Rather than apply each of these treatments to a different part of the city, the investigators decided to arrange matters so as to test a central economic issue: How much "circulation effect" can one expect in a program of this kind? To what extent can one depend on the population itself to spread the desired innovation, and how large an initial effort is required to prime the process? There has been substantial testimony that word-of-mouth diffusion played a large role in spreading ideas about family planning in the West and Japan; any such effect would clearly be of major importance to national efforts in the underdeveloped countries, which must influence large numbers of people and do so with limited resources.

In order to investigate this question of "spread" it seemed advisable to apply the four treatments in different concentrations in different parts of the city. Taichung was divided into three sectors roughly equivalent in urban-rural distribution, socioeconomic status and fertility, and designated as areas of heavy, medium and light "density." In the heavy-density sector the two "Everything" treatments were administered to half of the *lin's*, in the medium sector to a third of them and in the light sector to a fifth. In each sector the remaining *lin's* were assigned equally to the "Nothing" and the "Mail" treatment groups [see Table 1]. The *lin's* were assigned at random, although always in the proper proportion, and those designated for a particular treatment received exactly the same program regardless of their location in the city. They differed only in their environment; in the heavy-density sector, for example, "Nothing" *lin's* were much more closely surrounded by "Everything" *lin's* than were the "Nothing" neighborhoods in the two lighter-density sectors.

The program got under way in mid-February of 1963: the posters went up, meetings were held, 18 fieldworkers fanned out through the "Everything" *lin's* and the health stations prepared to receive inquiries. A set of educational materials was prepared for group and individual discussion, primarily visual aids dealing with the elementary facts about the physiology of reproduction, the reasons for practicing family planning and the major methods of contraception. The fieldworkers offered a wide choice of methods, encouraging couples to select whichever seemed most suitable: jelly, foam tablet, diaphragm, condom, rhythm, withdrawal, the oral pill and the new intra-uterine device. (The last is a recent

Table 1.

Treatment	Heavy (13,908)	Medium (11,154)	Light (11,326)	Total (36,388)
Nothing	232	243	292	767
Mail	232	244	292	768
Everything				
(wives only)	232	122	73	427
(wives and husbands)	232	122	73	427
Total *lin's*	928	731	730	2,389

Matrix shows the allocation of various "treatments" among the *lin's* in the three density sectors. The figures in parentheses give the total number of women 20–39 years old.

development that holds great promise for mass programs to reduce fertility because it does not require continued supply, sustained motivation or repeated actions on the part of the user. A plastic ring or coil is inserted in the uterus by a physician and remains there; it is extremely effective as a contraceptive, although its mode of action is still unclear.) Contraceptive supplies were provided at or below cost, or free if necessary; the pills sold for the equivalent of 75 cents for a cycle of 20. The same charge was made for the insertion of an intra-uterine device.

By the end of June fieldworkers had visited each of the nearly 12,000 designated homes at least once and more than 500 neighborhood meetings had been held. Between then and the middle of October follow-up visits were made to women or couples who had indicated interest and to women who had been pregnant or had been nursing infants earlier in the year. A final phase began in late October and is still continuing; direct action has been terminated, but services and supplies are still available at the health stations, and the momentum of the program is continuing to have effect as of this writing.

There are three ways in which the effectiveness of the whole program will be measured. One is through case records kept for all couples who were visited in their homes or came to clinics as a result of the action program. The second is a before-and-after survey of a random sample of 2,432 women of childbearing age. The final story will be told in fertility statistics to be compiled eventually from the official register.

So far one result has emerged from the before-and-after survey, and it is a key measure of the outcome: at the end of 1962, 14.2 percent of the women in the sample were pregnant, and at the end of 1963, 11.4 percent were pregnant, a decline of about a fifth.

Aside from this one statistic, only the case records are available. Even for the people directly involved it is too early to measure the effect of the program on fertility; an immediate effect would take at least nine months to begin to show up! A presumptive effect, however, can be gauged from the record of "acceptances," defined as the insertion of an intra uterine device or the receipt of instructions and the purchase of supplies for other methods, together with expressed intent to practice contraception. In the 13 months ending in mid-March of this year the action program was responsible for a total of 5,297 acceptances of family planning, 4,007 of which were from women living within Taichung proper. (The remainder came from outside the city even though no direct action was carried on there.)

How good is that record? There are different ways to appraise the figure of 4,000-odd acceptances within the city. First, the acceptors constitute 11 percent of the married women from 20 to 39. Not all the women in that age group, however, were "eligible" to accept family planning as a result of this program. About

16 percent were already practicing contraception to their own satisfaction. Another 16 percent had been sterilized or were believed to be sterile. Nine percent were pregnant, 3 percent lactating and 1 percent experiencing menstrual irregularities of one kind or another. If these women are eliminated, only about 55 percent of the 36,000 in the age group were "eligible." Of these 20,000 or so women, the program secured about 20 percent as family planners. Included in that definition of eligibility, however, are women who actively want another child—young wives who have not completed their families or those who want a son. If they are considered not really eligible for contraception at this time, the "currently eligible" category is reduced to some 10,000 women, and those who have taken up contraception in the first 13 months come to about 40 percent of this truly eligible population.

This arithmetic helps to define a "success" in the spread of family planning in the underdeveloped countries. At any given time somewhere between half and three-fourths of the target population is simply out of bounds for the purpose. If a program can get as many as a half—or even a third or a fourth of the remaining group to begin practicing contraception within a few years, it has probably achieved a good deal. In this kind of work, then, having an impact on 10 percent of the target population in a year or so is not a disappointing failure but a substantial success; one should report "Fully 10 percent," not "Only 10 percent"! Another way to appraise the Taichung results to date is to recognize that whereas in February, 1963, about 16 percent of the married women from 20 to 39 were practicing contraception, by March of this year about 27 percent were doing so, an increase of nearly 70 percent.

The impact of such a program is not felt immediately or at one time or evenly. At the outset the acceptance rate was remarkably constant, but after some seven weeks, when 40 percent of the home visits had been made and word-of-mouth reports of the program were well established, the curve began to climb steadily [see Fig. 5]. It hit a plateau in about four weeks and stayed there for about a month before declining. This was the height of the program, when two-thirds of the home visits had been completed and interest was strong. By the beginning of June, when nearly all the visits had been made, the cream had been skimmed: the women who were strongly motivated toward family planning had heard of the program and had decided what they would do about it. By the end of the summer follow-up visits were reaching less motivated women and the curve returned to its starting point. In the fall, when home visits ended but supplies and services were still available, the acceptances settled to a lower but steady rate.

A program of this kind, then, apparently starts off reasonably well, builds up quite rapidly and achieves roughly half of its first year's return within the first

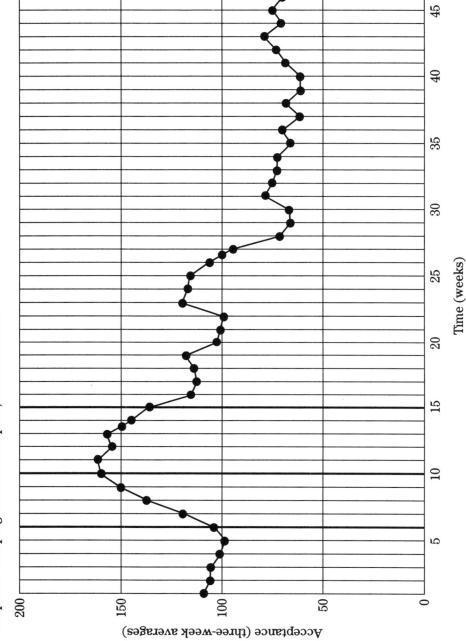

Figure 5. Progress of action program is traced by a curve showing the trend of "acceptances" of contraception in Taichung each week from the end of February 1963 to mid-January 1964. The three heavy vertical grid lines show (*left to right*) the points at which 40 percent, 62 percent, and 85 percent of the home visits had been completed. The program reached a peak, then leveled off.

Table 2.

Treatment	Heavy	Medium	Light	Total
Nothing	7	5	5	5
Mail	7	5	6	6
Everything				
(wives only)	16	13	11	14
(wives and husbands)	18	10	12	15
All treatments	12	7	7	9

Results of the program are given as of the end of last December. The figures show the acceptors as a percent of the married women aged 20–39, by "treatment" and density sector.

four months. The important thing is to develop a "critical mass" that can generate enough personal motivation and social support to carry on without further home visits. A poor country simply cannot afford visits to the entire population, so any realistic plan must rely heavily on personal and informal contacts from trusted sources; it may be that the job will have to be done by relatives, neighbors and friends or not at all. The task of a planned program will thus be to develop enough knowledgeable and convinced users of contraceptives to start a movement that reaches out to the ill-informed and unconvinced.

The indirect effects were extremely important in Taichung. The most dramatic indication is the fact that by the end of 1963 some 20 percent of the acceptances had come from women who did not even live in the city. (That figure has since risen to almost 25 percent.) Within the city about 60 percent of the acceptances were from "Everything" *lin's*; the other 40 percent were divided about equally between the "Nothing" and the "Mail" *lin's*. Even in the "Everything" neighborhoods about a sixth of those who accepted contraceptives actually came forward before their scheduled home visits had been made. Direct home visits, in other words, accounted for only some 40 percent of the acceptances by the end of December.

As for the effectiveness of various concentrations of effort, the proportion of those who accepted contraceptives was indeed higher in the heavy-density sector, but this effect was almost completely within the "Everything" *lin's* themselves [see Table 2]. The indirect effect—the "rub-off" from the home-visit areas to the "Nothing" and "Mail" *lin's*—was remarkably constant in the three sectors. Our tentative conclusion is that the maximum return for minimum expenditure can be obtained with something less than the heavy-sector degree of concentration. Finally, the added effect of visiting husbands as well as wives was not worth the expense, perhaps because in this program the preferred contraceptive method was one involving the wife alone.

Figure 6. Indirect diffusion of family planning was particularly marked in the case of the intra-uterine device. Almost all women who accepted contraception without home visits chose this device (*dark segments of bars*) rather than a traditional method (*light segments*).

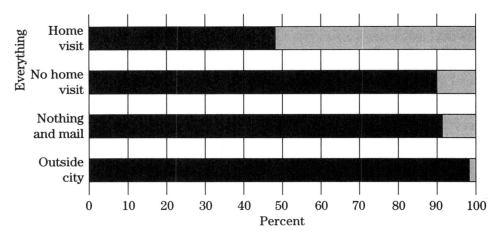

The nature of the contraceptive method, as a matter of fact, has more of an effect on the success of a program than may have been generally recognized. A "one-time" method requires far less field effort over a long term than a method dependent on resupply and sustained motivation. In Taichung the choice turned out to be overwhelmingly for the intra-uterine devices, which were preferred by 78 percent of those who accepted contraceptives; 20 percent selected one of the more traditional methods (mainly foam tablets or condoms) and 2 percent chose the oral pill (which was, to be sure, the most expensive method). The women themselves, in other words, elected the "one-time" method. This was particularly significant in view of the method's high effectiveness and what might be called its "accountability" through scheduled medical follow-ups. The six-month checkup shows that only some 20 percent of the devices have been removed or involuntarily expelled, whereas about 30 percent of the women who chose the traditional methods are no longer practicing contraception regularly.

The Taichung study revealed another significant advantage of the intra-uterine device: a striking tendency for information about it to be disseminated indirectly by word-of-mouth, obviating much of the task of communication and persuasion. Nearly 75 percent of the new devices were accepted without the necessity of a home visit, compared with only 15 percent in the case of the traditional methods. The intra-uterine devices "sold" themselves; what the home visits did, in effect, was to secure acceptance of the traditional methods [see Fig. 6]. Since last October, when the action program proper was terminated, more than

Figure 7. Acceptance of family planning varied in different groups. In this chart, the women are categorized according to various characteristics. The clear bars show the percent of the "currently eligible" women who fell into each category. The shaded bars show the percent of the new acceptors of contraception who fell into the same categories as of the end of 1963.

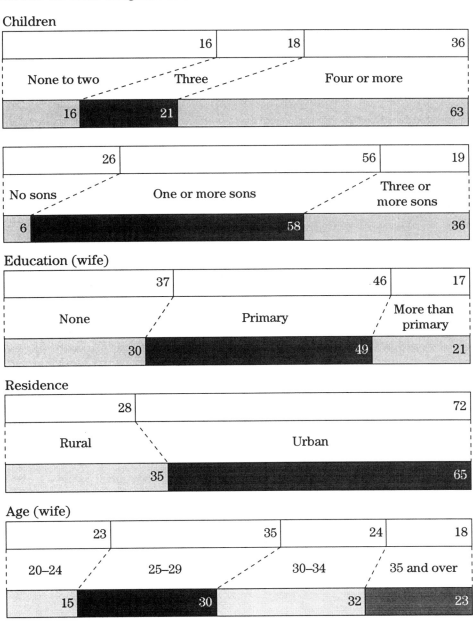

half of those who have accepted contraceptives have come from a widening circle around the city, and almost all of these women have chosen the new devices. This is presumably what happens when word of the method reaches women who are ready for family planning but want an easier and "better" way than they have heard of before.

Family planning does not, of course, diffuse evenly among the different kinds of people in a community. Acceptance varies with education and age and—in Taichung at least—above all with number of children and number of sons. When couples in Taiwan have four children, they have all they want and they are ready to do something about it—if there is something available that is reasonably effective, inexpensive and easy to use. The evidence here is that whereas the slow long-term "natural" spread of contraception through a population reaches the better-educated people first, a deliberate and accelerated effort like the Taichung program can quickly have a major impact on the families that already have large numbers of children.

Taiwan is one of many low-income countries where rapid increases in population thwart economic development and threaten to slow further improvements in the standard of living. In the long run, to be sure, it seems likely that economic and social pressures combined with personal aspirations will lead individuals to limit their families. The underdeveloped countries, however, cannot wait for a long-term solution to their present crisis. The program in Taichung suggests that fertility control can be spread by a planned effort—not so easily or so fast as death control, but nevertheless substantially, in a short period of time and economically. (The cost of each acceptance was between $4 and $8, far below the eventual economic value of each prevented birth, which has been estimated as being between one and two times the annual per capita income.)

A good deal of the story in Taiwan remains to be told, of course, including the results of the sample survey and the critical check of official birth statistics over the next months and years. Health agencies in Taiwan are now extending the program to a larger segment of the population, testing the Taichung results and trying out new approaches in the slum areas of cities and in poor fishing and mining villages. At this point one can at least say that fertility in Taiwan is changing and can be changed—changing over the long run as the result of unplanned social processes but, most significantly, changeable in the short run as the result of a planned effort to help people have the number of children they really want.

Acknowledgments

The authors wish to acknowledge the valuable contributions of their colleagues on the Taiwan project: S.C. Hsu of the Joint Commission on Rural Reconstruction in Taiwan; T.C. Hsu, Commissioner of Health; C.L. Chen and J.Y. Peng of the Maternal and Child Health Institute, and John Takeshita of the University of Michigan.

Bibliography

Colonial Development and Population in Taiwan. George W. Barclay. Princeton University Press, 1954.

The Growth of World Population. Publication 1091, National Academy of Sciences–National Research Council, 1963.

The Population Dilemma. Edited by Philip M. Hauser. Prentice-Hall, Inc., 1963.

Research in Family Planning. Edited by Clyde V. Kiser. Princeton University Press, 1962.

Operations and Other Types of Research in Taiwan's Family Planning History

Ronald Freedman

As a social demographer, I was privileged to observe almost the whole course of the demographic transition in Taiwan, from 1961 when Taiwan's total fertility rate (TFR) was 5.6 children per women to 1984, when it decreased to 2.1 and then to 1.7 by 1991. I participated in the Taichung Study, the preliminary report for which in the *Scientific American* (the article in this volume just preceding this essay) was the basis for the move to Taiwan's national family planning program. Our much more intensive analysis of the Taichung Study (Freedman and Takeshita, 1969) did not appear until the national program was well under way. In later years, I participated in or observed a large volume of additional research about the Taiwan family planning experience as the program moved to replacement fertility and beyond.

Some of that research fits easily into Foreit and Frejka's apt definition of operations research in the introduction to this volume: "The goal of operations research is to provide program managers with information they can use to make decisions to improve their programs' operations. . . . Independent variables in operations research are factors that can be manipulated by managers . . . dependent variables are indicators of program success." But other family planning research that does not fit that model neatly is important, too.

Theoretically, the definition covers both short-run and long-run research, and the wise manager should be concerned with both. However, the exigencies of running a program are likely to result in pressure to conduct research that produces early results. Much operations research has a short time horizon, although that need not be so.

I am in a good position to describe the variety of research that took place. Some projects were clearly operations research by Foreit and Frejka's definition; others were less clearly so; and others definitely were not. All of it was useful in various ways.

Some operations research results in the preliminary *Scientific American* report were issued quickly because our Taiwanese colleagues needed to use

---

This article was written for this volume. © 1998 by The Population Council, Inc.

valid results as quickly as possible. Such findings included: (a) that fieldwork contacts with both husbands and wives did not increase acceptance rates; (b) that letters to undifferentiated potential acceptors did not increase acceptance rates; (c)
that neighborhood meetings had a positive effect; (d) that a new IUD was very popular and swept the field; that strong documentation of this finding provided support
for an early decision to continue emphasis on this new method, but with careful
follow-up studies to monitor it; (e) that disadvantaged couples (for example, poor,
poorly educated, rural) accepted contraception at almost as high a rate as better-off
couples, a situation unlike that among those accepting before the program when the
disadvantaged lagged far behind. This finding bolstered a decision followed
throughout the national program to give special attention to disadvantaged
couples, a particularly important decision, because in the long run, the unexpect-
edly high acceptance rates among such couples was one of the most important
measurable effects of the program. The early decision to emphasize such couples
was already in the works, but the strong early evidence reported in the *Scientific
American* report reinforced the idea that this was feasible and productive.

The longer, more intensive, and complex report in our book-length treatment of the Taichung project covered the Taichung Study over a longer period
and included elements that also can be classified as operations research. For
example: (a) a follow-up study of IUD users over some years reported a fairly
high discontinuation of first IUDs and that nevertheless, IUD users had relatively
few pregnancies and even fewer births, because many of those who discontinued
use of first IUD insertions chose to have a second one before another pregnancy.
Some switched quickly to another method, and some who became pregnant had
an abortion. Careful follow-up of IUD acceptors was not only a desirable check
on side effects but also established that those with a first IUD insertion were
strongly motivated for birth limitation. This whole follow-up project (accompanied by reviews and reinstruction for both public and private doctors conducted
by noted IUD experts) strengthened the intention to provide service of as high a
quality as possible.

In India, where few significant follow-up studies were undertaken, the IUD
was simply dropped as a program method after the first signs of significant IUD
discontinuation rates appeared and rumors circulated of horrendous side effects.

The motto in Taiwan became, "Follow the woman, not just the method!"
These careful follow-ups in Taiwan were illustrative of a considerable effort to
stress quality of care. The follow-up studies in Taiwan bolstered the decision to
keep on emphasizing and monitoring the IUD.

In the de facto national program that fairly quickly followed the Taichung
Study, a program of short-run "experiments" clearly included operations research. These were organized mainly by George Cernada and Robert Gillespie,

consultants who worked with the Taiwanese on their program operations. The experiments (Cernada, 1970) involved deliberately short-term projects that could yield early results: a program to test the acceptability of the pill for younger women; mailings to new mothers—a success compared to the failure of mailings to general couples in the Taichung Study; a test of the effect of a marketing idea—"free contraceptives for a limited time only"—another success, and finally, a large mass media program in Taiwan's second-largest city that was followed by a large increase in acceptance rates.

I turn now to research projects for which a classification as operations research is doubtful. Some of them were, nevertheless, important for the success of the program:

One of the main purposes of the Taichung Study was to demonstrate to political leaders that a large-scale family planning effort could be carried out according to plan with measured results without political repercussions and in such a way as to provide a secure basis for an island-wide program. Indeed, the political leaders were impressed that the unmet need measured in earlier surveys was real and that meeting that need had popular support.

Similar effects resulted from early pilot programs in several countries (for example, Bangladesh, Korea, and Thailand) that had this important political and bureaucratic effect.

In Taiwan, the political sensitivity about family planning before Taichung was exemplified by the euphemistic designation "prepregnancy health" for a small program preceding Taichung. This euphemism was intended to avoid potential problems with national leaders believed to be unenthusiastic about "family planning" or "birth control."

Before actually launching the Taichung Project, S.C. Hsu, an important and charismatic public health leader who needed no persuasion, helped to obtain the essential approval of the Provincial Commissioner of Health. That the Commissioner still had trepidations just before the study began was indicated when, before the study was launched, he insisted on cancelling a large mass media plan, initially part of the study. His timidity seemed anomalous in view of the large public effort that he accepted: 12,000 home visits, thousands of revisits, 2,713 before and after survey interviews, 894 neighborhood meetings, and 50,000 posters! When the program proved to be a huge popular success, the Commissioner became its champion and talked often of "his" program.

In retrospect, I marvel at the courage of our Taiwan collaborators who not only helped with the design of a large, potentially risky project but who also were responsible for planning and executing in detail its complex logistics.

Even before the Taichung Study was completed, Hsu used such early results as those reported in *Scientific American* as a "scientific" basis for beginning what he called an "experimental" extension of the family planning program to 100 of Taiwan's 361 local areas.

Then, as early as 1964, K.T. Li, Taiwan's chief economic planner and the architect of Taiwan's Economic Miracle, announced a de facto five-year plan to provide 600,000 women with IUDs and to reduce family size by 0.5 births—all accomplished, although no official population policy or program existed. Both only came a few years later. Li was favorable to population work at an early point, and he was kept informed regularly as the activity progressed.

Persuading important political figures through a successful pilot that extension on a national level is feasible does not quite fit the operations research definition, although it is certainly good for the goal of national family planning. Perhaps whether the pilot is successful or not is the independent variable and persuading (or not) the political figures to support the family planning extension is the dependent variable.

The finding that diffusion was an important element in Taichung acceptances was important to understanding what was happening. This finding also did not fit neatly the definition of operations research, however, because what a program manager could do to produce diffusion beyond conducting a good program was not clear. The use of the mass media for such a purpose was not important then in Taiwan's program, but it was used successfully later in what was clearly operations research.

The strong diffusion findings were used sometimes to inform political leaders concerned with population policy and program budgets that a considerable multiplier of measurable program results from the large diffusion effects had been documented. We were certain, also, that an acceptance of contraception in the private sector was partly, perhaps substantially, influenced by diffusion from program efforts. Acceptance of contraception was considerable in the private sector. In retrospect, I am surprised and chagrined that we did not measure that additional effect, although doing so would not have been easy.

Finally, research that definitely was not program research is, nevertheless, very important for understanding fertility decline in Taiwan.

Some of the important findings were not explicit parts of the experimental design. An advantage of such a complex design is that many "inadvertent" findings come to light. One such was that 40 percent of acceptors in the Taichung Study had previously used and given up methods that were presumably unsatisfactory, so that the reduction of their fertility that could be attributed to the program may have been minimal. The major gain may have been in terms of these families' health, happiness, and greater feelings of personal security and in terms of better quality of care. This finding was not planned, but we greeted it with satisfaction.

The excellent population registration data in Taiwan enabled us to determine that 30 percent of the fertility decline from very high to replacement levels was a result of the decrease in proportions married, especially of those married at younger ages, a clear trend to later marriage. The remaining 70 percent was due to declines in age-specific fertility for married women. The decline to total fertility rates as low as 1.6–1.7 children per woman after that was almost entirely the result of nuptiality changes. Nearly all efforts in Taiwan and many other places, first to decrease and later to increase the rate of marriage,[1] have failed, except for that of China, which relied on compulsion. Such failures might be considered failed operations research projects in terms of their effect on fertility.

Socioeconomic change was rapid in the 23 years between 1961 and 1984, when the TFR fell from 5.6 to 2.1 children per woman. By way of illustration, income per capita increased by a factor of 4.5; junior-high-school enrollment more than doubled; consumption of electricity per capita increased 60 times; the number of households with telephones increased 60-fold; and the number of automobiles in the country increased from 9,000 to 800,000.

During approximately the same period, however, the proportion of young married couples who began married life together living with available parents fell from about 85 percent to about 65 percent. Therefore, about two-thirds of these couples were still beginning married life within a traditional configuration when the TFR reached 2.1 children. Although by 1984 substantial differentials were found in coresidence between the best- and least-educated wives and between those with the least and most premarital familial experience,[2] in about 1984, a majority still coresided with their husbands' parents at marriage in every educational category and even among wives with the least premarital traditional familial experience.

In 1984, the TFR was 2.1 children and 78 percent of married women of childbearing years were using contraceptives.

Such analyses (including multivariate analysis) were possible because the frequently repeated benchmark surveys included comparable data on familial forms on a cohort basis. As a social demographer, I had asked for and received assurances that we could include the necessary questions needed for such analyses as I have described here briefly.

This research on important sociological issues in Taiwan obviously is not operations research in terms of the Foreit and Frejka definition. However, for a considerable period of time it gave Taiwan program managers and their political superiors assurance that they could proceed without anxiety about presumed cultural barriers.

Taiwan's program, because it was an early success, was visited by thousands of people concerned with programs in developing countries. A frequent question was whether in their own settings they could expect to overcome cultural barriers. We always replied that only pilot empirical tests could determine that, but that experience elsewhere was encouraging.

One important function of the Matlab study in Bangladesh that was conducted much later was to demonstrate once again that the distinctive cultural barriers of Bangladesh were not insuperable problems, as some distinguished social demographers had thought.

Good program research is important to program managers and to their political superiors, but understanding the relevant social and cultural setting also has an important function in helping designers of new programs in different settings understand that pilot tests can replace speculation and anxiety about such issues.

A number of different kinds of research efforts in the Taiwan program confirmed and elaborated in various ways the Taichung finding that the program was especially effective in bringing disadvantaged strata to contraceptive use and lower fertility. Hermalin (1978) undertook an important multivariate areal analysis for 1966–1972. The principal independent variable was program input and the principal dependent variable was fertility, with controls for the rapid socioeconomic development during this period. Tests of different models revealed that the program contributed to the decline in fertility. The effect was the strongest in the least modernized areas, which had the highest levels of preprogram fertility. In retrospect, it is unfortunate that this analysis was not repeated at later times.

The Taiwan surveys found that the contraceptive-use levels for illiterate women increased from 11 to 78 percent in just 11 years (1965–1976), and that their fertility fell by 31 percent in just eight years. That this might have happened so quickly without the program's special interest in such women is possible but not plausible. This conclusion requires an inference from the documented emphasis that the program reached the lower-status couples and enabled them to the use of contraceptives. The record indicates that the program was much more successful in helping couples initiate the practice of contraception than in changing their preferences for number of children.

An important issue is whether the program could and did act successfully to reduce family-size preferences. Te-Hsiung Sun, the very competent Director of the Taichung Family Planning Institute for many years, believes that, after an initial period of about ten years when the supply of "ready" acceptors was reduced by rapid adoption of contraception, the program had to seek clients elsewhere and was able to work successfully to reduce family-size preferences (Sun, 1997). He points especially to the effects of an intensive education campaign in 1971 when "many disadvantages of having too many children were emphasized through home visits, meetings, and mass media." As Sun indicated, between the 1970 and 1973 surveys, a decrease in family-size preferences occurred that was greater than that in the periods immediately preceding or following. Although the intensive educational effort may, indeed, have played a role in producing this effect, the evidence for other influences includes: (1) survey data for 1970–1971 for women aged 20–29 that indicate that at least for these younger married women, most of their preference reduction occurred before the education campaign; (2) continuing rapid economic development that certainly played a role; and (3) the rapid increase in contraceptive use in the preceding period, which increased the proportion of small family planners in the social environment of most women.[3]

Ming-Cheng Chang, the Director of the Taichung Family Planning Institute from 1988 to the present and on the staff before that, strongly supports Sun's view of program effect on preferences.

> In the early stages of the program . . . [its] success was dependent on existing demand . . . However, the program [later] put much of its effort to persuade people of lower status to have fewer children through home visitings or mass media campaigns. There are many stories from our field reports saying that rural women who wanted more children accepted sterilization right after our fieldworkers' home visits . . . I think our program has reduced demand for children and created demand for family planning through these efforts. (Chang, 1988)

Although the program certainly may have had some effect on the preferences of the poor and poorly educated rural women, its possible effect on their use of contraceptives is much more notable. Between 1970 and 1985 the percentage decline in preferences was less among the poorly than among the better educated. Furthermore, on the one hand, the correlation rates (eta) between education and mean reproductive preferences increased during this period among both younger and older women. On the other hand, use of contraceptives increased faster among the poorly educated than among the well educated, so that the correlation ratio (eta) between contraceptive use and education for both younger and older women decreased rapidly. By 1980–85, contraceptive use was similar—at saturation levels—at all educational levels (Chang et al., 1987).

In recent years, I have come to believe that a decrease in family-size preferences does not always automatically result in contraceptive use, as some economists believe (for example, see Pritchett, 1994; Freedman, 1996). Often an intervening step is necessary—the creation of contraceptive demand. A family planning program (and other societal influences) may be needed to facilitate the change from a decline in preferences to a demand for contraception to its actual practice. These intermediate steps after the preference change are hastened by the provision of additional information, legitimation, and appropriate services and supplies.

A program may not always be needed for the progression from changed preferences to contraceptive use, but clearly situations arise where it plays an important role. I cite two examples:

In the Matlab, Bangladesh, study, approximately the same decline in reproductive preferences occurred in the control and experimental areas, but the increase in contraceptive use was substantially greater in the experimental area
with its intensive household visitation program. The same pattern is reported for
the Matlab "Extension Area," in which results were tested in an area using normal program resources. Phillips et al. (1996), Koenig et al. (1987), and Arends-
Kuenning et al. (1996) all interpret these patterns as crystallization of latent demand, rather than as the creation of it.

The important Potharam Study (1971) in Thailand also demonstrated that
a program could foster quick, substantial adoption of contraception in a rural
area in which considerable pre-existing demand had not, by itself, led to any significant use of contraceptives. This result did not involve or require family-size
preference change. Such change had already occurred independently.

Concerning Taiwan, I suspect that the principal effect of the field-workers
was to help women who had ambiguous feelings about having no more children
to crystallize their sentiments, but more particularly, to enable those who were
almost ready to use contraceptives to do so. This enabling was an important
accomplishment, even if it accounted for only part of the substantial increase in
contraceptive use, especially among the poor.

I respect my Taiwan colleagues' view that the field-workers were instrumental in reducing family-size preferences. This reduction probably happened in
some cases but, unfortunately, no systematic evidence exists concerning whether
preferences or readiness to use contraceptives or both were changed. In retrospect, interviews with systematically selected samples of both field-workers and
their clients would have been desirable for gathering information about how they
came to their decisions about family size and whether to use contraceptives. The
field-workers may have believed that they changed couples' preferences. Follow-
up interviews with clients could have strengthened the evidence one way or the
other. Questions about this issue on the recurrent knowledge, attitudes, and
practice (KAP) surveys would have helped, too. I don't remember that we, as
consultants, ever suggested such studies, nor do I know of any other programs
that conducted such crucial evaluation studies.

Because the reader may wonder whether the measures of family-size preferences and of proportions wanting no more children were sufficiently stable
and meaningful to justify this discussion, I hasten to point out that longitudinal
and cohort studies demonstrated that in this period, the preferences were not
only stable for individual women but were predictive of their later use of contraceptives and abortion (Sun et al., 1978; Freedman et al., 1974; Jejeebhoy, 1981).

I conclude with an example of how a specific operations research investigation was embedded in a larger data-gathering system in Taiwan's program. The

specific operations research was an effort to reduce family-size preferences especially among poor and poorly educated couples by means of a powerful combination of mass media messages, clinic messages, group meetings, and household visits. Before-and-after measurements for this major piece of program research could be obtained from two of the regular KAP surveys that systematically covered a much wider range of pertinent variables for long-range evaluation studies. The regular before-and-after surveys seemed to suggest that the short-run operations research effort was successful. By happenstance, however, a survey covering only young respondents indicated that at least for this youthful group, the unusual decrease in preferences occurred before the stimulus intervention—not during or immediately after.

At the same time, the broad, long-range gathering of a whole battery of relevant variables enabled me to report much later that program (and nonprogram) stimuli had a much greater effect on contraceptive use than on preferences. This finding has enabled me to use the data for the entire longer period as probable evidence for the view that this program and others did not primarily reduce preferences, but instead, had the major effect of increasing couples' acceptance of the idea of contraception and then to its practice (Freedman, 1998).

Initially, I came to this view when I wrote a large-scale review of whether programs affect reproductive preferences. The evidence was overwhelming that they did not (Freedman, 1996 and 1997). Some new evidence came to light, however, just as I was completing the review suggesting that mass media projects might, under some circumstances, be an exception.

These ideas came to the fore long after Taiwan reached a TFR of 2.1 and below and have not been relevant to Taiwan's current population policy and research, which deals now with family planning issues for young people, but primarily addresses issues and problems of aging.

In retrospect, Taiwan's family planning history has significant value, however, for other countries in the early stages of their demographic transitions.

Insofar as the Taiwan program was responsible for the trends I have reported, the patterns described were consistent with my view that programs have relatively little effect on preferences, but that they can have a considerable effect on converting demand for fewer children first into a demand for contraception and then to its practice. This view suggests much more than the idea that programs provide access. I believe that in Taiwan, decreased family-size preferences came about mainly as a result of considerable social and economic development that affected all social strata. The next stage still required the development of social support, especially for the disadvantaged, for the idea that contraception was a legitimate and safe way to have fewer children and that the program (or the private sector) could provide the information, supplies, and services needed.

For this complex set of ideas, evidence from various sources is required, supplemented by inferences where precise empirical data are not available to verify every point. Some examples from the Taiwan experience provide useful information derived from operations research and for other examples, research had a different character. Both sorts of research were useful to the implementation of the family planning program, but in different and complementary ways.

Notes

1. In Taiwan, when the net reproduction rate fell and remained below one, the Executive Yuan (1992) deplored the prospect of negative growth and called for measures to increase the marriage rate and the birth rate. The only actions taken were rhetorical statements made in the media and by family planning workers during their household visits, but these failed to produce change. For example, the mean and median age at marriage continued to increase fairly steadily (Taiwan, Ministry of the Interior, 1992 and 1997) and the total fertility rate remained around 1.7.

    Singapore is, perhaps, a better example, because it designed and implemented a strenuous program to increase nuptiality, which also did not succeed. Mui Teng Yap (1995) claimed a success in this promarriage program, because the number of marriages "among single women increased substantially from 1987 to 1992 . . . probably because of the promarriage and profamily environment created by the government's marriage promotion effort." However, he did not take into account the variation in the number of eligible spinsters. The marriage rate for such spinsters actually decreased from 1987 to 1992 (Singapore, Department of Statistics, 1996). Demeny (1986) and Gauthier (1992), after a survey of European pronatalist programs, had already concluded that they were uniformly of little or no effect.

2. Premarital familial experience was measured by work in nonfamilial enterprises, social interaction with other young people without parental supervision (especially independent dating and choice of a mate without parental supervision). For a detailed study with multivariate analyses for a whole complex of issues about changes in the Taiwan family, see Thornton and Lin, 1994. This book won awards as the best volume on the family and on human ecology for the year after it was published.

3. Current use of contraceptives increased from 24 to 44 percent between 1965 and 1970, and the proportion of users among those wanting no more children increased from 39 to 64 percent.

References

Arends-Kuenning, Mary, Mian Bazle Hossain, and Barkat-e-Khuda. 1996. "The effects of family planning programs on fertility preferences: Evidence from Bangladesh." Paper presented at the Population Association of America annual meeting, New Orleans 9–11 May.

Cernada, George (ed.). 1970. *Taiwan Family Planning Reader*. Taichung: Chinese Center for International Training in Family Planning.

Chang, Ming-Cheng. 1998. Personal communication, February 6.

Chang, Ming-Cheng, Ronald Freedman, and Te-Hsiung Sun. 1987. "Trends in fertility, family size preferences, and family planning practice: Taiwan, 1961–85." *Studies in Family Planning* 18, 6: 320–337.

Demeny, Paul. 1986. "Pronatalist policies in low-fertility countries: Patterns, performance, and prospects." *Population and Development Review* 12 (Supplement): 335–358.

Executive Yuan, Republic of China. 1992. "Implementation of Population Policy." Taipei, October (in Chinese).

Freedman, Ronald. 1996. "Do family planning programs affect reproductive preferences?" *Working Paper of the Evaluation Project.* Chapel Hill: University of North Carolina, Carolina Population Center.

———. 1997. "Do family planning programs affect fertility preferences? A literature review." *Studies in Family Planning* 28, 1: 1–13.

———. 1998. "Observing Taiwan's demographic transition: A memoir." *Working Paper of the Population Studies Center.* Ann Arbor: University of Michigan.

Freedman, Ronald and John Y. Takeshita. 1969. *Family Planning in Taiwan: An Experiment in Social Change.* Princeton: Princeton University Press.

Freedman, Ronald, Lolagene C. Coombs, Ming-Cheng Chang, and Te-Hsiung Sun. 1974. "Trends in fertility, family size preferences, and practice of family planning: Taiwan, 1965–73." *Studies in Family Planning* 5, 9: pp. 270–288.

Gauthier, Anne H. 1992. "Consequences of fertility decline: Cultural, social, and economic implications—the European experience." Paper prepared for the seminar on "Impact of Fertility Decline on Population Policies and Programme Strategies: Emerging Trends for the 21st Century." Seoul: Korea Institute for Health and Social Affairs.

Hermalin, Albert I. 1978. "Spatial Analysis of Family Planning Program Effects in Taiwan, 1966–72." *Papers of the East-West Population Institute*, 48, April. Honolulu: East-West Population Institute.

Jejeebhoy, Shireen J. 1981. "Cohort consistency in family size preferences: Taiwan, 1965–73." *Studies in Family Planning* 12, 5: 229–232.

Koenig, Michael A., James F. Phillips, Ruth S. Simmons, and Mehrab Ali Khan. 1987. "Trends in family size preferences and contraceptive use in Matlab, Bangladesh." *Studies in Family Planning* 18, 3: 117–127.

Phillips, James F., Mian Bazle Hossain, and Mary Arends-Kuenning. 1996. "The long-term demographic role of community-based family planning in rural Bangladesh." *Studies in Family Planning* 27, 4: 204–219.

"The Potharam Study." 1971. Bangkok: Chulalongkorn University, Institute of Population Studies, Research Report No. 4.

Pritchett, Lant H. 1994. "Desired fertility and the impact of population policies." *Population and Development Review* 20, 1: 1–55.

Singapore, Department of Statistics. 1996. *Singapore Statistical Highlights, 1965–1995.* Singapore: Department of Statistics.

Sun, Te-Hsiung. 1997. Personal communication, December 17.

Sun, Te-Hsiung, Hui-Sheng Lin, and Ronald Freedman. 1978. "Trends in fertility, family size preferences and family planning practice: Taiwan, 1961–76." *Studies in Family Planning* 9, 4: 54–70.

Taiwan, Ministry of the Interior. 1992 and 1997. *Taiwan-Fukien Demographic Fact Book, 1991, 1997.* Taipei: Taiwan, Ministry of the Interior.

Thornton, Arland and Hui-Sheng Lin (eds.). 1994. *Social Change and the Family in Taiwan.* Chicago: University of Chicago Press.

Yap, Mui Teng. 1995. "Singapore's 'three or more policy': The first five years." *Asia-Pacific Population Journal* 10, 4: 39–52.

Effects of a Family Planning Program on the Fertility of a Marginal Working-Class Community in Santiago

Aníbal Faúndes-Latham, Germán Rodríguez-Galant, and Onofre Avendaño-Portius

Programmatic issue: *In the early 1960s, family planning programs were being organized and implemented. However, evidence and documentation of their impact was scarce. "[A] number of family planning programs were going on in Santiago with the purposes of fighting induced abortion and of reducing fertility and maternal-child mortality and morbidity, but no data were available to show the effects of the programs..., even though some date back to 1959.... This problem...was observed in many Latin American countries and throughout the world."*

Research design: *A family planning program and a research and evaluation project were designed simultaneously. The family planning program involved the provision of information about the risks of induced abortion and contraceptive options as well as the free distribution of IUDs and oral contraceptives, and the availability of sterilization in a community of 32,000 inhabitants. A baseline (March/April 1965) and a follow-up (January/March 1967) were conducted. The latter involved interviews with women, mainly a detailed pregnancy history, of women aged 15–49 in a stratified sample of 892 dwellings.*

Findings: *The total fertility rate of the community was almost 20 percent lower in 1966 than in 1964. A detailed and informed analysis of the data revealed that 90 percent of the decline could be ascribed to the family planning program.*

Program response to findings: *No program response is discussed in the paper, but this project clearly contributed to the expansion of family planning programs and to their legitimization in Chile and throughout Latin America*

Discussion: *The authors state the purpose of the project clearly at the outset, which may seem the logical and right thing to do, but which is frequently omitted. They claim that they will evaluate "the demographic,* *medical, and social effects of family planning." In this paper, however, they document and analyze only the demographic effects. The medical and social effects are discussed in subsequent papers, in particular the achievements with regard to one of the main objectives of the project, namely the prevention of induced abortions. In the short run, that is between 1964 and 1966, the total fertility rate (TFR) declined by 19 percent, whereas the total abortion rate (TAR) by 39 percent. The longer-term effect was similar; between 1964 and 1968 the TFR declined by 45 percent and the TAR by 63 percent (see Faúndes et al., 1970, "Evaluación de los efectos de un programa de planificación familiar sobre la fecundidad en una población marginal de Santiago, Chile," in IUSSP, 1970, Conferencia Regional Latinoamericana de Población, Mexico, pp. 429–437).*

Effects of a Family Planning Program on the Fertility of a Marginal Working-Class Community in Santiago

Aníbal Faúndes-Latham, Germán Rodríguez-Galant, and Onofre Avendaño-Portius

In late 1964, a number of family planning programs were going on in Santiago with the purposes of fighting induced abortion and of reducing fertility and maternal-child mortality and morbidity, but no data were available to show the effects of the programs on these variables, even though some date back to 1959. This lack of objective evidence on the effectivity of family planning programs was discouraging for the people engaged, and, at the same time, was reinforcing the opinions of some groups against family planning. Under these conditions, it was difficult to justify either the maintenance or improvement of the existing programs or the initiation of new programs in other areas. This problem, moreover, was observed in many other Latin American countries and throughout the world.

The Project

In order to face the problem of evaluating the demographic, medical, and social effects of family planning, a pilot project was designed on the following lines:

1. To choose a small community in Santiago, slightly or not at all affected by any family planning program, which was as representative as possible of other communities with demographic, medical, and social problems, and which presented as many other advantages for the development of a family planning research and action program as possible.

2. To initiate in that community a family planning program designed in accordance with the experience achieved in other programs in Chile and Latin America.

3. To develop a proper research design for the measurement of the possible effects of that family planning program on (a) the birth and abortion

Reprinted with the permission of the Population Association of America from *Demography* 1968. 5,1: 122–137.

rates, (b) maternal-child mortality and morbidity, and (c) some related social and psychological variables.

The San Gregorio Community

The San Gregorio community, located in the southern part of Santiago, was chosen for the development of the Pilot Project. San Gregorio has approximately 32,000 inhabitants who are distributed in 5 defined sections, each of which is characterized by a different, well-known type of dwelling. These dwellings range from wooden houses of poor construction, with two bedrooms, a cesspool, and with no sanitary facilities, up to modest apartments and houses with three bedrooms, brick walls, wooden floors, equipped kitchens, and sanitary facilities. The number of inhabitants per dwelling usually ranges between 5 and 9, the average being 7 persons.

The inhabitants are almost evenly distributed in number of males and females. As is characteristic of fast-growing communities, more than one-half of the people are aged under 15 years. Almost 70 percent of the women in the age group 15–49 years are married. Married women have 4 children on the average. They have a low educational level (less than 4 years of basic education for the great majority), but few are illiterate. Many women work, preferably in their own homes (sewing, ironing, and working for better-off families).

Married men are mainly unskilled workers, with a low educational level (less than 6 years of basic education for most) and a very low income: the average is 200 escudos (=U.S. $30) per month. The per capita income in the community is insufficient for the satisfaction of the most basic needs of these people. Most of the inhabitants are Catholics, but they do not attend church very often.

This community was not under the direct influence of any family planning program until 1964. There were no reasons for suspecting any important difference between it and any other marginal working-class community in Santiago, and it presented three advantages for the development of the project.

First, it has exact boundaries within which there is no risk of construction of new dwellings, because all the land is either occupied or destined for specific purposes to serve the community. Since migration in this area occurs mainly through the construction of new dwellings and communities, this characteristic limits the possibility of in-migration. Out-migration may still occur when young couples get married and leave San Gregorio, but most of these couples remain in the community, living in their parent's homes. Second, a maternal child-health clinic is located approximately at the geographic center of the community, which was created at the same time as the community itself. Third, and finally, a map of the community with each block and dwelling numbered is available, and this made the selection of samples easier.

The Family Planning Program

The experimental family planning program, initiated March 9, 1965, includes education and services. Information and education center on the risks of induced abortion and on the possibilities of modern contraception. Physicians, midwives, nurses, and social workers give information at the clinic, when women attend for pre-natal and child care. Information is given, too, at the mother's centers in the community and at the Barros Luco Hospital which takes care of this area, and where most of these women deliver their babies.

The services available at the maternal and child health clinic are free. The most used contraceptive is the IUCD although many women use pills, and a few others are advised to attend the Barros Luco Hospital for sterilization.

Research Design

The basic Research Design of the project includes three steps. First, an initial baseline survey—March and April, 1965—investigated fertility and abortions in 1964, as well as knowledge of, attitudes towards and practice of modern contraception, and other variables which could influence these factors (such as age, marital and educational status, and so forth). Second, the administration of the experimental treatment—the family planning program—was initiated at the same time as the field work of the 1965 survey. And, third, later fertility and KAP surveys which permitted the evaluation of the family planning program were conducted. The first of these was completed in January–March, 1967.

Since the 1967 survey investigated fertility and abortion in 1966, as well as knowledge of, attitudes towards and practice of modern contraception, its comparison with the 1965 survey will provide a before-after measure of the possible effects of the first year of the family planning program. Currently, we are working on this comparison, the results of which will be ready to publish this year.

A complete record of all pregnancies experienced by the sample was obtained in the 1967 survey, following Bogue's suggestion for the study of fertility through the collection of pregnancy histories.[1] This method has provided a new set of data to measure the possible effects of the first year of the program.

In this paper, the results obtained through the pregnancy history method will be presented and discussed. Special emphasis will be placed on the analysis of the cause-effect relationship between the program and the changes observed.

Methodology

The design we have used for the measurement and analysis of the possible effects of the program, through the pregnancy history approach considers (1) the measurement of the fertility of the community in 1966, the year in which the effects of the first year of the program were expected, and the fertility of the four previous years (1962–1965), in order to obtain a one-year-after and a 4-years-before measure of fertility; and (2) the analysis of the cause-effect relationship between the program and the change—if any—of the fertility in 1966 with respect to the four previous years.

The measure to be used for reporting changes in fertility will be the "total fertility rate," the total number of children that a hypothetical cohort of 1,000 women would bear in the age group 15–44 years, if they bore children throughout these years according to the specific pattern of age-specific fertility rates which prevail in the community at a given moment. For the analysis of the cause-effect relationship between the program and the change in fertility, the sample will be classified in terms of attendance at the family planning clinic and use of contraceptives, and a method will be suggested for analyzing the participation of "patients" of the family planning clinic in the change of fertility in 1966. Both the classification and the method will be introduced below. (See "Results.")

The Pregnancy History Method

The pregnancy history method consists in obtaining the full record of all pregnancies experienced by a cross section of women during all their lives, and in computing, on the basis of these data, age-specific, general, and total fertility rates.

The procedure for computing rates has four steps. (1) Construct a matrix in which the rows represent single years of age, and the columns represent single calendar years. (2) Compute the number of months each woman spends in each age for each calendar year; that is, entering "person-months" in the matrix. (3) Accumulate the person-months for the whole sample, and divide by 12 to convert to person-years, in order to obtain the denominators of the age-specific fertility rates for various years. (4) Construct a matrix identical to the last, and classify in it each birth experienced by every woman in the sample, according to the year of delivery and the age of the mother at the time. The numerators for the age-specific fertility rates are obtained by adding all births for each age and calendar year.

Population and sampling. The population was defined as all women in the age group 15–49 years who were living for at least 6 months in San Gregorio when the survey was taken, irrespective of their marital status or position in the house.

A stratified random sample of 892 dwellings proportionally distributed in the different sections of the community was taken, but the units of analysis were women who lived in those dwellings and who were aged 15–49 years in 1966.[2] However, the age group 45–49 years could not be considered in the comparison of the fertility for the years 1962–66 because the oldest women interviewed (who were aged 49 years in 1966) were aged only 48 years in 1965, 47 in 1964, and so forth. For this reason we have no data for 49-year-old women in 1965, for 49- and 48-year-old women in 1964, and so on. The study, then, includes only women who were aged 15–44 years in the five years that are analyzed.

The size of our sample is estimated to assure sampling errors not greater than 2 percent for the principal variables investigated in the total sample.

Questionnaires and pre-test. The Pregnancy History questionnaire used was the same that the Latin American Center for Demography (CELADE) has used for its rural fertility studies in Latin America.

A questionnaire was prepared, asking for knowledge, opinion, and use of contraceptives during the last 4 years (1963–66), as well as for knowledge of and attendance at the family planning clinic at San Gregorio. A trial run of these questionnaires was made in a sample of 60 dwellings. This initial survey helped to predict potential difficulties and problems in the questionnaires, and to make the necessary revisions. It was of particular help in preparing more specific instructions for the interviewers.

Selection and preparation of the interviewers. The interviewers were preferably midwives. Chilean midwives are highly qualified university graduates, and are held in high regard by the members of the community. Owing to the nature of their work and to the high level of confidence they enjoy, midwives are most suited to talk with the women of San Gregorio about their births, abortions, and experiences in the use of contraceptives.

The interviewers were trained in four group sessions, and one or more individual sessions in which they received instructions about the purpose of the survey, the questionnaires being used, and general aspects of interviewing, and in turn, discussed difficulties they had encountered during the first interviews.

Field work and supervision. The field work took two and one-half months, and was completed in March, 1967. During this phase, special emphasis was placed on everyday close supervision of the interviewers, and some of the interviewers were checked in the field by the supervisors.

The supervision was done in such a way that in any one day it was possible, for each dwelling in the sample, to tell exactly in which of six stages the interview was.

1. Interview not yet assigned
2. Interview assigned to a given person
3. Some women in the dwelling interviewed
4. All women interviewed
5. Interviews supervised with objections (back to field)
6. Interviews checked

Through this procedure it was intended to assure that the interviews were conducted as connectedly as possible.

Table 1. Age-specific fertility rates, by age; general fertility rates; total fertility rates; and percentage change, for the total sample of the San Gregorio Community, Santiago, Chile, 1962–66

Age	1962			1963				1964				1965				1966			
	W	LB	ASFR	W	LB	ASFR	% Ch	W	LB	ASFR	% Ch	W	LB	ASFR	% Ch	W	LB	ASFR	% Ch
15–19	192	31	161.5	225	43	191.1	+18.3	249	43	168.7	−11.7	287	40	139.4	−17.4	302	40	132.2	−5.0
20–24	130	50	384.6	133	55	413.5	+7.5	143	44	307.7	−25.6	153	45	294.1	−4.4	151	43	317.9	−5.1
25–29	155	55	354.8	140	53	378.6	+6.7	134	39	291.0	−23.1	144	45	312.5	+7.4	152	31	203.9	−34.8
30–34	225	56	248.9	225	58	257.8	+3.6	214	51	235.3	−7.6	196	47	239.8	+0.5	174	36	206.9	−13.7
35–39	165	40	242.4	169	35	207.1	−14.6	191	36	188.5	−9.0	190	39	205.3	+8.9	208	23	110.5	−10.1
40–44	103	17	165.0	120	11	91.7	−44.4	125	7	56.0	−38.9	134	16	119.4	+113.2	145	8	55.2	−53.8
GFR	970	249	256.7	1012	255	252.0	−1.8	1056	219	207.4	−17.7	1104	232	210.1	+1.3	1132	186	164.3	−21.8
TFR			7,786.0			7,699.0	−1.1			6,251.0	−18.8			6,552.5	+4.3			5,132.5	−21.6

The pregnancy history data were coded during June and July. This work was done by the same people who supervised the field work. In this way, they were acquainted with the characteristics of the survey as well as with the most common difficulties which they might encounter when coding.

Results

Age-Specific Fertility Rate (ASFR), General Fertility Rate (GFR), and Total Fertility Rate (TFR) of the Total Sample, 1962–66

In order to simplify the presentation of the results, the number of births and person-years by each year of age were grouped in five-year intervals for each calendar year, 1962–66. The ASFR, GFR, and TFR for these years were computed according to standard formulas and to the previous definitions. For each rate computed for the years 1963–66, the change with respect to the year before was expressed in percentage, and these data, rates, and percent changes are shown in Table 1.

The fertility of San Gregorio was at a very high level in 1962. The TFR for this year was 8,286; that is, a woman bearing children according to the ASFR for this year was expected to bear 7.8 children before her forty-fifth birthday.

A small decline (–1.1 percent) can be observed in the fertility of 1963 (7,699), and a more marked fertility reduction (–18.8 percent) occurred in 1964 (6,251.5). While the only mild increase (+4.8 percent) occurred in 1965 (6,552.5), the largest decline (–21.6 percent) observed in the period studied took place in 1966 (5,134.5).

The ASFR allows us to see in which age groups these changes occurred. But it should be noted that these rates are affected by sampling errors greater than the error of the TFR, and, thus, they cannot be considered in their literal value. Moreover, because they are based on a small number of women, some of their variations may represent periodic fluctuations of fertility in which increases and decreases alternate every year (as we suspect is the case for the age group 40–44 years.) However, a significant change occurred in most of the ASFRs both in 1964 and in 1966.

The fertility decline observed in 1966 will be preferentially considered because it is the largest, and might be an effect of the family planning program. The changes observed in 1964 will be discussed below.

Classification of the Sample

According to our research design, the sample will be classified in terms of attendance to the family planning clinic and use of contraceptives, and a comparative analysis of the fertility of the groups resulting from this classification will be made, in order to discover if the 1966 fertility decline is an effect of the family planning program.

If we assume that births occur in the tenth month after conception, the babies born in 1966 should have been conceived between April, 1965 and March, 1966. According to this assumption the use of effective contraception between these dates is defined as *protective*. Only the IUCD, pills, and sterilization are included as effective contraceptives in this definition.

Three groups were defined: "patients," "other protected women," and "non-protected women."

Patients. This group comprises all women in the sample who attended the family planning clinic between April, 1965 and March, 1966,[3] whether or not they used some effective contraceptive during that time. Since the fertility of these women in 1966 was under the direct influence of the program, the extent to which they may have caused the 1966 fertility decline will represent the extent to which that decline is an effect of the program.

Other protected women (OPW). This group comprises all women who used effective contraceptives for any period of time between April, 1965 and March, 1966. Since they regulated their fertility in 1966, though not by the program, they represent another potential source of explanation for the 1966 fertility decline.

Non-protected women (NPW). This group comprises all the remaining part of the sample. Since these women did not use contraceptives during the period April, 1965 to March, 1966, they are not expected to explain any part of the 1966 fertility decline. If they do, then that decline should be explained by factors other than the adoption of family planning.

The information required to classify each woman in one of the three previously defined groups, was obtained from their answers to questions on the use of contraceptives and attendance at the clinic.

Sixteen percent of the total sample was classified in the patient's group. Most of these women were IUCD users, some of them used pills, and very few did not use any effective contraceptive at all during April, 1965–March, 1966.

Twelve percent of the total sample was classified in the OPW group, sixty percent were sterilized, and the rest were mainly pill users. Most (85 percent) became users of effective contraceptives before April, 1965 and even before the family planning program started. Accordingly, most of the OPW were also protected from having births in 1965, and, moreover, some of them were protected from having births in 1964, 1963, and so on.

It should be noted that this is not necessarily true for the other two groups; some patients may have been protected in 1965 or before, and some may not have been protected for those years. Similarly, some NPW may have been protected for 1965 or before and others may not have been protected for those years. This fact will be recalled later on when we discuss the 1964 fertility decline.

ASFR, GFR, and TFR, 1962-66, for Patients, OPW and NPW

For each of the three groups in which the sample was divided, the ASFR, GFR, and TFR for each year during 1962–66 were computed using a procedure similar to that described in the section on methodology.[4] For each rate for the years 1963–66, the change with respect to the year before was expressed in percentage. These data and rates are shown in Tables 2, 3, and 4. The TFRs for these groups as well as for the total sample are better illustrated in Figure 1.

The patients had a very high fertility in 1962 and small fluctuations during 1962–63. The TFR is in the 12,000–14,000 level during all these years. In 1966, the fertility of patients presents a very sharp and significant reduction, in which the TFR comes down to the 3,000 level.

The amount of change may be better understood if it is considered that the 1962–65 ASFRs imply that a woman would bear 12-14 children before her forty-fifth birthday, while if she were to have followed the 1966 ASFR pattern, she would be expected to bear only 3 children before that birthday.

The OPW group presents a high fertility for 1962 and 1963. The TFR for these years is 10,000–11,000. Though high, this value is lower than the TFR of patients for those years. In 1964 the OPW present a reduction of fertility in which the TFR comes down to 7,000—a level which is almost maintained in 1965. But, a new decline appears in 1966, but not as important as the reduction of patients' fertility in that year. The TFR of OPW for 1966 is in the range of 5,000.

In comparison to the former groups, the NPW group presents a low fertility for 1962, and during the following four years, its fertility shows small fluctuations. The most important change is a decline observed in 1964. Its TFR is around the level of 5,000–6,000 for the five years studied. The low fertility of this group may be explained because the group is formed mainly by single women, widows, and women who belong to infertile couples. Conversely, patients and OPW groups are mainly married women of proven fertility. The hypothesis may be suggested that they are protected precisely because of their higher fertility and that the NPW groups do not use contraceptives because most of them do not need to be protected. This line of reasoning will be further pursued in the discussion.

Figure 1 illustrates the changes in the fertility of the three groups and in the total sample during 1962–66. The participation of each of the three groups in the decline of the fertility of the total sample in both 1964 and 1966 is clearly visualized.

The 1966 fertility decline is composed of a slight increase (+13.2 percent) in the fertility of the NPW, a moderate decrease (–24.4 percent) of the OPW's fertility, and a dramatic decrease, (–78.3 percent) of the patients' fertility.

Even though patients are only 16 percent of the total sample, the importance of their decline suggests that they are mainly responsible for the fertility decline observed in the total sample in 1966. Since the OPW have a moderate

Table 2. Age-specific fertility rates, by age; general fertility rates; total fertility rates; and percentage change, for the "patients" of the San Gregorio Community, Santiago, Chile, 1962–66

Age	1962 W	1962 LB	1962 ASFR	1963 W	1963 LB	1963 ASFR	1963 % Ch	1964 W	1964 LB	1964 ASFR	1964 % Ch	1965 W	1965 LB	1965 ASFR	1965 % Ch	1966 W	1966 LB	1966 ASFR	1966 % Ch
15–19	29	12	413.8	31	13	419.4	+1.4	25	11	392.9	−6.3	19	11	578.9	+47.3	14	3	214.3	−63.0
20–24	48	16	400.0	38	21	617.6	−54.4	29	11	379.3	−38.6	31	16	516.1	+36.0	29	1	34.5	−93.3
25–29	43	19	441.9	42	19	452.4	+2.4	45	20	444.4	−1.8	45	23	511.1	+15.0	43	8	186.0	−63.6
30–34	45	23	511.1	44	16	363.6	−28.9	46	17	369.6	+1.6	42	10	238.1	−35.6	42	6	142.9	−40.0
35–39	16	9	562.5	26	7	269.2	−52.1	26	8	307.7	+14.3	35	17	485.7	+57.8	40	1	25.0	−91.9
40–44	2	1	500.0	4	2	500.0	0	8	4	500.0	0	9	4	444.4	−11.1	13	0	0	−100.0
GFR	175	80	457.1	181	78	430.9	−5.7	182	71	390.1	−9.5	181	81	447.5	+14.7	181	19	105.0	−76.5
TFR			14,146.5			13,111.0	−7.3			11,969.5	−8.7			13,871.5	+15.9			3,013.5	−76.3

Table 3. Age-specific fertility rates, by age; general fertility rates; total fertility rates; and percentage change, for the other protected women of the San Gregorio Community, Santiago, Chile, 1962–66

Age	1962 W	1962 LB	1962 ASFR	1963 W	1963 LB	1963 ASFR	1963 % Ch	1964 W	1964 LB	1964 ASFR	1964 % Ch	1965 W	1965 LB	1965 ASFR	1965 % Ch	1966 W	1966 LB	1966 ASFR	1966 % Ch
15–19	6	2	333.3	5	3	600.0	+80.0	4	2	500.0	−16.7	3	2	666.6	+33.3	2	1	500.0	−25.0
20–24	17	8	470.6	15	10	666.0	+41.6	12	5	416.7	−37.5	9	3	333.3	−20.0	6	2	333.3	0
25–29	25	14	560.0	23	9	391.3	−30.1	20	6	300.0	−23.3	23	2	87.0	−71.0	22	3	136.4	+56.8
30–34	49	11	224.5	48	10	208.3	−7.2	47	7	148.9	−28.5	41	5	122.0	−18.1	32	1	31.3	−74.3
35–39	32	12	375.0	38	8	210.5	−43.9	40	4	100.0	−52.5	42	8	190.5	+90.5	45	4	88.9	−53.3
40–44	21	3	142.9	21	2	95.2	−33.4	24	2	83.3	−12.5	24	1	41.7	−49.9	30	0	0	−100.0
GFR	150	50	333.3	150	42	280.0	−16.0	147	26	176.9	−36.8	142	21	147.9	−16.4	137	11	80.3	−45.7
TFR			10,531.5			10,859.5	+3.1			7,744.5	−28.7			7,205.5	−7.0			5,449.5	−24.4

Table 4. Age-specific fertility rates, by age; general fertility rates; total fertility rates; and percentage change, for the non-protected women of the San Gregorio Community, Santiago, Chile, 1962–66

Age	1962 W	1962 LB	1962 ASFR	1963 W	1963 LB	1963 ASFR	1963 % Ch	1964 W	1964 LB	1964 ASFR	1964 % Ch	1965 W	1965 LB	1965 ASFR	1965 % Ch	1966 W	1966 LB	1966 ASFR	1966 % Ch
15–19	157	17	108.3	189	27	142.9	+31.9	217	29	133.6	−6.5	265	27	101.9	−23.7	286	36	125.9	+23.6
20–24	73	26	356.2	84	24	285.7	−19.8	102	28	274.5	−3.9	113	26	230.1	−16.2	116	45	387.9	+68.6
25–29	87	22	252.9	75	25	333.3	+31.8	69	13	188.4	−43.5	76	20	263.2	+39.7	87	20	229.9	−12.7
30–34	131	22	167.9	133	32	240.6	+43.3	121	27	223.1	−7.3	113	32	283.2	+26.9	100	29	290.0	+2.4
35–39	117	19	162.4	105	20	190.5	+17.3	125	24	192.0	+0.8	113	14	123.9	−35.5	123	18	146.3	+18.1
40–44	80	13	162.5	95	7	73.7	−54.6	93	1	10.8	−85.3	101	11	108.9	+908.3	102	8	78.4	−28.0
GFR	645	119	184.5	681	135	198.2	+7.4	727	122	167.8	−15.3	781	130	166.5	−0.8	814	156	191.6	+15.1
TFR			6,051.0			6,333.5	+4.7			5,112.0	−19.3			5,556.0	+8.7			6,292.0	+13.2

Figure 1. Changes in total fertility rate for the total sample of the San Gregorio community, Santiago, Chile, 1962–1966.

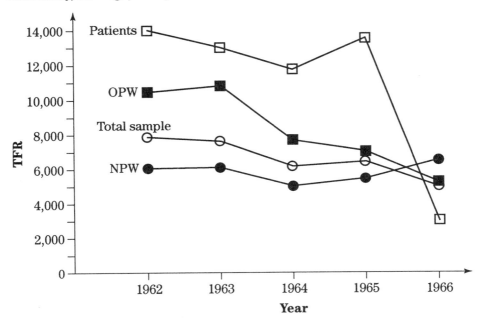

decline and are relatively few (12 percent of the sample), their reduction in fertility does not seem sufficient, on the one hand, to explain an important part of the total decline in fertility. On the other hand, there is no doubt that the NPW cannot be responsible for the decline, because they present a small increase of their fertility in 1966. This reasoning favors the hypothesis that the program is the principal cause of the 1966 fertility decline, and this hypothesis will be carefully tested in the section on the analysis of the 1966 fertility decline.

As to the 1964 fertility decline, it is composed of a slight decrease (–8.7 percent) in the patients' fertility, a marked decline (–19.3 percent) of NPW fertility, and a more marked reduction (–28.7 percent) of OPW fertility.

Since the patients' decline is slight, they do not seem to be responsible for an important part of the 1964 decline. Though the OPW have an important reduction, they are relatively few; thus, they do not seem to be responsible for the greatest part of the decline. The hypothesis is suggested that the NPW group is the principal one responsible for the decline, because its reduction is considerable and it is a large group (72 percent of the sample). This hypothesis will be further analyzed in the discussion.

Analysis of the 1966 Fertility Decline

Theoretical statement of the model used for the analysis. A method has been developed to measure the proportion of the total fertility decline observed in

1966 that may be attributed to each of the groups into which the sample was divided,[5] as well as to measure the amount of change induced by each group.

The method consists in separating each of the possible components of the total variation observed.[6] In our case, the total decline will be divided into two additive components: (1) patients' effect, or the part of the total change that would not have been observed if patients had not changed; (2) OPW effect or the part of the total change that would not have been observed if OPW had not changed That is,

Total effect = Patient's Effect + OPW Effect[7]   (1)

Definition and computation of the effects. In order to compute the total effect as well as its two components, two or three estimates of fertility have to be defined and computed.

We will estimate the TFR that the total sample would have presented in 1966 if patients had maintained the fertility they had in previous years instead of decreasing it by adopting family planning. The estimate will be symbolized by E_1 $(TFR)_t$ or, briefly, E_1. The difference between E_1 and the value actually presented by the TFR or the total sample in 1966 measures the effect of patients on the fertility of the total sample. If we symbolize the actual value of the TFR of the total sample in 1966 as R (for "real"), the effect of the patients is as in formula (2).

Patient's Effect = $R - E_1$ (2)

The computation of E_1 and the method followed are presented in Table 5.

Now, E_1 is 6,866.4; that is, the TFR for the total sample in 1966 would have been 6,866.4 instead of 5,134.5 if the program had not reduced the fertility of the patients in 1966.

The effect of the program then is:

Patient's Effect = 5,134.5 − 6,866.4 = −1,731.9   (3)

This means that the patients have reduced the fertility of the total sample in 1966 by 1,731.9 points.

We will now estimate the TFR that the total sample would have presented in 1966 if the OPW had maintained in 1966 the fertility they had in 1965 instead of decreasing it as actually occurred. This estimate will be symbolized by E_2 $(TFR)_t$ or briefly, E_2.

The difference between E_2 and the real value of the TFR of the total sample in 1966 (R) measures the effect of OPW on the fertility of the total sample. That is,

OPW Effect = $R - E_2$ (4)

The computation of E_2 and the method followed are presented in Table 6. There, E_2 is 5,340.4; that is, the TFR for the total sample in 1966 would have been 5,340.4 instead of 5,134.5 if the OPW had not reduced their fertility in 1966. The effect of the OPW then is as follows.

Table 5. Computation of total fertility rate, E_1

| Age | Patients | | Total sample | |
	$E(ASFR)_p$	$E(LB)_p$	$E_1(LB)_t$	$E_1(ASFR)_t$
15–19	451.24	6.32	43.32	143.44
20–24	478.27	13.87	60.87	403.11
25–29	462.45	19.89	42.89	282.17
30–34	370.61	15.57	45.57	261.90
35–39	406.28	16.25	38.25	183.89
40–44	486.11	6.32	14.32	98.76

$E_1(TFR)_t = 6,866.4$

Note: The ASFR of each age group of the patients in 1966 was assumed to be equal to the average of the ASFR of the same age group during 1962-66 (see note in Table 6). These averages were entered in col. E $(ASFR)_p$. Multiplying them by the corresponding number of patients in each age group in 1966 (W from Table 2) and dividing by 1,000, the estimated number of livebirths in 1966 in each age group of the patients ($E[LB]_p$) was obtained. These values were added with the corresponding number of livebirths for 1966 in the OPW and the NPW groups (LB from Tables 3 and 4), thus giving the estimate 1 of the number of livebirths for the total sample in 1966: $E_1(LB)_t$. By dividing these values by the corresponding number of women in each age group in the total sample in 1966 (W from Table 1) and multiplying by 1,000, the estimate 1 of the ASFR's for the total sample in 1966 $E_1(ASFR)_t$ were obtained. In terms of these rates, the estimate 1 of the TFR for the total sample in 1966 was calculated.

Table 6. Computation of total fertility rate, E_2

| Age | Other protected women | | Total sample | |
	$E(ASFR)_{opw}$	$E(LB)_{opw}$	$E_2(LB)_t$	$E_2(ASFR)_t$
15-19	666.67	1.33	40.33	133.54
20-24	333.33	2.00	48.00	317.88
25-29	86.96	1.91	29.91	196.77
30-34	111.95	3.90	38.90	223.56
35-39	190.48	8.57	27.57	132.54
40-44	41.67	1.25	9.25	63.79

$E_2(TFR)_t = 5,340.4$

Note: The ASFR of each age group of the OPW for 1966 was assumed to be equal to the ASFR of the same age group in 1965 (ASFR from Table 3). The fertility of patients presented an increase in 1965 reaching almost their highest level in four years. Accordingly a natural small decline was expected for 1966 without any exterior influence. For this reason, the average fertility for the years 1962-65 was used to estimate the 1966 fertility of patients. But the case of the OPW was different. These women show a clear continuous tendency to decline in 1963-65, and there were no reasons to expect a natural increase in 1966. For this reason, their 1965 fertility was used to estimate their fertility in 1966, instead of the average of the four previous years.

These values were entered in col. $E(ASFR)_{opw}$. By multiplying them by the corresponding number of OPW in each age group in 1966 (W. from Table 4) and dividing by 1,000 the estimated number of livebirths in each age group of the OPW in 1966. $E(LP)_{obv}$ was obtained. These values were added with the real numbers of livebirths in 1966 in each age group of the patients and the NPW (LB from Tables 2 and 4) to obtain estimate 2 of the number of livebirths in each age group of the total sample in 1966: $E_2(LB)_t$. Dividing these values by the number of women in each age group of the total sample in 1966 (W. from Table 1) and multiplying by 1,000 gave estimate 2 of the ASFR's for the total sample in 1966: $E_1(ASFR)_t$. In terms of these rates, estimate 2 of the TFR for the total sample in 1966 was calculated.

OPW Effect = 5,134.5 − 5,340.4 = −205.9   (5)

This means that the OPW have reduced the fertility of the total sample in 1966 by 205.9 points.

According to the additive nature of the model, the total change observed is

Total Effect = −1,731.9 + −205.9 = −1,937.8   (6)

This means that the combined effect of the patients and the OPW has been to reduce the TFR of the total sample in 1966 by 1,937.8 points. This makes it clear that the major part of the decline is an effect of the program, but let us proceed further in the elaboration of these data.

The total effect represents the difference between the real value observed for the TFR of the total sample in 1966 (R) and the TFR that would have been observed in the total sample in 1966 if neither the patients nor the OPW had reduced their fertility in 1966. If we call this last estimate E_3, the total effect may be now computed as

$$R − E_3 \tag{7}$$

But, E_3 may be computed directly from the data, as was done in Table 7 where the method followed is explained. In this way, E_3 is 7,072.3; that is, the TFR for the total sample in 1966 would have been 7,072.3 instead of 5,134.5 if neither the patients nor the OPW had reduced their fertility in 1966. The total effect is 5,134.5 − 7,072.3 = −1,937.8.

This procedure has led us to check the consistency of the model and to check former computations. But it has also provided a baseline in terms of which the effects may be interpreted.

The total effect of 1,937.8 points may now be interpreted as a decline from an estimated fertility under conditions of no change of 7,072.3, to a real fertility produced by the changes of the two groups of 5,134.5. This may be expressed as a percentage change:

$$\text{Total Percentage Decline} = \frac{1,937.8}{7,072.3} \bullet 100 = 27.4 \text{ percent} \tag{8}$$

In other words, a 27.4 percent fertility decline has been observed in the total sample in 1966.

The patients' effect of 1,731.9 points may be interpreted as a decline from the estimated fertility under conditions of no change—7,072.3. Expressing this as a percentage change, we have:

Patient's Percentage Decline of TFR of Total Sample

$$= \frac{1,731.9}{7,072.3} \bullet 100 = 24.5 \text{ percent} \tag{9}$$

Table 7. Computation of total fertility rate, E_3

Age	E_3 (LB)$_t$	E_3 (ASFR)$_t$
15-19	43.65	144.54
20-24	60.87	403.11
25-29	41.80	275.00
30-34	48.47	278.56
35-39	42.82	205.87
40-44	15.57	107.38

E_3(ASFR)$_t$ = 7,072.3

Note: The estimated number of livebirths for 1966 in each age group in the patients and the OPW, $E(LB)_p$ and $E(LB)_{opw}$ (from Tables 5 and 6) were added to the corresponding real number of livebirths in each age group of the NPW in 1966 (LB from Table 4) to obtain Estimate 3 of the number of livebirths in each age group of the total sample in 1966: $E_3(LB)_t$. Dividing these values by the number of women in each age and multiplying by 1,000 the estimate 3 of ASFR's for the Total Sample $E_3(ASFR)_t$ were obtained and in terms of them the estimate 3 total fertility rate for the total sample.

Patients have produced a 24.5 percent decline of the fertility of the total sample. Similarly, we have:

OPW Percentage Decline of TFR of Total Sample

$$= \frac{205.9}{7,072.3} \bullet 100 = 2.9 \text{ percent} \tag{10}$$

The OPW have produced a 2.9 percent decline of the fertility of the total sample.

Up to this point, we have been measuring the absolute and percentage magnitude of each effect, but we have not yet computed "the proportion of the total effect that is caused by each group." Let us proceed with this computation.

Since the patients have produced a decline of 1,731.9 points of a total decline of 1,937.8, we have:

Patient's Proportion of Total Decline = $\frac{1,731.9}{1,937.8} \bullet 100 = 89.4$ percent (11)

The patients are responsible for 89.4 percent of the total decline of the fertility of the total sample observed in 1966. Similarly the OPW who have produced a decline of 205.9 points from a total decline of 1,937.8 points, are responsible for 10.6 percent.

OPW Proportion of the Total Decline = $\frac{205.9}{1,937.8} \bullet 100 = 10.6$ percent. (12)

From these last computations it is clear that the main responsibility for the fertility decline observed in the total sample in 1966 is that of the patients, or in other words, that the principal cause of the fertility decline observed in 1966 is the family planning program.

Discussion

Our data demonstrate that a family planning program has markedly reduced the fertility of a working—class community in Santiago after only 13 months of operation. But, we are aware that this result and the method through which it was obtained may arouse several objections, some of which will be discussed here.

Relative Number of Women Protected by the Program

The amount of change may seem surprisingly high for a program that has protected only 16 percent of the women in childbearing age (15–44 years). But the relative number of women protected by a program is not the only factor that determines the amount of change that the program may induce in the total population. At least two other factors should be considered: the effectiveness of the prescribed contraceptives and the previous fertility of the adopters. On the one hand, the higher the effectiveness of the contraceptive used, the greater the number of births that will be prevented in a given group. On the other hand, births in a community do not occur equally distributed among women of all ages, marital statuses, educational levels, and so on, but concentrate in women aged 20–35 years with less education. Consequently, the protection of a given number of married women in the ages 20–35 years will prevent a much larger number of births than will the protection of the same number of widows in ages 40–49 years or of single girls aged under 20 years.

The 181 "patients" in San Gregorio, had 81 livebirths in 1965 and only 19 in 1966; thus, their protection resulted in the prevention of 62 live births in the community. The same number of women in the NPW group had only 5.6 live births in 1965, and even if protected with 100 percent effective contraception, their protection would have resulted in the prevention of only 5.6 live births.

The relative number of women who were protected by the program (16 percent) was computed in terms of the total number of women in the sample instead of in terms of the number of women who need protection.

In the sample we found 465 single, widowed, or infertile women who do not need protection, all of whom belonged to the NPW group. Accordingly, the number of women who need protection is equal to the total sample minus 465. That is $1,132 - 465 = 667$. Now the percentage of women protected by the program may be computed as $\frac{181}{667} \cdot 100 = 27.1$ percent. We believe that the reader will get better information if we say that the program protected 27.1 percent of the women who need to be protected, instead of saying that the program protected 16 percent of all women in childbearing age in the sample.

All this tends to prove that the San Gregorio Family Planning Program was able to reduce the fertility of the community in 1966 because it gave only highly effective contraceptives to the women who attended the clinic and succeeded in selecting the women with the highest previous fertility in the community (Figure 1, Tables 1–4), and thus presented a considerable number of births through the protection of relatively few women.

The Pregnancy History Approach

The fertility data obtained through the pregnancy-history approach may be affected by errors of recall which run in the line of under-reporting of births (particularly of those babies who lived only a few months). If births were under-reported by errors of recall, the error should be greater for the years 1962-65 than for 1966. Consequently, the method would have underestimated the fertility decline observed in 1966, and the program would be responsible for a percentage decline even greater than 24.5 percent. On the other hand, our 1965 survey gave a TFR for 1964 for the total sample of 5,474 while the 1967 pregnancy history (based on a different sample) gave a TFR for 1964 for the total sample of 6,251. Both values are only slightly different since they are lower than the TFR obtained through the pregnancy history approach.

Consequently, the pregnancy history data were only slightly or not at all affected by errors of recall, at least for three years before the date of the survey, and if the data were affected, the effect of the program would have been greater than reported in this paper.

The 1964 Fertility Decline

The fertility of the total sample dropped in 1964, in the absence of a family planning program, in a rate similar to that observed in 1966. It has to be noted that whatever the validity of this objection and the significance of the 1964 fertility decline, the results presented in this paper demonstrating that the family planning program reduced the fertility of San Gregorio in 1966 are not invalidated. This objection only shows that the fertility of a community may change without an organized family planning program.

In trying to search for the factors that influenced the 1964 fertility decline and its significance, a deeper analysis of that change was made.

In order to measure the magnitude of the 1964 decline, we estimated the TFR that the total sample would have presented in 1964 if neither the patients, nor the OPW, nor the NPW had reduced their fertility in that year. This value is 7,801.0.[8] Since the real value of the TFR for 1964 is 6,251.0, the total decline observed is 1,550 points or 19.9 percent. This result shows that the 1964 decline is not as important as the reduction observed in 1966 which was 27.4 percent.

The total effect was subdivided in three components which correspond to the three groups that were classified according to attendance at the clinic and use of contraceptives in the period April, 1965–March 1966.[9] It was observed that the patients are responsible only for a 4.4 percent decline, the OPW account for a 6.5 percent decline, and the NPW account for the main responsibility—9.0 percent.

This confirms that the 1964 decline was mainly produced by the NPW as was suggested when we presented Figure 1. It may be better understood how this group may be responsible for a fertility decline in 1964 if we recall that the NPW were not necessarily unprotected before 1964.

In Figure 1 it may also be noted that both patients and NPW recovered the fertility they had before 1964 in the next years, while the OPW were the only group who continued fertility reduction.

San Gregorio and the rest of Santiago may have been under the influence of mass communication supporting family planning and modern contraception for the first time in 1963. The hypothesis may be suggested that the 1964 fertility decline was produced by some women in the three groups who started using contraceptives in 1963 without an organized program. As should be expected, only a small group continued using contraceptives in the next years (the OPW), and the others discontinued contraception after a first failure. Some of these women initiated the use of contraception again when the organized program of San Gregorio became available.

If this explanation were to be valid, the 1964 fertility decline would have been, to a great extent, a temporary change produced by the first trial in the use of modern contraceptives by a large number of women in San Gregorio. On the other hand, the reduction in fertility in 1966 is a larger decline produced by the full adoption of family planning by relatively few women.

It can be argued that patients will also recover their previous fertility in the years after 1966. The new survey to be taken in 1969 will give us data to answer this and other questions on the effect of the second and third year of the family planning program on the fertility of the community.

Assumptions Underlying the Estimation of the Effect of the Program

The effect of the program was estimated assuming that without its influence the patients would have maintained the fertility they had in the previous years. But we have seen that organized family planning programs are not the only source of fertility change. The fertility decline of the OPW in 1966, for instance, may be the result of extra-program factors, such as the general change in attitudes towards and practice of modern contraception that has been observed in Santiago in the last few years. To the extent that these factors may have influenced the patients, it has to be assumed that in the absence of the family planning program they would have reduced their fertility in a rate similar to that of the OPW, instead of maintaining it.

This objection led us to estimate the TFR that the total sample would have presented in 1966 if the patients had reduced their fertility in 1966 in the same rate as the OPW since 1963 (provided that the NPW and the OPW behaved as they actually did).

The computation of this estimate gave 6,411.0; that is, the TFR for the total sample in 1966 would have been 6,411.0 instead of 5,134.5 if patients had reduced their fertility in the same rate as OPW instead of at the rate they really did under the family planning program.

The difference between 6,411.0 and 5,134.5, which is 1,276.5, or 19.9 percent decline, provides our most conservative estimation of the change induced by the program on the TFR of the total sample in 1966. However, this fertility estimated for 1966 assumes that the patients reduced their TFR from 13,871.5 in 1965 (Table 2) to 10,301[10] in 1966 without an organized family planning program. This is hard to believe because the reduction observed in the previous years never reached a third of the decline assumed for 1966.

Even accepting this objection, the family planning program would have caused a 19.9 percent decline of the fertility of the total sample, and the program would still have the main responsibility for the change in fertility observed in 1966.

Notes

1. D. J. Bogue, "Inventory, Explanation, and Evaluation by Interview of Family Planning Motives-Attitudes-Knowledge-Behavior" (paper presented to the International Conference on Family Planning Programs, Geneva, Switzerland, August 23–27, 1965).
2. The sample design corresponds then to a stratified cluster sample with proportional allocation.
3. The first patient attended the contraceptive clinic at San Gregorio on March 9, 1965. All patients who attended the clinic from March 9 to March 31, 1965 returned later and are included, consequently, as patients. The patients' group includes then all women who attended the clinic in the first thirteen calendar months of operation of the family planning program.
4. A slight approximation was introduced in the computation of the person-years: each woman was classified directly as 1 person-year in the age group corresponding to the age at which she was at the end of each calendar year.
5. The method may be used to study the causes of any fertility change on the basis of a subdivision of a sample into different groups which represent potential sources of fertility change, and which are determined by the hypothesis that the study is based on.
6. In the development of the method, we have borrowed some terms from variance analysis terminology. We hope this will not result in confusion. Although a "total effect" is subdivided into "additive effects" due to different "sources of variation," no variances are computed nor subdivided in our method.
7. The NPW group could have been included as a source of variation, but we have omitted it because we are interested in explaining the "decline," and this group has no participation in the decline. The NPW effect was of slight importance in any case. Its omission has the advantage of simplifying the analysis.
8. The correponding tables are omitted to save space.
9. We are aware that the group should be classified according to use of contraception in the period April, 1963–March, 1964, but that is out of the scope of this paper. We are more interested in the evolution in time of the three groups into which the 1966 sample was subdivided.
10. The TFR that patients would have presented in 1966 if they had reduced their previous fertility in the same rate as the OPW is 10,301. It was computed by applying the average percentage reduction of the ASFR of OPW since 1963 to the ASFR of the patients estimated as in Table 5.

Auxiliary Midwife Prescription of Oral Contraceptives: An Experimental Project in Thailand

Allan G. Rosenfield and Charoon Limcharoen

Programmatic issue: *The issue that prompted the design of this project was the shortage of physicians and health personnel in general, a serious obstacle in the delivery of health and family planning services in the developing countries. Some evidence was found that nurses and auxiliary personnel were sufficiently competent to prescribe IUDs and oral contraceptives.*

Programmatic processes/components: *The National Family Planning Program in Thailand was initiated in 1968 using the existing health-care system, facilities, and personnel. Because a shortage existed of physicians and of nurses together with a relative abundance of auxiliary midwives, in 1969 a project was designed to test the use of midwifes to prescribe oral contraceptives to replace physicians' services in rural Thailand.*

Research design: *The project was designed to test whether clients would experience any health risks if auxiliary midwives were to prescribe pills, and whether midwives' proximity to rural couples would increase the number of contraceptive acceptors. Of 17 provinces where the family planning program was in place, four were selected in which midwives would have the right to prescribe pills and the remaining 13 were assigned as control provinces. The midwives were trained to use a checklist to review the client's relevant health history and present status. If any of the almost 20 items on the checklist, such as severe headaches, nipple discharge, high blood pressure and sugar in urine, were positive, the midwife referred the woman to a physician.*

Findings: *In the six months after the project started the number of acceptors of oral contraceptives increased by 395 percent in the four study provinces, four times as many as in the six previous months. In the 13 control provinces, the comparable increase was 29 percent. In addition, the six- and 12-month continuation rates of OC acceptors were higher among women who were serviced by auxiliary midwives, compared with those serviced by physicians. Their continuation rates were also higher than before. Furthermore, no increase in side effects or complications was recorded.*

Program response to findings: *The results of this project prompted the Ministry of Public Health to decide that trained auxiliary midwives throughout* *the country could prescribe oral contraceptives using the checklist. Thus in mid 1970, the number of clinics offering an effective family planning method increased from 350 to 3,500. The number of monthly pill acceptors grew from 8,800 in April 1970 to 31,000 in December 1971; OC acceptors accounted for 71 percent of total acceptors.*

Discussion: *Rosenfield and Limcharoen conclude that the results of the study are "a most compelling demonstration of the effect of bringing services closer to the people." They also assert that this procedure is justified taking into account risks of OCs compared with risks of pregnancies: "The health of mothers and children will be improved since it is clear that maternal and infant morbidity and mortality rates are higher in high-parity women, particularly when there are many children with little or no spacing." Finally, the authors emphasize that the increased use of nursing and paramedical personnel is an absolute necessity for widespread delivery of family planning services.*

Auxiliary Midwife Prescription of Oral Contraceptives: An Experimental Project in Thailand

Allan G. Rosenfield and Charoon Limcharoen

One of the great problems in the delivery of both health and family planning services, in countries throughout the world, has been the shortage of physicians.[11] This is particularly true in developing countries where as many as 80 per cent of the population reside in rural areas, while the vast majority of physicians live and work in the few urban centers. In Thailand, for example, there is one physician per 7,000 people, as compared to the United States where the ratio is 1:700. But even these figures are misleading, since half of the total number of Thai doctors live in Bangkok where the ratio is 1:1,000, and most of the rest are in other cities or large towns. In the rural areas, there is approximately 1 physician per 110,000 people.

Much attention has been given to the development of medical assistants, who can provide many needed health services in place of physicians.[5, 6, 12] Medical assistants of various types are presently being utilized in several areas of the world including China, Russia, and a number of African countries. In the United States, in recent years, there has been a great deal of discussion about the use of such personnel, and a number of training programs have been developed.[8, 9, 15]

Family planning programs are presently being given high priority in countries throughout the world, but there are many who feel that the programs are not moving fast enough to offset the critical consequences of the present high population growth rates.[3, 4] The serious shortage of medical personnel certainly makes the implementation of a family planning program based on the more effective methods of contraception, such as the pill and the intrauterine contraceptive device (IUD), extremely difficult. A recent paper reviewed experiences in a variety of countries of the use of nurses and auxiliary health personnel to prescribe hormonal contraception and to insert intrauterine devices.[13] The conclusion was reached that it was both safe and practical to allow persons other than physicians to do these jobs. The report suggested that, in the absence of facilities and personnel to handle cytologic smears and in the face of very limited health care

Reprinted with permission from Mosby-Year Book, Inc. from *American Journal of Obstetrics and Gynecology* 1972. 114,7: 942–949.

systems, a pelvic examination could safely be omitted prior to the prescription of oral contraceptives, although use of a special checklist was recommended.

Family planning activities in Thailand were first initiated on a national scale in 1968, and were introduced within the existing health services, with the use of existing personnel rather than full-time family planning workers.[14] No incentives are given to the field staff or to acceptors; to the contrary, a small donation is requested from those patients who can afford to pay (up to 25 cents for a cycle of pills, $1.00 for an IUD, and $7.50 for a tubal ligation).

In 1969, a research project was developed by the National Family Planning Program of the Ministry of Public Health to test the concept of the use of auxiliary midwives to prescribe oral contraceptives, because of the totally inadequate number of physicians in rural Thailand to provide the needed services. There are similar shortages of nurse-midwives in the rural areas, but there is a relative abundance of auxiliary midwives, who are women with 10 years of basic education, recruited from predominantly rural areas. They receive an 18 month training course in midwifery and various aspects of public health nursing, with emphasis being given to service in rural areas, outside of hospital facilities. There are, at present, over 3,500 of these auxiliary midwives, producing a ratio of one such midwife per 8,000 rural inhabitants. They have a tendency to remain in the village or town of their assignment, preferring, it appears, to live near their families rather than moving to the larger cities where work is more difficult to find (the majority of urban deliveries occur in hospitals in which there are no positions for auxiliary midwives). Thus, auxiliary midwives are relatively close to the people, closer, certainly, than most other health personnel. And, of great importance, they continue to work after marriage and after having children.

The research project was designed primarily to attempt to prove two hypotheses, namely, that it was safe for auxiliary midwives to prescribe the pill and that the accessibility of the midwives to rural couples would significantly increase the number of oral contraceptive acceptors. It was also hoped that this same proximity of the auxiliary midwife would help to improve pill continuation rates.

Material and Methods

During 1969, the first year of the Ministry of Public Health's National Family Planning Program, personnel were trained and family planning clinics were opened in existing facilities of 17 provinces in the northeast and southern regions of Thailand. Four of these provinces were chosen at random to take part in this study, with the remaining 13 provinces serving as a control.

Table 1 presents the population data for the 4 study provinces and the 13 control provinces, as well as data on the health facilities in the provinces. Provincial hospitals are located in the capital town of each province, and, in addition, one of the control provinces also had a second hospital located in a large district town. In the hospital family planning clinics, physicians are responsible for prescription of the pill as well as insertion of the IUD. Health centers are located in the rural areas, those with a physician being in larger district towns. For comparison purposes, Table 1 also shows the ratio of the 3 categories of health facilities per 1,000,000 people, and, as can be seen, there were significantly fewer health centers without a physician in the 4 study provinces than in the control provinces while the ratio of health centers with a physician was similar throughout.

In the 4 study provinces, there were over 160 auxiliary midwives who had previously attended the basic one-week family planning training course in which emphasis had been placed on the two most important methods of contraception used in the national program (intrauterine devices and oral contraceptives), as well as on sterilization procedures. The material stressed contraindications, side effects, and common rumors and fears related to the IUD and the pill. It was felt that this basic training should have been sufficient and that no special further training would be necessary. Thus, the auxiliary midwives were simply called together for a one-day meeting in each province, at which time the project to study the prescription of oral contraceptives by auxiliary midwives was explained in detail. In the 13 control provinces, there were 783 midwives who had received family planning training, but they were not allowed to prescribe the pill.

The special checklist, mentioned previously, was modified and prepared in Thai for use by the auxiliary midwives (Table 2). The list included a simple history and examination, designed to rule out contraindications to the use of the pill. If the answer to any of the questions was positive, the patient was not to receive the pill but was, instead, to be referred to a physician for a decision concerning prescription of the pill. During the one-day briefing session, the use of the questionnaire was explained in detail to the auxiliary midwives and to their

Table 1. Population data and health facilities in the four study and thirteen control provinces (1969)

	Four study provinces	Thirteen control provinces
Total population	2,231,500	8,940,000
Eligible female population	280,000	1,540,000
Hospitals		
No.	4	14
No. per 1,000,000	1.8	1.6
Health centers with MD		
No.	13	36
No. per 1,000,000	5.8	4.0
Health centers without MD		
No.	139	764
No. per 1,000,000	62.3	85.5

Table 2. Checklist for personnel prescribing oral contraceptives*

	Yes	No
History: Ask if the patient has had a history of any of the following:		
Yellow skin or yellow eyes		
Mass in the breast		
Discharge from the nipple		
Swelling or severe pains in the legs		
Severe chest pains		
Unusual shortness of breath after exertion		
Severe headaches		
Excessive menstrual periods		
Increased frequency of menstrual periods		
Bleeding after sexual intercourse		
Examination: Check the following:		
Yellow skin and yellow eye color		
Mass in the breast		
Nipple discharge		
Varicose veins in the legs		
Blood pressure (yes = above 160)		
Pulse (yes = above 120)		
Urine for sugar		
Urine for protein		

*Instructions: If all the above are answered in the negative, the patient may receive oral contraceptives, but, if any are answered in the positive, the patient must first be seen by a physician.

nurse supervisors, these latter personnel having the responsibility of supervising the activities of the auxiliary midwives. The government rural health physicians in each province also took part in the session, so that they, too, were fully informed.

After the meeting, the auxiliary midwives in the 4 provinces, the majority of whom worked in health centers without a physician, were then allowed to prescribe the pill. The study began in April, 1969, and a follow-up survey of family planning acceptors was conducted in 1970. In this study, acceptors were randomly selected from the 4 study provinces and the control provinces. Interviews were conducted in the villages and supervised by staff from the central evaluation unit of the national program. Continuation rates were compared between women receiving the initial prescription of pills from auxiliary midwives and those receiving them from physicians.

The pills used were ethynodiol diacetate, 1 mg., and mestranol, 0.1 mg. (Ovulen, G.D. Searle & Co., Chicago, Illinois), and norgesterol, 0.5 mg., and ethinyl estradiol, 0.05 mg. (Ovral, Wyeth Labs., Philadelphia, Pennsylvania), which were the drugs used in the national program. In general, one cycle was given the first time, and anywhere from one to three cycles were given at the times of resupply. Motivational efforts were limited to face-to-face communication because public informational activities in the field of family planning were not allowed by the Thai Government at the time of this study. The auxiliary midwives in all 17 provinces had earlier been supplied with flip-charts, simple motivational leaflets, and pamphlets with instructions for the use of the pill and IUD.

In presenting the results, only data from health centers are reported because there were no policy differences between hospitals in the study provinces and the control provinces. Furthermore, the hospitals do not have auxiliary midwives on their staff.

Results

The number of pill acceptors in rural health centers of the 4 study provinces, for the period of April to September, 1969, was greater than the total number of pill acceptors in the 13 control provinces during the same period (Table 3). Similarly, the increase in pill acceptors, noted in these 4 provinces, between the 6 months before and after initiation of the study, is dramatic. Table 4 presents the percentage of married, fertile women between the ages of 15 and 45 who accepted an IUD or pill in a rural health center in the study and control provinces during the first 6 months of the study. The percentage of women accepting the pill in the 4 study provinces was significantly higher than in the control provinces, and this increase was so great that it produced a much higher percentage of women who had accepted family planning services in general.

Of interest in this study was the comparative continuation rates. Because of time constraints, only 6 and 12 month rates could be calculated, although

Table 3. Acceptors in rural health centers by method 6 months before and after the onset of the study

	Four study provinces		Thirteen control provinces	
	IUD	Pill	IUD	Pill
October, 1968 to March, 1969	1,940	1,129	3,927	4,298
April, 1969 to September, 1969	1,348	5,590	3,297	5,559
Percent change	−31	+395	−16	+29

Table 4. Percentage of married, fertile women accepting contraception or sterilization in the study and control provinces between April and September, 1969

	Study provinces		Control provinces	
Method/institution	Acceptors	Percent of eligible women	Acceptors	Percent of eligible women
IUD/H.C.*	1,348	0.5	3,297	0.3
Pill/H.C.	5,590	2.0	5,559	0.5
IUD/Hospital	629	0.2	1,946	0.2
Pill/Hospital	55	<0.1	1,013	<0.1
Sterilization/Hospital + H.C.	166	<0.1	736	<0.1
Total	7,788	2.8	12,551	1.1

*H.C.=Health center.

Table 5. Continuation rates and reasons for termination of oral
contraceptives prescribed by doctors and by auxiliary midwives

	6 Months		12 Months	
	Pill/doctor	Pill/midwife	Pill/doctor	Pill/midwife
Continuation rate	76.0	84.5	66.7	75.8
Reasons for termination				
Pregnancy	—	0.3	—	0.3
Medical reason	15.8	11.0	22.1	14.3
Personal reason	8.2	4.2	11.2	9.6

another follow-up study is planned in order to obtain rates for 24 months and longer. As can be seen in Table 5, the 12 month rate for women accepting the pill from an auxiliary midwife was higher than that for women receiving services from a physician, although the difference may not be significant since the rates were not cross-tabulated with the various patient characteristics of the two groups of acceptors. The discontinuation of usage for medical reasons was lower in the pill/midwife cases, and there were no reports of serious complications related to the pill in either study or control provinces. Similarly, discontinuation for personal reasons was also lower in the study provinces.

Table 6 presents the incidence of side effects, most of which were minor, in the 4 study provinces. A detailed study was not conducted in the control provinces, but the incidence in the study provinces was lower than that found in a study of side effects in a large Bangkok hospital family planning clinic[2] for all complaints but vomiting and face pigmentation. As in most studies, decreased menstruation, weight gain, and nausea were the most common complaints. Other than face pigmentation, however, these were all subjective complaints, and the difference in incidence, therefore, could simply be related to more sophisticated questioning by doctors in the urban Women's Hospital as compared to auxiliary midwives in rural health centers.

Comment

The major purpose of this study was to demonstrate the safety and the effectiveness of the use of auxiliary midwives to prescribe oral contraceptives. While it is obviously too early to make definitive statements about side effects and complications, it is fair to state that there was no increase in the incidence of either during the first year of study.

The fact that there were more pill acceptors in the 4 study provinces than in the 13 control provinces, in spite of the fact that there were approximately 6 times as many health centers and health personnel in the control provinces, is a most dramatic demonstration of the effectiveness of the use of auxiliary midwives to prescribe the pill. The remarkable increase in the number of pill accep-

Table 6. Percentage of oral contraceptive acceptors having side effects in the 4 study provinces and at Women's Hospital*

Side effect	Women's hospital	Study provinces
Decreased menstruation	44.2	28.1
Amenorrhea	3.0	2.0
Weight gain	46.5	20.0
Nausea	18.5	18.4
Vomiting	2.1	9.9
Headache	14.4	7.3
Face pigmentation	3.0	10.0

*A Bangkok hospital with large maternity and family planning services (unpublished data).

tors in the first 6 months after the study was initiated as compared to the 6 months immediately before, together with the significantly higher percentage of eligible women accepting contraception in the study provinces, further demonstrates the tremendous potential impact of the adoption of this concept on a nationwide scale.

More specifically, the acceptor targets in the 5 year plan of the National Family Planning Program make the assumption that approximately 8 per cent of the eligible population will accept family planning services each year. In the study provinces, during the first 6 months of the study, almost 3 per cent of the eligible women accepted family planning as compared to only 1 per cent in the control provinces. Thus, based on the experience in these 17 provinces, it seems clear that the national target would be extremely difficult to reach without the use of auxiliary midwives.

There was concern that there might be more acceptors but lower continuation rates. The opposite occurred, and the pill continuation rates in the 4 provinces in which midwives prescribed the pill were actually higher than in those provinces in which pills were prescribed by doctors. It is hypothesized that auxiliary midwives, who are located in much closer proximity to the village women than are the clinics with a physician, and who are also much closer in terms of socioeconomic background, are perhaps able to develop a better relationship with the women than can a physician.

The implications of this study were of great significance to the National Family Planning Program of the Ministry of Public Health.[14] By the end of 1970, over 4,000 personnel (doctors, nurses, and auxiliary midwives) had received training in the fields of population and family planning. There were 84 provincial hospitals with clinics outside Bangkok and over 250 other clinics with a physician offering family planning services in Bangkok hospitals and governmental health centers throughout the country. Thus, there were only approximately 350 clinics offering the pill or the IUD to a married, fertile female population, aged 15 to 45, of over 4,300,000 people.

In mid-1970, as a result of the apparent success of this pilot study, the Ministry of Public Health ruled that all auxiliary midwives who had received the basic family planning training course could prescribe the pill, making use of the checklist, as in the study. This meant that the total number of clinics offering an effective method of contraception immediately jumped from approximately 350 to almost 3,500.

Fig. 1 presents the 6 month totals of family planning acceptors nationwide in Thailand. The pill and the IUD were approximately equal in numbers in late 1969 and early 1970, but a dramatic increase in the number of pill acceptors can be seen beginning in June, 1970, as a result of the Ministry ruling; the monthly totals increased from approximately 8,800 in April, 1970, to almost 31,000 in December, 1971. In 1971, there were 404,187 new acceptors of family planning services, with the pill accounting for 73 per cent of the total, the great majority being prescribed by auxiliary midwives in rural health centers. This was over 100,000 more than the original 1971 target and allowed the national program to reach the 1973 target of over 8 per cent of the eligible population in one year, two years earlier than expected.

Figure 1. Family planning acceptors by 3 month periods, 1969 to 1971.

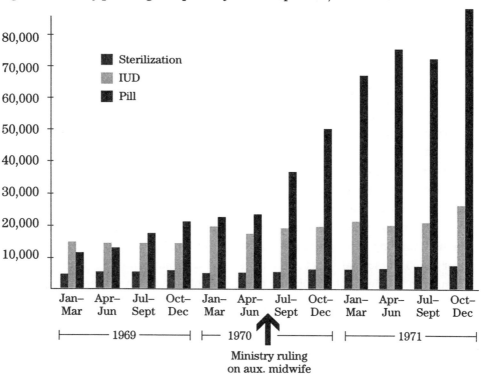

Although a national population policy was declared in March, 1970, and there was increasing government commitment to family planning thereafter, the only major change in program activities during this period was the ruling concerning auxiliary midwives. Major efforts in the field of public information are only beginning in 1972. This, then, is a most compelling demonstration of the effect of bringing services closer to the people. Furthermore, it is clear that the national program would have had great difficulty in reaching its targets without the ruling concerning midwife prescription of the pill.

Conclusion

There is little hope of being able to provide family planning services to the vast numbers of women living in the rural areas of the world if we rely on physicians alone. This study has shown that auxiliary midwives can, indeed, prescribe oral contraceptives safely and that acceptance rates will dramatically increase when services are made more readily accessible to potential acceptors. Similarly, continuation rates also appear to increase, although the difference noted may not be significant.

The fact that a pelvic examination was not performed by the auxiliary midwives prior to the prescription of the pill is a somewhat dramatic departure from presently accepted medical practice. It is generally recommended, for example, that all potential pill acceptors should have a Papanicolaou smear taken prior to the prescription of the drug. Unfortunately, in the rural areas of most developing countries, this is impossible because there simply are insufficient personnel and facilities available to prepare and read the slides. Thailand has recently embarked on a program to produce cytotechnicians, although the question of health priorities must be taken into consideration. The opinion was stated in an earlier paper that ". . . in many countries, the priority for such a program may be relatively low compared to other pressing health needs,"[13] as well as compared to the critical pressures developing due to the population problem.

There is ample evidence that paramedical personnel can be taught to perform pelvic examinations and to insert intrauterine devices.[1, 7, 10, 13, 16] Not only will this help to further the aims of family planning programs when there are shortages of physicians, but it will help to improve basic health care. The problem, however, is that it is relatively simple to train auxiliary personnel to use a medical checklist, such as the one described in this paper, but it is much more difficult to train these personnel to do pelvic examinations and to insert the IUD properly. In Thailand, for example, it was considered that the basic one-week family planning course sufficiently prepared the auxiliary midwife to utilize the pill checklist. A pelvic examination and IUD insertion training course unfortunately takes much longer.

Recently, the National Family Planning Program has developed an IUD insertion training program for nurse/midwives in which the techniques of pelvic examination are emphasized. This course will take a minimum of 6 weeks, and only a relatively small number of personnel can be trained together at one time. While there is the hope that eventually the training can be carried out at a number of clinics, where the local physician, trained in the technique of IUD insertion, will serve as the instructor of personnel under his jurisdiction. At the present time, however, the training is only being carried out in major institutions, and, during the first year (1972), only 60 nurse/midwives will be trained. It will be necessary to accelerate this training if we are to hope to have an effect similar to that already seen with the pill. Eventually, training in the techniques of pelvic examination and IUD insertion (as well as in other areas of medical care, previously restricted to physicians only) will be introduced into schools for nurses and for auxiliary midwives, so that, in the future, all graduates of these schools will already be prepared to provide these vital services.

In the interim period, while waiting for nurse/midwives and auxiliary personnel to receive the appropriate training to perform pelvic examination, and considering the risk of oral contraception as compared to the risk of the pregnancy which the pill prevents, it is the opinion of the authors that it is perfectly justified to allow the pill to be prescribed simply with the use of the checklist. This is particularly so in rural areas where it is estimated that the maternal mortality rate is as high as 500 per 100,000 live births. Readily available family planning services will obviously help to lower the critically high rates of population growth. In addition, the health of mothers and children will be improved since it is clear that maternal and infant morbidity and mortality rates are higher in high-parity women, particularly when there are many children with little or no spacing.[17] Similarly, the contact with the women in a family planning clinic provides the opportunity for improving other related health services as well.

The delivery of health and family planning services is severely limited in the rural areas of the developing world, areas in which the majority of the people live. The problems of improved services are immense. The increased utilization of nursing and paramedical personnel is an absolute necessity; "It behooves the medical profession to remove unnecessary and unrealistic roadblocks from improved delivery of presently available contraceptive *(and health)* services."[13]

References

1. Beasley, W. B. R.: Am. J. Obstet. Gynecol. 98: 201, 1967.
2. Banharnsupawat, L., and Limtrakarn, J.: Unpublished data.
3. Berelson, B.: Stud. Family Planning 38: 1, 1969.
4. Davis, K.: Science 158: 730, 1967.

5. Fendall, N. R. E.: Pub. Health Rep. 78: 977, 1963.

6. Fendall, N. R. E.: Pub. Health Rep. 82: 471, 1967.

7. Hartfield, V. J.: Contraception 3: 105, 1971.

8. Hellman, L. M.: Obstet., Gynecol. 30: 883, 1967.

9. Hellman, L. M.: Yankauer, A., Jones, S. H., et al.: Internat. J. Gynaecol. Obstet. 8: 732, 1970.

10. Jafarey, S. A., Hardee, J. G., and Saterthwaite, A. P.: Demography 5: 666, 1968.

11. King, M.: *In* King, M., editor: Medical Care in Developing Countries, London, 1966, Oxford University Press, p. 1.1.

12. King, M.: *In* King, M., editor: Medical Care in Developing Countries, London, 1966, Oxford University Press, p. 7.1.

13. Rosenfield, A. G.: Am. J. Obstet. Gynecol. 110: 1030, 1971.

14. Rosenfield, A. G., Hemachudha, C., Asavasena, W., and Varakamin, S.: Stud. Family Planning 2: 181, 1971.

15. Smith, M. R., Bradley, S., Soderstrom, R., and Hayden, G. E.: Obstet. Gynecol. 38: 308, 1971.

16. Valliant, H. W., Cummins, G. T. M., Richart, R. M., and Barron, B. A.: Br. Med. J. 3: 671, 1968.

17. Wray, J. D.: *In* Revelle, R., editor: Rapid Population Growth: Consequences and Policy Implications, Baltimore, 1971, Johns Hopkins Press, p. 403.

The Demographic Impact of the Family Planning–Health Services Project in Matlab, Bangladesh

James F. Phillips, Wayne S. Stinson, Shushum Bhatia,
Makhlisur Rahman, and J. Chakraborty

Programmatic issue: *The need to test the hypothesis that "contraceptive service programs can increase the prevalence of contraceptive use by fulfilling a latent demand for services.....meeting this demand will change fertility significantly by increasing the prevalence of birth spacing and limitation behavior."*

Programmatic processes/components: *Appropriately selected literate, young married village women were recruited, most of them members of influential families in the villages where they were to work. They underwent six weeks of special training to conduct frequent and regular visits to all women whether practicing contraception or not. A wide choice of methods was conveniently available as were ancillary health services.*

Research design: *Continuous (quarterly and annual) monitoring of the use of contraceptives and of fertility measures was feasible because of to the existence of a demographic surveillance system at Matlab. At the time the project was designed the system covered a population of 168,000 in 149 villages. Treatment and control areas were established.*

Findings: *The central finding of the project was the confirmation of the main hypothesis, namely that "contraceptive services can initiate a fertility change in a poor rural traditional population." In other words, unmet demand for contraception exists in rural Bangladesh that can be served by an intensive field program. Specifically, during the first 15 months of implementation contraceptive use increased from 10 percent in October 1977 to 34 percent by the end of 1978. During the first two project years, 1978 and 1979 (July 1978–June 1980) fertility in the treatment areas was 25 percent lower than in the areas of comparison. Possible contamination of the findings by an earlier project, the Contraceptive Distribution Project (CDP), was recognized and results from that project were isolated by the help of a sophisticated statistical analysis showing that the fertility-decline effect of this effort was about 22 percent compared with that of the CDP of 8 percent.*

Program response to findings: *A hypothesis is discussed, namely that the poor performance of the national program could be the result of incomplete program implementation rather than of the absence of motivation among rural Bangladeshi couples to limit or space births. During the 1980s, Matlab experience was used in the national family planning program.*

Discussion: *A number of meaningful policy implications are discussed in the paper. Apparently fertility can be reduced significantly in Bangladesh by making contraceptives readily available. Several conditions, such as appropriately trained field workers and systematic follow-up, must be fulfilled for the proposition to apply. Further a user-oriented program with a wide choice of methods, skilled counseling, rigorous follow-up, treatment of side-effects and ancillary health services, will be substantially more effective than a program based on one or two methods distributed by unskilled workers. Also pertinent research issues are raised, such as: Do reproductive motives change after accepting contraception? Are they affected by programs? What are the determinants of program success, considering that it varies substantially from one village to another?*

The Demographic Impact of the Family Planning–Health Services Project in Matlab, Bangladesh

James F. Phillips, Wayne S. Stinson, Shushum Bhatia, Makhlisur Rahman, and J. Chakraborty

Demographic research has shown that fertility has declined in a variety of settings where there has been concomitant proliferation of contraceptive use. This has suggested to many observers that organized contraceptive service programs have contributed to the observed trends.[1] Yet the causal role of contraceptive service programs in inducing and sustaining fertility reduction in developing countries continues to be the subject of discussion and debate, principally because establishing causality requires rigorous experimental designs. Field experiments appropriate for a test of service program effects require large-scale field operations, treatment and control areas, and accurate longitudinal demographic data—conditions that can rarely be met in practice.[2] This report analyzes the demographic effects of a study in Matlab Thana of Bangladesh that meets these conditions.

The Family Planning–Health Services Project Hypothesis

The Family Planning–Health Services Project (FPHSP) was launched by the Cholera Research Laboratory (CRL)[3] in October 1977 and continues to the present. The FPHSP followed an earlier study, the Contraceptive Distribution Project (CDP).[4] Although these studies differed in their service strategies, they shared an underlying hypothesis—namely, that contraceptive service programs can increase the prevalence of contraceptive use by fulfilling a latent demand for services. According to this hypothesis, meeting this demand will change fertility significantly by increasing the prevalence of birth spacing and limitation behavior.

The Matlab Setting

Matlab was selected for contraceptive field experiments because of the demographic data resources of the CRL. In 1963, a demographic surveillance system (DSS) was established for evaluating cholera vaccines. At the time the FPHSP

Reprinted with the permission of the Population Council from *Studies in Family Planning* 1982. 13,5: 131–140.

was launched in 1977, the DSS encompassed 149 villages and a population of approximately 168,000. Since research had shown that the DSS data are complete and accurate, contraceptive service effects could be evaluated by simply tabulating vital data for the Matlab area and updating census data for 1974 with birth, death, and migration data for successive years. Since the population under surveillance was large and the mobility of families is limited, it was possible to designate treatment and comparison areas.

The value of Matlab as a social research laboratory is greatly enhanced by features of the geographic and social setting that mitigate the prospect of confounding effects from social or economic change. The geography of the area tends to insulate treatments from one another and from the outside world. Matlab is a totally rural, riverine area intersected by tributaries of the Gumoti and Megna rivers. As such it is largely inaccessible by road or other forms of modern transportation and communication, and is therefore an area where the potentially contaminating effects of intervillage trade and contact are less than would prevail in most other rural areas of Asia.

The social setting in Matlab can also be viewed as relatively free of potentially contaminating factors. In much of Asia rural populations have been increasingly exposed to nontraditional economic institutions and values in recent years. Mass communication and transportation, for example, have penetrated most rural areas of South East Asia, with effects on values and aspirations that greatly complicate the assessment of the net effects of contraceptive services. While it would be incorrect to posit that conditions in Matlab have been altogether static in recent years, there is no evidence of systematic economic, social, or political improvements of the sort that would contribute significantly to demographic change. In fact, most analysts stress the worsening of conditions in rural Bangladesh: landlessness has grown markedly in recent years;[5] illiteracy, though high, has not declined;[6] and health conditions, while improved in this century owing to control of infectious diseases, may have deteriorated over the past decade from the combined effects of political crises and famine.[7] The changes that have occurred are therefore not of a sort that demographers regard as prerequisites or corequisites of demographic transition.[8] Even if change were occurring, it is reasonable to argue that trends would affect treatment and comparison areas similarly.[9] Since the pre-experimental population was noncontracepting and dramatic socioeconomic development is lacking, the prospect that secular fertility changes would confound results is remote. Matlab is thus in many respects an ideal site for testing the latent-demand hypothesis.

Experimental Design

The FPHSP design was intended to address issues that arose from an earlier study, the CDP. The CDP employed largely illiterate and elderly female workers, who distributed pills and condoms to women in their homes.[10] After an initial three month period of success, prevalence declined. Demographic effects were limited to the first project impact year.[11] Since the project was initially successful, the CDP findings suggested an unfulfilled demand. Since effects were temporary, however, the CDP findings suggested that a residual unfulfilled demand for contraception persisted in 1977 despite two years of CDP services—a demand that could be better served by a wider battery of methods and more intensive follow-up and care of users. Certain operational problems of the CDP approach underscored this conclusion. Although workers were knowledgeable about their villages, they were too old to have practiced contraception, and they were not trained to deal with side effects. Thus they lacked credibility as family planning workers and were only infrequently relied upon for contraceptive advice. This situation was exacerbated by their relatively low social status among villagers, who accorded them too little prestige for them to be effective agents of social change.

The limitations of the CDP led to a restructuring of contraceptive research in Matlab into the Family Planning–Health Services Project (FPHSP).[12] CDP treatments were partitioned into cells of the FPHSP and subsequently collapsed into new treatments. The populations of village groups of the new design are shown in Table 1.

Although the FPHSP work began in October 1977, CDP household distribution activity continued in CDP treatment areas until March 1978, when fieldworkers provided acceptors with a six-month supply and advised them to contact local government family planning workers for their future supplies. In the remaining half of the CDP distribution area and in half of the comparison area, a new FPHSP field structure was developed.[13] Literate, young, married village workers were recruited, most of whom were members of influential families. All were recruited from households in the village in which they were to

Table 1. Populations of village groups in the CDP-FPHSP experimental design

	FPHSP villages					
	Treatment			Comparison		
	Number of villages	1974[a] population	1978[b] population	Number of villages	1974[a] population	1978[b] population
Former CDP treatment	39	42043	44682	54	43742	45020
Former CDP comparison	31	42731	44668	25	39134	40576
Total FPHSP[c]	70	84774	89350	79	82876	85596

[a]Midyear population, 1974. [b]Year-end population. [c]Note that the DSS surveillance area was contracted to 149 villages in 1978 owing to cost constraints. Thus CDP cell populations do not correspond to the presentation of CDP treatments in Stinson et al., in this issue.

work. These female village workers (FVWs) were given six weeks of intensive training in contraception, field visitation methods, and basic reproductive physiology. In the first 12 months of the project weekly meetings were convened to train FVWs in the treatment of minor ailments, basic nutrition, tetanus toxoid injection methods, and other MCH work.

The administrative system incorporated two forms of supervision: technical supervision for treatment and referral of MCH/FP problems, and administrative supervision to ensure that work was being done on schedule at all levels. This system involved recruitment of lady family planning visitors (LFPVs), who were government-certified paramedics with 18 months of formal training, and male supervisors, senior health assistants (SHA). One SHA and one LFPV were assigned to districts of 20 villages, each encompassing a population of 20,000. SHAs served as male motivators and community organizers. One medical officer was assigned to the project, to supervise tubecotomies in Matlab,[14] conduct medical rounds in the field, and train paramedics continuously.

Day-to-day management of the FPHSP was conducted by an administrator-paramedic and two assistants. Field staff were accountable to them for both service and research activities.

This service system was maintained continuously over the period October 1977 to October 1981. The overall goal of the FPHSP service system was to shift from the emphasis of the CDP on contraceptive technology to an emphasis on comprehensive contraceptive care, to include frequent and regular visits to all women whether contracepting or not, a wide choice of methods conveniently available, and ancillary health services. The initial emphasis was on comprehensive family planning services rather than MCH. The most important change was the addition of Depo Medroxyprogesterone Acetate (DMPA) to the battery of methods available in the village. At the subcenters paramedics inserted Copper T intrauterine devices and performed menstrual regulation.[15] The principal link between health and family planning services was a three-tiered referral system for the detection and treatment of side effects. All FVWs treated minor side effects and referred more serious problems to LFPVs, based in stationary subcenters, for treatment. LFPVs, in turn, were trained to conduct further referral to the physician in the Matlab clinic.

Methodology

The most salient feature of the methodology that follow is its simplicity: direct unadjusted fertility measures can be used owing to the availability of accurate and complete census and vital data for the period from 1968 to the present.[16] The DSS system has included birth, death, and migration registration since 1966 and marriage registration since 1975. Although intervillage migration is recorded in the field, only migration into and out of the surveillance areas is computerized. Thus information is not available on local migration, most notably among younger women who migrate for marriage. Resulting biases, if any, accumulate with time, but they are likely to be concentrated among women under age 20 or 25. A critical assumption of the research reported below is that net migration across treatment boundaries was sufficiently inconsequential to permit reliable birth rate comparisons.

This study presents quarterly and annual births for various village groups[17] for the period between mid-1974 and mid-1980.[18] The number of births was obtained from the vital registration data, although it should be noted that 1980 figures are preliminary.[19] The denominator was estimated for each period after mid-1974 by the lexis method of advancing a portion (in this case one-tenth) of each age group for each semester,[20] adjusting for deaths and net migration. Because project impact assessment begins at mid-years, all annual rates are expressed in July to June project years (PY). Denominators for annual birth rates of each PY use the estimated December 31st population, while midquarter denominators were interpolated for quarterly rates.

Three fertility measures are emphasized in this analysis. The first is the general fertility rate (GFR), which is calculated by dividing total births during a particular time period by the estimated number of women aged 15 to 44. Quarterly rates were annualized by multiplication. Since younger women typically have higher fertility rates than older ones, this measure is only appropriate if the areas and time periods being compared have approximately the same age distribution, as they do in this study.[21] Since project effects seemed to vary by age, we also calculated age-specific rates for women aged 15 to 29 and for women 30 and over. Five-year age-specific rates were calculated by year but not by quarter, owing to marked random fluctuation in quarterly rates for small populations. The total fertility rate (TFR) is not used extensively because the computational assumption of equal numbers of women in each five-year age group spuriously accentuates fertility impact if effects are pronounced among women aged 35 and over.

Results

Trends in Contraceptive Use Prevalence

Introduction of the FPHSP system was followed by a dramatic rise in contraceptive prevalence from 10 percent in October 1977 to 34 percent by the end of 1978, where use prevalence has remained to date. This trend in prevalence is illustrated in Figure 1. Contraceptive use was initially dominated by DMPA, but as alternative methods were developed—most notably tubectomy and the Copper T—the proportion of users protected by DMPA declined. But more significant, perhaps, than the declining proportion of DMPA users is the finding

Figure 1. Trends in prevalence of contraceptive use among married women of reproductive age by method, FPHSP treatment area, 1977–81

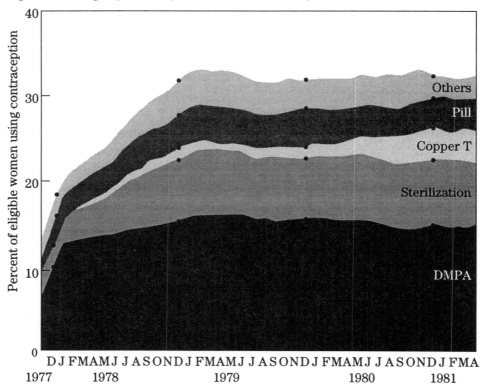

that absolute prevalence of DMPA has been roughly constant. Thus, as more methods were added to the cafeteria, more women were protected. This suggests that a wider choice of methods contributes to overall levels of contraceptive protection.

The Demographic Impact of the FPHSP

Table 2 presents fertility measures for the FPHSP for four years prior to the program and for two years in which program effects are possible. Since services were launched in the fourth quarter of 1977, July of 1978 was the earliest date for which effects were possible.

The data in Table 2 demonstrate that fertility patterns and levels were similar prior to PY 1976. By PY 1976 and PY 1977 treatment area fertility was approximately 8 percent lower than control area fertility, although age-specific rates show no consistent trend over time. We thus conclude from the table that fertility levels were essentially similar before the FPHSP, although minor differences arose in 1976 and 1977. We analyze the differences below.

Table 2. Age-specific fertility rates, total fertility rates (TFR), and general fertility rates (GFR) for the comparison and treatment areas of the FPHSP, preproject and project periods

	Preproject period												Project period					
	1974[a]			1975[a]			1976[a]			1977[a]			1978[a]			1979[a]		
Age group	T	C	% diff.	T	C	% diff.	T	C	% diff.	T	C	% diff.	T	C	% diff.	T	C	% diff.
15–19	152.1	155.1	−1.9	114.7	122.8	−6.6	171.9	181.3	−5.2	135.6	161.0	−15.8**	125.5	146.1	−14.1**	148.3	156.1	−5.0
20–24	259.8	260.4	−0.2	186.1	185.4	+0.4	303.0	337.6	−10.2*	232.2	248.6	−6.6	216.1	269.0	−19.7**	235.6	308.6	−23.7**
25–29	275.4	267.9	+2.6	188.1	207.8	−9.5	294.7	331.6	−11.1**	241.9	259.6	−6.8	185.3	236.1	−21.5**	215.7	281.7	−23.4**
30–34	213.9	231.2	−7.5	181.1	184.8	−2.0	315.6	328.2	−3.8	236.4	274.4	−13.8**	184.5	253.7	−27.3**	168.7	260.5	−35.2**
35–39	122.4	122.1	+0.2	91.2	100.5	−9.2	170.2	156.8	+8.5	150.8	154.6	−2.5	95.6	186.3	−48.7**	114.1	199.9	−42.9**
40–44	46.1	53.9	−14.5	41.9	47.9	−12.5	64.7	72.7	−11.0	69.9	70.2	−0.4	29.4	66.3	−55.6**	41.0	66.1	−37.9**
TFR	5.4	5.5	−1.8	4.0	4.3	−5.4	6.6	7.0	−6.2	5.3	5.8	−8.7	4.2	5.8	−27.8	4.6	6.4	−28.1
GFR	185.4	186.6	−0.6	138.5	145.0	−4.5	225.2	239.9	−6.2*	180.2	198.6	−9.3*	147.3	196.5	−25.0**	164.1	217.8	−24.7**

T = FPHSP treatment area. C = FPHSP comparison area. [a] All years are project years (July to June) of the specified year. * Statistically significant at p<.05.
** Statistically significant at p<.01. TFR differences were not tested.

The PY 1978 data contrast markedly with the level and pattern of fertility in the preproject period. Overall fertility in the treatment area was 25 percent lower than comparison area rates, a difference that accrued principally from marked reductions in fertility among women aged 30 and over. Among women aged 30–34 in Table 2, the birth rate is 27 percent lower in the treatment area than in the comparison area. Among women 35 and over the treatment area fertility level is nearly 50 percent lower—a differential that was unprecedented in recent years. The data thus suggest that fertility effects of the FPHSP were significant, substantially so among women aged 30 and over. The data, moreover, demonstrate a direct relationship between age and program impact: between-treatment differentials (i.e., percent difference between the CDP and FPHSP treatment and comparison areas) range over all age groups and increase monotonically with age.

The time series in Figures 2–5 further elucidate the impact of the FPHSP. Figure 2 depicts the GFR time series for the FPHSP areas. Fertility levels were closely comparable across the FPHSP treatment and comparison areas prior to

Figure 2. Quarterly GFRs in FPHSP treatment and comparison areas, 1974–80

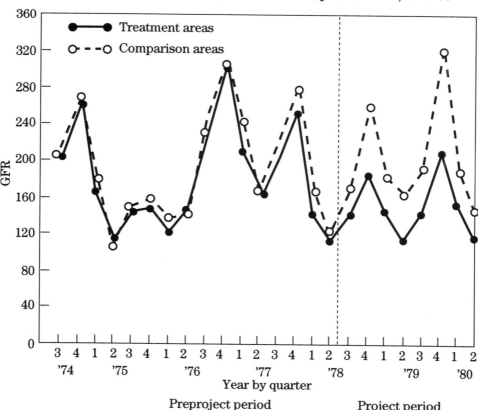

the time of CDP impact. The timing of the onset of lower FPHSP treatment area fertility suggests that a differential impact of the CDP across the areas apportioned to treatments of the FPHSP may have contaminated the FPHSP. Thus FPHSP fertility may have been lower at the outset than it would have been in the absence of the CDP because areas where the CDP was most effective were assigned in the treatment area of the FPHSP. The trajectory of the GFR over time nevertheless suggests that a more pronounced differential emerged during the FPHSP and that the magnitude of the differential was unprecedented in recent years.

As Figure 2 illustrates, natural fertility in rural Bangladesh is subject to marked seasonal variation that can obfuscate the short-term effects of fertility control.[22] We therefore compute seasonally adjusted fertility rates in order to elucidate FPHSP effects in the context of long-term fertility trends. These seasonally adjusted rates are depicted in Figure 3.[23] The Figure 3 time series shows more clearly than Figure 2 the hypothesized contaminating effect of the CDP and the pronounced effect of the FPHSP in the project period. Viewed in terms of the

Figure 3. Quarterly seasonal adjusted GFRs in FPHSP treatment and comparison areas, 1974–80

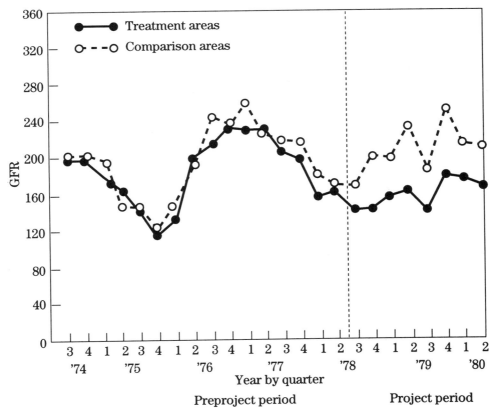

long-range cycles in fertility, the FPHSP impact period commenced at a time
when fertility was unusually low owing to the "ripple effect" of the 1974 famine.
An unusually large proportion of women were at risk of conception in 1975
owing to the low fertility in that year. Birth rates were therefore high in 1976,
which, in turn, reduced the proportion of women at risk of conception in the
subsequent year. Although the FPHSP did not reduce fertility below the already
low 1978 levels, it averted a rise in treatment area fertility that would have occurred in the absence of FPHSP services. This is illustrated in Figure 3 by the
sustained increase in comparison area fertility over the 1978 to 1980 period.

Figure 4 shows that the FPHSP had a sustained effect on fertility among
women under age 30 that was not restricted to the peak fertility season. Figure
5 shows the more pronounced impact of the program among women aged 30 and
over and the tendency of the program to dampen seasonal fertility swings among
older women. This is not surprising since seasonality is a natural fertility phenomenon.[24]

Figure 4. Quarterly fertility rates among women aged 15–29 in FPHSP treatment
and comparison areas, 1974–80

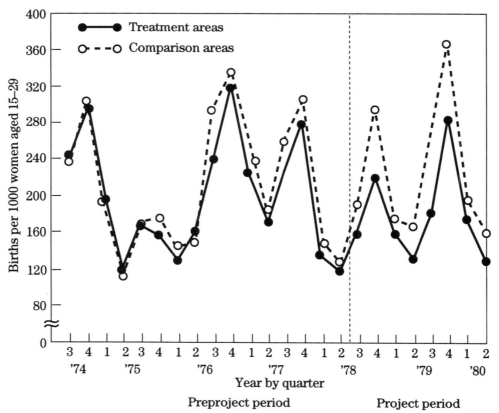

Figure 5. Quarterly fertility rates among women aged 30–44 in FPHSP treatment and comparison areas, 1974–80

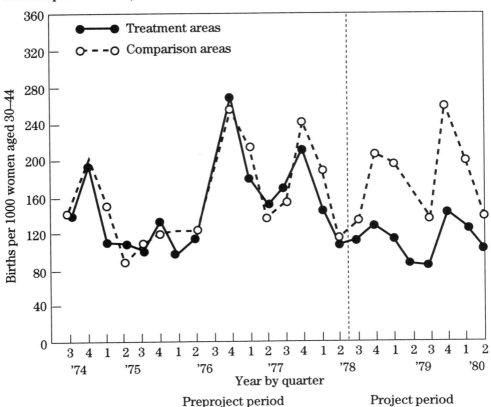

Preproject period   *Project period*

Adjustment for Contamination

Figures 2–5 show fertility trends that are consistent with the hypothesis that the CDP contaminated the FPHSP. It is therefore appropriate to model the fertility levels for the project periods of the CDP and the FPHSP for the four cells of the CDP-FPSHP design. The objective of modeling is to adjust the effects of one project for concomitant effects of the other. Since seasonality is pronounced, it is also useful to examine net effects of services controlling for fertility cycles unrelated to service activities. A model that achieves this is the following:

$$Y_t = \phi Y_{t-i} + \ldots + \phi_p Y_{t-p} + \alpha + \Sigma \beta_i + \gamma + \delta \qquad (1)$$

where,

Y_t = the general fertility rate at time t,

ϕ_i = a lag coefficient for time lag i for p specified lags,

α = an intercept equivalent to the mean GFR for quarter 4,

β_i = seasonality effects,

γ = the additive effect of the CDP, and

δ = the additive effect of the FPHSP.

The sample for estimation of (1) consists of 64 quarterly observations of GFRs for the four village groups of the CDP-FPHSP design over the 1976–80 period. Estimation uses the method of Box and Jenkens.[25]

The estimated parameters of this model are reported in Table 3. Coefficients attest to the predominant independent effects of seasonal variation. This suggests that variation in natural fertility determinants such as the timing of marriage, coital frequency, spouse separation, and the like accounts for substantially more of the variation in Matlab fertility than variables defining the presence or absence of FPHSP or CDP conditions. Tests on coefficients nevertheless suggest that both service strategies had fertility effects, substantially so among couples in the FPHSP areas. Over 80 percent of the variance is explained by the regression, the unexplained portion being secular trends or "famine ripple" effects discussed above.

The expected GFRs in Table 3 show the predicted Y under different conditions. The intercept row (202.8) is the predicted GFR when all independent variables are set at their mean—the sample grand mean of the GFRs. The GFR for the seasons is the predicted GFR when all seasonal effects are set at their means and CDP and FPHSP effects are zero. Thus the CDP and FPHSP coefficients express the additive effect of services adjusting for seasonality. The predicted CDP GFR (203.0) represents an 8.3 percent impact on fertility, on the average.[26] The FPHSP GFR, 172.7, represents a net decline of 22 percent. Thus the coefficients suggest an effect of the FPHSP that is nearly three times the effect of the CDP.

Additional regressions were estimated to test the hypothesis that program effects are subject to seasonal variation. Since interaction terms were insignificant, regressions fail to support the hypothesis that treatment effects vary with

Table 3. First-order autoregressive analysis of the relative impact of the CDP and the FPHSP

Coefficient name	Coefficient	Standard error	t ratio	Predicted GFR
φ	-0.5	0.1	-4.4**	—
Intercept[a]	290.5	9.3	31.1**	202.8[b]
Quarter 1 effect	-87.7	7.4	-11.8**	
Quarter 2 effect	-129.8	8.2	-15.8**	221.4[c]
Quarter 3 effect	-80.8	6.8	-11.9**	
CDP effect	-18.4	11.0	-1.7*	203.0[d]
FPHSP effect	-48.7	11.8	-4.5**	172.7[e]

Multiple R = 0.910. R^2 = 0.828.   F = 55.92**   d.f. = K/N-K-1/58
*p<.05 (one tail).   **p<.001 (one tail).   N = 64.
[a]Since quarter 4 is omitted, the intercept is the quarter 4 mean.   [b]GFR = Y = the grand mean.
[c]GFR = Y = α +$\Sigma\beta_i\overline{X}_i$ [d]GFR = Y = α + $\Sigma\beta_i\overline{X}_i$ + y   [e]GFR = Y = α + $\Sigma\beta_i\overline{X}_i$ + δ

fertility seasonality.[27] Effects of programs are thus additive: contraceptive services have altered the level of fertility but not the seasonal variation infertility.

We conclude, in summary, that both projects had a net effect on fertility. Seasonality has more pronounced effects than contraceptive services—effects that are dampened in absolute, but not relative terms by widespread fertility control. The FPHSP, under the assumptions employed, reduced fertility by an amount ranging between 22 and 25 percent in its first two project years.

Implications

Much of the international literature on population policy in the past decade has been addressed to a debate on the efficacy of contraceptive service programs.[28] Two positions have achieved prominence in this debate, although it could be argued that a third has emerged in recent years.

The first position holds that the effects of contraceptive services are a consequence of prior changes in reproductive motives. In this view contraceptive service effects are an outcome of social and demographic changes that influence reproductive motives. Once motives have been affected by social change, fertility limitation behavior will change, because traditional alternatives to contraception exist wherein some measure of fertility control can be exercised. Modern contraception can substitute for traditional birth planning behavior, but it can never induce demographic change.[29]

The second position holds that contraceptive services have effects because a latent demand exists for efficient birth planning methods. In this view there are gradations in reproductive motives such that convenient, inexpensive, and effective services can to some extent obviate the need for strong fertility control motives. In the absence of widespread birth limitation behavior, service programs can initiate fertility change.[30]

A third view emerges from the study of contemporary demographic trends: namely, that contraceptive service programs do not initiate fertility change, but can nevertheless satiate a growing demand for fertility control more efficiently than traditional means and can stimulate diffusion of contraceptive innovation in traditional societies. Thus as demographic changes occur, fertility declines are more pronounced in the period following the introduction of services than in the prior period.[31]

The data from the Matlab contraceptive services studies support the second position. The findings appear to show that contraceptive services can initiate a fertility change in a poor rural traditional population. Thus it appears that an unmet demand for contraception exists in rural areas of Bangladesh that can be served by an intensive field program.

Six policy implications emerge from this research with specific relevance to Bangladesh.

First, fertility can be significantly reduced in Bangladesh by making contraceptives readily available to households. Effects are likely to be temporary, however, unless distribution involves trained workers who systematically follow-up users and attend to their needs. Since poverty and chronic ill health are widespread in rural Bangladesh, users are incapable of distinguishing side effects from other illnesses and cannot afford treatment for minor ailments. Although rural couples will experiment with new contraceptive technology, they will not sustain its use unless both real and perceived contraceptive and health problems are attended to by trained and sympathetic village-based paramedics.

Second, a user-oriented program with a wide choice of methods, skilled counseling, rigorous follow-up and treatment of side effects, and ancillary health services will be substantially more effective than one based on one or two methods distributed by unskilled workers. Moreover, effects can be sustained over time. It is difficult, in an analysis of the FPHSP, to determine the extent to which the project's success relates to family planning strategies (home-administered DMPA, follow-up, improved training, etc.) or to ancillary health services (treatment and referral of side effects, MCH care, etc.). It is useful to note, however, that dramatic increases in prevalence were attained prior to development of MCH services. Thus integration of MCH with family planning seems to have improved program performance through its direct effects on family planning care. A health service approach has enabled ICDDR,B workers to provide couples with a wider choice of methods and better contraceptive care than would be possible in a vertical family planning campaign. (The question of whether comprehensive MCH services aimed at reducing morbidity and mortality can indirectly affect fertility is a question to be addressed in future research.)

Third, seasonality of fertility is pronounced even in areas served by the FPHSP. This feature of fertility needs investigation and recognition in policy planning. Intensive campaigns, for example, will be much more effective if launched in the months from December to March than in April to November. Intensive education and promotional campaigns should coincide with seasons when conception rates are high. More research should be addressed to developing our understanding of natural fertility dynamics and their policy implications.

Fourth, trends in reproductive motives require further research. We have no evidence that reproductive motives have been affected by the two projects. We have observed that use prevalence in Matlab has remained constant at 34 percent for three years. This prevalence of use agrees well with the preproject proportion of women who said they were either using a method or would use one in future if contraceptives were provided. While this may suggest that we have met the existing demand for contraception in Matlab and that, by so doing, our project has had substantial fertility effects, we must study this question formally to determine whether reproductive motives have changed *after* acceptance of contraception. We recognize that further increases in the impact of the FPHSP may require changes in reproductive motives. Whether such motives can be influenced by health service interventions or other policies is thus a critical question to be investigated in Matlab in the next few years.

Fifth, more research is needed on the determinants of program success. Several villages in Matlab have use prevalence rates exceeding 50 percent; others have rates of less than 10 percent. The question of why the project succeeded in some villages but failed in others is an important research issue.

Sixth, the success of the Matlab experiment presents a challenge to researchers and administrators to discover ways in which project results can be translated into further action. In particular, it must be recognized that the ability of the ICDDR,B to train, field, supervise, and support a comprehensive contraceptive service program is the principal difference between the program in the FPHSP service and comparison areas. This operational ability needs careful scrutiny, with a view toward implementation of its elements elsewhere in Bangladesh. Future research should test implementation in the context of the government service system, and focus on identifying and understanding the critical barriers to replicating the Matlab experience.

The Matlab contraceptive service experiments demonstrate that rural Bangladesh holds considerable promise for achieving demographic development and that effective services can produce substantial fertility declines. The paucity of evidence of demographic effects resulting from the national program may thus relate more strongly to incomplete program implementation than to an absence of motivation among rural Bangladesh couples to limit or space births.

References and Notes

1. See, for example, W. P. Mauldin and B. Berelson, with a section by Z. Sykes, "Conditions of fertility decline in developing countries, 1965-75," *Studies in Family Planning* 9, no. 5 (May 1978): 89–147.

2. A critical review of family planning experiments and their limitations is found in D. J. Hernandez, "The impact of family planning programs on fertility in developing countries: A critical evaluation," *Journal of Social Research* 10 (1981): 32–66.

3. In 1979, the CRL became the International Centre for Diarrhoeal Disease Research, Bangladesh (ICDDR,B).

4. The CDP is discussed in M. Rahman, W. H. Mosley, A. R. Khan, A. I. Chowdhury, and J. Chakraborty, "Contraceptive distribution in Bangladesh: Some lessons learned," *Studies in Family Planning* 11, no. 6 (June 1980): 191–201; and its effects are assessed in Wayne S. Stinson, James F. Phillips, Makhlisur Rahman, and J. Chakraborty, "The demographic impact of the Contraceptive Distribution Project in Matlab, Bangladesh," in this issue.

5. M. Alamgir, "Some aspects of Bangladesh agriculture: Review of performance and evaluation of policies," *Bangladesh Development Studies* 2 (1975): 737–818.

6. Bangladesh Bureau of Statistics, National Volume: 1974 *Bangladesh Population Census Report* (Dacca: Statistics Division, Ministry of Planning, Government of the People's Republic of Bangladesh, 1977).

7. See, for example, G. T. Curlin, L. C. Chen, and S. B. Hussain, "Demographic crisis: The impact of the Bangladesh civil war (1971) on births and deaths in a rural area of Bangladesh," *Population Studies* 30 (1976): 87–105.

8. A useful review of the development situation in Bangladesh and its demographic consequences appears in W. B. Arthur and G. McNicoll, "An analytic survey of population and development in Bangladesh," *Population and Development Review* 4, no. 1 (March 1978): 23–80. Recent research in Indonesia has shown that areas with the greatest economic adversity are those most receptive to contraception: R. Freedman, Siew-Ean Khoo, and B. Supraptilah, "Modern contraceptive use in Indonesia: A challenge to conventional wisdom," *International Family Planning Perspectives* 7, no. 1 (1980): 3–15. Clearly the social and economic context of the Matlab study bears further investigation.

9. The question of possible contaminating effects of social and economic change in Matlab is difficult to assess because this has not been the subject of systematic investigation over time. Tabulation of the Matlab CRL census of 1974 has shown, however, that across-treatment socioeconomic status differentials were inconsequential: J. F. Phillips, S. Bhatia, and A. I. Chowdhury, "*Differentials* in social and economic characteristics of treatment and comparison areas of the Family Planning–Health Services Project, 1974 Cholera Research Laboratory Census, Matlab," unpublished manuscript, 1981.

10. Rahman et al., cited in note 4.

11. Stinson et al., cited in note 4.

12. A comprehensive review of the FPHSP is found in S. Bhatia, W. H. Mosley, A. S. G. Faruque, and J. Chakraborty, "The Matlab Family Planning–health Services Project," *Studies in Family Planning* 11, no. 6 (June 1980): 202–212. Although the project has included maternal and child health services, only tetanus immunization and oral therapy for diarrhea have been fully implemented. Workers were trained to advise pregnant women on delivery practices, to provide nutritional information, and to train households on hygiene and sanitation. Since health work is mainly oriented to the treatment and care of contraceptive users, however, the approach is more one of comprehensive family planning services delivery than an integrated health service approach.

13. See Bhatia et al., cited in note 12, and J. F. Phillips, P. Claquin, and J. Chakraborty, "A case study in the integration of health with family planning services in Matlab Thana, Bangladesh," paper presented at the Regional Seminar on Evaluation of Schemes and Strategies for Integrated Family Planning Programmes with Special Reference to Increased Involvement of Local Institutions (United Nations: ESCAP, Bangkok, June 1981).

14. All tubectomies are performed by paramedics in Matlab, with a physician attending.

15. Menstrual regulation (MR) is not actively promoted in the field. Rather, it has served primarily as a backup method for contraceptive failures. Accordingly, only 250 MRs were performed in three years.

16. This census and vital data system is known as the Demographic Surveillance System (DSS). A useful review of the DSS appears in *Cholera Research Laboratory, Demographic Surveillance System–Matlab*, Vol. 1, *Methods and Procedures* (mimeographed, March 1978); and K. M. A. Aziz, "The methodology of vital events registration in rural Bangladesh," in *Statistics—The Essential Tool for Research and Planning*, proceedings of the First National Statistical Conference of the Bangladesh Sta-

tistical Association, March 1977, pp. 98–101.

17. Births to women under 15 or over 44 were added to the adjacent age groups.

18. In mid-1978, 84 villages were dropped from surveillance. Only the included villages are used in FPHSP tabulations. Thus FPHSP analyses of 1974–78 data use the reduced DSS area villages to ensure comparability with tabulations of post-1978 data.

19. Mortality and migration data for 1980 are incomplete. Incomplete mortality data introduced only minor spurious reductions in 1980 rates, however, because mortality among women in the childbearing ages is low. The 1980 data presented below are nevertheless tentative and subject to revision.

20. Denominators for five-year age groups are somewhat distorted by age heaping and by discontinuities in the size of individual age groups. We advanced a constant one tenth of each five-year age group per semester, although a graduated method using a parabolic curve would have been more valid. Most analyses in this paper are based on 15-year age groups or on the general fertility rate, and it is doubtful whether results would have been significantly affected by this refinement.

21. Age differentials do not affect our areal comparisons, but the fall in the median age by approximately 15 months from 1974 to 1979 has a slight impact on chronological comparisons.

22. Seasonality was first documented in J. Stoeckel and A. K. M. A. Chowdhury, "Seasonal variation in births in rural East Pakistan," *Journal of Biosocial Science* 4 (1972): 107–116, and has been observed in other areas of Bangladesh. See, for example, the reports of fertility dynamics in Campanigonj in N. Alam, A. Ashraf, and A. H. Khan, "Land, famine, and fertility," a report from the Research and Evaluation Unit of Companigonj Health Project (Dacca: Christian Commission for Development in Bangladesh, 1980, mimeo). Becker has analyzed and modeled seasonal variation for the 1968–74 period and found a corroborating pattern in which peaks and troughs varied 40 percent from the mean, a level of variation that is "more pronounced than social, economic, or geographic differentials that have been observed in the Bangladesh population"; S. Becker, "Seasonality of fertility in Matlab, Bangladesh," *Journal of Biosocial Science* 13, no. 1 (1979): 97–105. Seasonality of coital behavior is the most frequently cited explanation for this pattern (see H. D. Gupta, "Climate and conception rates in Punjab India," *Indian Journal of Public Health* 19 (1975): 122; and K. M. A. Aziz, *Sex Socialization and Philosophies of Life in Relation to Fertility Behavior: An Anthropological Approach*, Ph.D. dissertation, Rajshahi University, (1981), although seasonality in spouse separation contributes to the observed pattern; L. C. Chen, S. Ahmed, G. Gesche, and W. H. Mosley, "A prospective study of birth interval dynamics in rural East Pakistan," *Population* 28 (1974): 277–297. The harvest season, which precedes the peak conception period, reduces nutritional adversity, thereby increasing fecundability at a time when coital frequency is relatively high owing to the cool weather at that time of year; S. L. Huffman, A. K. M. A. Chowdhury, W. H. Mosley, and J. Chakraborty, "Nutrition and post partum amenorrhea in rural Bangladesh," *Population Studies* 32, no. 2 (1978): 251–260.

23 In Figure 3 seasonality was adjusted by the following procedure: Let F define an adjustment factor for quarter i of age group m. Then

$$F_{im} = \frac{\sum\limits_{i=1}^{4} \sum\limits_{j=2}^{6} B_{ijm}}{\left[\sum\limits_{j=2}^{6} B_{ijm} \right]} \qquad (2)$$

where B_{ijm} is the number of births to mothers age m in quarter i of year j annualized by multiplying by four. The adjusted GFR was calculated using quarterly factors for each age group as follows:

$$GFR_{ij} = \frac{\left[\sum_{m=4}^{9} F_{jm} B_{ijm} \right] \cdot 100}{P_{ij}} \qquad (3)$$

where the GFR_{ij} is the adjusted general fertility rate for quarter i of year j and P_{ij} is the number of women 15–44 at risk in midquarter i of year j. An implicit assumption of this approach is that seasonality. A useful discussion of alternative factors is found in C. Chatfield, *The Analysis of Time Series: An Introduction* (London: Chapman and Hall, 1980).

24. As Figure 1 shows, contraceptive use prevalence is not seasonal in Matlab.

25. G. E. P. Box and G. M. Jenkins, *Time Series Analysis, Forecasting and Control* (San Francisco: Holden-Day, 1976).

26. Stinson et al (in this issue) have shown that a single fertility-impact estimate for the two years of the CDP is inappropriate because effects occurred in the first year only. The lasting impact of the CDP was thus nil.

27. Second-order interactions with age were not tested. It is possible that program effects are seasonal among women over age 30.

28. A useful review of positions in this debate can be found in R. Freedman and B. Berelson, "The record of family planning programs," *Studies in Family Planning* 7, no 1 (January 1976): 1–40. Positions in the debate are well represented by Amy Ong Tsui and Donald J. Bogue, "Declining world fertility: Trends, causes, implications," *Population Bulletin 33*, no. 4 (Washington, D.C.: Population Reference Bureau, 1978), and a critical review of that paper in Paul Demeny, "On the end of the population explosion," *Population and Development Review* 5, no. 1 (March 1979): 141–162.

29. J. Blake and P. Das Gupta, "Reproductive motivation versus contraceptive technology: Is recent American experience an exception?" *Population and Development Review* 1, no. 2 (December 1975): 229–250.

30. D. J. Bogue, "The end of the population explosion," *The Public Interest* 7 (Spring 1967): 11–20.

31. Mauldin and Berelson, cited in note 1.

ACCESS

Introduction

James R. Foreit

Access to contraception is the ability of people to obtain family planning from a service-delivery system. Family planning program goals of the 1960s and 1970s emphasized reaching underserved rural and poor urban populations. Virtually all current service-delivery modalities and supporting information, education, and communication (IEC) programs were developed during those years. The modalities developed include the use of paramedical personnel, community-based distribution (CBD) of contraceptives, workplace-based services, postpartum and postabortion family planning, social marketing, and integration of family planning into other health and community development activities (Taylor and Berelson, 1971; Foreit et al., 1978).

Access is traditionally understood to encompass four dimensions, all of which can be influenced by program managers: *geographic access* refers to the number, type, and location of services; *economic access* refers to the costs of obtaining services incurred by prospective users; *administrative access* refers to program norms and procedures that may facilitate or restrict a client's ability to obtain services; and *information access* refers to the amount of information available to prospective users about services, contraceptives, and the need for family planning (Park et al., 1977; Foreit et al., 1978; Bertrand et al., 1995). A fifth dimension of access, *psychosocial access*, refers to factors such as social approval, stigma, or individual attitudes that can facilitate or prevent potential clients from using program services (Bertrand et al., 1995).

Geographic Access

Physical placement of family planning facilities is often correlated with contraceptive use. Contraceptive prevalence in rural Thailand and the Philippines has been found to decline with distance from a contraceptive source (Akin and Rous, 1997). Family planning program managers cannot influence where their target populations live; however, they can locate services so that they can be reached by many potential users. Operations research to increase geographic access in rural and periurban areas has studied the effectiveness and safety of non-physician distribution, as an alternative to physician-centered, usually urban-based services.

Among the first studies of non-physician prescription were the training of nurse-midwives to insert IUDs in Korea (Bang et al., 1968) and the use of auxiliary nurses to provide oral contraceptives in Thailand (Rosenfield and Limcharoen, in this volume). Because the greatest obstacle to the use of paraprofessionals has been the opposition of local physicians, studies of the safety of using non-physician service providers have had to be replicated in country after country. Consequently, studies on the safety and use of non-physicians forms one of the largest bodies of work in the OR literature (Foreit, 1991). The classic article by Rosenfield and Limcharoen about the training and use of non-physician service providers is found in the Impact section.

Historically, once the feasibility of using non-physician health professionals to prescribe contraceptives was established, attention shifted to the possibility of using non-health workers to distribute temporary supply methods. Community-based distribution programs are probably the best-known application of this approach. These programs recruit and train nonprofessionals such as housewives and market traders to distribute pills, condoms, and spermicides. OR has often demonstrated that CBD programs can increase contraceptive prevalence, usually at fairly low per-user costs. Many variations on the CBD model have been tested, including household distribution, in which program workers make recruiting visits to prospective clients and resupply visits to continuing users of contraceptives, and commercial distribution in areas without pharmacies where nontraditional outlets such as hairdressers and grocery stores sell pills and condoms (Foreit et al., 1978).

Operations research on CBD programs continues to be an important activity, especially in Africa, where the existence of large rural populations who live beyond the reach of health centers, coupled with a limited supply of health workers, has created a need for nonprofessional providers. Research on African CBD programs has mainly reported the effectiveness of programs in reaching target populations, but more recent work in Africa (Bertrand et al., 1993), has also begun to report CBD program costs. The first selection in this section (Doucoure et al.) is the report of a CBD demonstration project conducted in 52 rural villages in Mali. Like much earlier work on impact and access, this study was instrumental in convincing the national government and an international donor, USAID, to support an extensive family planning effort in rural areas.

Economic Access

Program managers cannot improve the incomes of their users, but they can affect the prices of the services they provide. The goal of most early family planning programs was to minimize economic costs to users. Contraceptives were commonly made available free of charge or at nominal prices (Foreit et al., 1978), and, in many cases, free contraceptives were also delivered to households, thereby eliminating other user costs such as transportation, as well. A literature review by Lewis (1986) found that lowering prices of contraceptives increased the quantity distributed. Such reductions, however, did not always result in a net increase in contraceptive use. In some cases, such reductions resulted only in existing consumers' substitution of lower-priced sources for higher-priced outlets (World Bank, 1993). Similarly, evidence has emerged suggesting that users with higher income receive the greatest share of contraceptive subsidies (Haaga and Tsui, 1995).

In the 1990s, with demand for contraception increasing and international donor funding for family planning programs stagnant or decreasing, providers began charging increasingly larger fees for contraceptive services. A widespread concern has developed that price increases will result in the poorest users being denied access to family planning. As a result of reduced subsidies for users, the economic access problem has changed from one of maximizing access to family planning by reducing prices to one of minimizing reductions in access caused by the need to raise prices.

So far, a clear picture of the actual impact of user fees on contraceptive use has yet to emerge. However, some evidence has been gathered from Peru and Bangladesh (APROPO, 1991; Janowitz and Bratt, 1996) suggesting that source substitution occurs when prices are increased, and that reductions in program use resulting from price increases are often only temporary.

The study of issues related to price elasticity in the demand for family planning services is relatively new. In this section, we present a diagnostic study that estimates the effect of IUD price increases on family planning program use and revenues in an Ecuadorian nonprofit organization, APROFE (León and Cuesta).

Administrative Access

At the service-delivery point, administrative restrictions to contraceptive use include demands for excessive documentation, inconvenient clinic hours, long waiting times, and overcrowded services. Instruments such as patient-flow analysis have been developed, and both diagnostic and intervention studies have been conducted to improve service organization. A handful of intervention studies have been conducted to improve the organization of services at the service-delivery-point level (see, for example, Solari et al., 1989). More common are diagnostic studies that seek to describe a problem and, ideally, suggest potential solutions (see, for example, Lassner et al., 1986).

Medical barriers—scientifically unjustified medical restrictions on contraceptive provision to prospective users—have been identified as administrative access problems (Bertrand et al., 1995). Physicians themselves are the source of medical access problems, and their knowledge and behaviors are a major challenge for the international family planning and reproductive health community. Our example of the use of OR to improve administrative access to family planning is a diagnostic study that examined medical barriers to oral contraceptive use in Senegal (Stanback et al.).

Information Access

Contemporary family planning programs typically have large promotional components and seek to reach many different audiences, including policymakers, the general public, current users, and potential users (Piotrow et al., 1997). The papers in this section focus more narrowly on the problem of providing information to potential users of family planning. (The problem of providing information to current contraceptive users is touched on in León et al. in the Resources section.)

Potential users require a wide range of information to make informed choices about contraceptive use, including its benefits, available methods, method characteristics, and location of services. Early investigators (Rogers and Shoemaker, 1971 and Rogers, 1973) argued that the most important type of communications process in the diffusion of family planning in developing countries was interpersonal communication. Other researchers (Lin and Hingson, 1974) suggested that in many circumstances, mass and/or local (lectures, billboards, village theater) media could be more effective and more cost-effective than interpersonal communications in creating family planning awareness. In fact, evidence suggests that all three types of communication can be effective in changing behavior related to family planning (Piotrow et al., 1997), and most programs regard them as complementary rather than competing channels: "Whereas the mass media provide information quickly and repeatedly to large audiences, interpersonal communication leads to more in-depth understanding, addresses individual concerns, and gives immediate feedback" (World Bank, 1993: 77).

Information access research is usually conducted at two stages of a communications campaign, first during the design of the intervention, and later in testing the intervention. Information, education, and communications (IEC) research specialists refer to the diagnostic studies that are conducted at the first phase of an IEC initiative as audience analysis. An audience analysis is conducted to determine the size, information needs, and media habits of the target population. An audience analysis may be conducted in many ways, for example, by using published data, focus groups, or surveys. Once an intervention has been decided upon, the messages, presentation, and content is pretested using members of the target audience (Piotrow et al., 1997).

After an IEC campaign has been launched, research is often conducted to determine the effect of the message or communications medium on a family planning output or outcome. A large number of publications have documented the effects of IEC interventions on program outputs and outcomes. In this book, we include selections on the effects of both mass media and interpersonal communication efforts. Our mass media selection (K. Foreit et al.) is one of several studies (see also, Kincaid et al., 1996) demonstrating the effectiveness and cost-effectiveness of using the mass media, in this case mass circulation magazines, to promote vasectomy. The study was conducted by Pro-Pater of Sao Paulo, Brazil.

Operations research on interpersonal communication includes numerous examples of studies of professional providers, peer promoters (adolescents who promote methods to their schoolmates, and the like), and satisfied users (individuals who agree to promote the method they use in the community). Although peer promoters and satisfied users can help potential users decide to use a contraceptive, the provider plays the key role in communicating with the client. Not only does a provider furnish information that helps a potential user decide if she or he wants to practice contraception; she/he also helps clients who have decided to adopt select a specific method; and, finally, she/he provides the new user with instructions for correct use of the method selected. As an example of interpersonal promotion, we have included an article on sterilization promotion by hospital-based providers in Nigeria (Omu et al.).

Most applied research has been conducted concerning information campaigns the goal of which was to inform potential users of the benefits of family planning or to promote a specific method or source (as in the case of the two sterilization articles in this section). The effect of promotional campaigns can be measured in terms of new users, attitudes about family planning, and changes in knowledge about the existence of methods and sources. However, many communications materials are designed to help current users employ their methods correctly and more effectively. Little is known about the effect of these materials on outcomes such as contraceptive continuation or method failure. Testing the effect of communications materials explaining method use should become an urgent priority for future OR.

Psychosocial Access

Few operations research studies deal with the problem of psychosocial access to family planning, even though, in some environments, these factors may be of critical importance in constraining contraceptive use. Psychosocial problems may include issues such as a fear of modern medicine, women's confinement to the home, or religious beliefs. The role of managers is to find ways to remove or work around these barriers. For instance, an information campaign can be launched to better inform potential clients about the efficacy and safety of modern medicine and about which contraceptive methods are approved by religious authorities. Household delivery can be used to bring contraceptives to secluded women.

More OR should be directed at removing psychosocial barriers. As programs become better at increasing the number of locations where contraceptives can be obtained, and at providing information about family planning, an ever-larger proportion of the reasons for nonuse of family planning can be attributed to psychosocial access problems (Bongaarts and Bruce, 1995).

Among the psychosocial problems amenable to solution by family planning programs is "social distance," which occurs when clients and providers are of different ages, classes, castes, or ethnic groups (Huntington et al., 1990; Schuler et al., 1985; Cospin and Vernon, 1997). In Latin America, operations research on reducing social distance has focused on problems created by gender differences. Family planning services are organized to meet the needs of women rather than men, and substantial evidence has accumulated that men are not comfortable receiving services from female providers in women-oriented settings. Vernon et al. (1991) found that clinics that separated services for men and women, either physically or temporally, performed greater numbers of vasectomies than did clinics that did not separate services. Studies in Guatemala (Bertrand et al., 1987) have also shown the effectiveness of using men to recruit other men to use contraceptives. Our example of OR undertaken to overcome a psychosocial access problem is a study conducted in two Peruvian CBD programs to test the effectiveness of using male distributors to attract men as clients and increase condom use (J. Foreit et al.).

References

Akin, John S. and Jeffrey J. Rous. 1997. "Effect of provider characteristics on choice of contraceptive behavior: A two-equation full-information maximum-likelihood estimation." *Demography* 34, 4: 513–24.

Apoyo al los Programas de Poblacion (APROPO). 1991. *A Study to Increase the Availability and Price of Oral Contraceptives in Three Program Settings.* INOPAL II Final Report. New York: The Population Council.

Bang, S.S. et al. 1968. "Improving access to the IUD: Experiments in Koyang, Korea." *Studies in Family Planning* 27: 4–11.

Bongaarts, John and Judith Bruce. 1995. "The causes of unmet need for contraception and the social content of services." *Studies in Family Planning* 26, 2: 57–75.

Bertrand, Jane et al. 1987. "Evaluation of a communications program to increase adoption of vasectomy in Guatemala." *Studies in Family Planning* 18, 6: 361–370.

————. 1993. "Community based distribution of contraceptives in Bas Zaire." *International Family Planning Perspectives* 19, 3: 84–91.

————. 1995. "Access, quality of care and medical barriers in family planning programs." *International Family Planning Perspectives* 21, 2: 64–69 & 74.

Cospin, Gloria and Ricardo Vernon. 1997. *Reproductive Health Education in Indigenous Areas Through Bilingual Teachers in Guatemala.* INOPAL III Final Report of a project with the Asociacion Guatemalteca de Educación Sexual y Desarrollo Humano (AGES). New York: The Population Council.

Foreit, James R. 1991. "Reaching More Users: More Methods, More Outlets, More Promotion." In Myrna Seidman and Marjorie C. Horn, *Operations Research: Helping Family Planning Programs Work Better. Proceedings of an International Conference and Workshop on Using Operations Research to Help Family Planning Programs Work Better, held in Columbia, MD. June 11–14, 1990. Progress in Clinical and Biological Research*, vol. 371. New York: Wiley-Liss.

Foreit, James R. et al. 1978. "Community based and commercial contraceptive distribution, an inventory and appraisal." *Population Reports* Series J, 19 (March).

Haaga, John and Amy Tsui. 1995. *Resource Allocation for Family Planning in Developing Countries: Report of a Meeting.* Washington, DC: National Academy Press.

Huntington, Dale et al. 1990. "User's perspective of counseling training in Ghana: The 'mystery client trial.'" *Studies in Family Planning* 21, 3: 171–177.

Janowitz, Barbara and John Bratt. 1996. "What do we really know about the impact of price changes on contraceptive use?" *International Family Planning Perspectives* 22, 1: 38–40.

Kincaid, D. Lawrence et al. 1996. "Impact of a mass media vasectomy promotion campaign in Brazil." *International Family Planning Perspectives* 22, 4: 169–175.

Lassner, Karen J. et al. 1986. "Sterilization approval and follow-through in Brazil." *Studies in Family Planning* 17, 4: 188–198.

Lewis, Maureen A. 1986. "Do contraceptive prices affect demand?" *Studies in Family Planning* 17, 3: 126–135.

Lin, Nan and Ralph Hingson. 1974. "Diffusion of family planning innovations: Theoretical and practical issues." *Studies in Family Planning* 5, 6: 189–194.

Park, C.B. et al. 1977. "The Euiryong experiment: A Korean innovation in household contraceptive distribution." *Studies in Family Planning* 8, 3: 67–78.

Piotrow, Phyllis Tilson et al. 1997. *Health Communication: Lessons Learned from Family Planning and Reproductive Health.* Westport, CT: Praeger Publishers.

Rogers, Everett M. 1973. *Communication Strategies in Family Planning.* New York: The Free Press.

Rogers, Everett M. and F.F. Shoemaker. 1971. *Communication of Innovations: A Cross-Cultural Approach.* New York: The Free Press.

Rosenfield, Allan and Charoon Limcharoen. 1972. "Auxiliary midwife prescription of oral contraceptives." *American Journal of Obstetrics and Gynecology* 114,7: 942–949.

Schuler, Sidney Ruth et al. 1985. "Barriers to effective family planning in Nepal." *Studies in Family Planning* 16, 5: 260–270.

Solari, Andres et al. 1989. *Operations Research to Improve Ministry of Health Family Planning Services in the Departments of Ayacucho and Huancavelica, Peru.* INOPAL I Final Report. New York: The Population Council.

Taylor, Howard C. and Bernard Berelson. 1971. "Comprehensive family planning based on maternal/child health services: A feasibility study for a world program." *Studies in Family Planning* 2, 2: 21–50.

Vernon, Ricardo et al. 1991. "Making vasectomy services more acceptable to men." *International Family Planning Perspectives* 17, 2: 55–60.

World Bank. 1993. *Effective Family Planning Programs*. Washington, DC: World Bank.

The Effect of a Family Planning CBD Project in Mali

Arkia Doucoure, Diane Djeneba, Fanta Toure,
Amadou Traore, Seydou Doumbia, Diouratie Sanogo,
Dale Huntington, and Claire Viadro

Programmatic issue: *The problem confronting program managers was how to provide services in an area where family planning was not available and the expansion of clinical services was not feasible.*

Programmatic processes/components: *The study examined the effectiveness of an entire community-based distribution package including provider selection, training, and compensation, methods distributed and supervision, rather than a single process or component. Two distributors, one man and one woman, were trained per village. They provided condoms, spermicide, and, eventually, oral contraceptives. Distributors kept a portion of the selling price to reimburse them for their efforts. Promotion was done through home visits and educational meetings in the villages.*

Research design: *Two studies were conducted. The first was a comparison of contraceptive use with and without the CBD program. This study was a demonstration project that used a simple one-group design with pre- and postintervention measurement of contraceptive prevalence in the study villages. The second study used an experimental design to evaluate the effect of adding oral contraceptives to the barrier methods offered by the program. Villages were assigned to a barrier + oral condition or a barrier-method-only condition, and contraceptive prevalence rates between the two groups were compared*

Findings: *Within 12 months, prevalence of contraceptive use among women of fertile age in the villages had increased from 1 percent to almost 12 percent.*

Program response to findings: *On the basis of the results, USAID Mali developed a $9 million program to expand CBD to the entire country. The CBD project was still operational in 1998, six years after the termination of the original OR demonstration.*

Discussion: *A demonstration project using a pretest-post-test design usually does not permit imputation of causality because it does not control for maturation—the possibility that the change would have occurred without* *the intervention. However, our knowledge of rural Mali—a place where no other sources of contraception existed other than the demonstration program—suggests that although the possibility that prevalence would have increased without the CBD program cannot be ruled out, that it would have done so is extremely improbable. Therefore, the "weak" design appears adequate to provide an estimate of the effectiveness of a rural CBD program in the Mali setting.*

The Effect of a Family Planning CBD Project in Mali

Arkia Doucoure, Diane Djeneba, Fanta Toure,
Amadou Traore, Seydou Doumbia, Diouratie Sanogo,
Dale Huntington, and Claire Viadro

The Republic of Mali, a West African country of approximately ten million people, is beginning the demographic transition from high fertility and mortality to low fertility and mortality. In 1991, the total fertility rate (TFR) was seven children per woman, and contraceptives were used by only 5 percent of married women of reproductive age. Life expectancy at birth was 45 years, and infant mortality was estimated at 162 deaths per 1,000 live births. Mali is more than 80 percent rural, and the population is poor, with little access to education or health services. Real annual gross national product per capita is estimated at US$570. Only 32 percent of adults are literate, and just 43 out of every 1,000 inhabitants owns a radio. Access to health services is severely limited, with only one doctor for every 23,500 residents (United Nations Development Program, 1993).

This paper reports the results of an operations research project to determine the feasibility and acceptability of using the community-based distribution (CBD) approach to promote the use of modern family planning methods in rural Mali. To improve the health status of the population and to lower fertility, the Government of Mali began family planning programs in 1990, including a CBD program to help serve people living in rural areas. Prior to this project, the few family planning services that were available were limited almost exclusively to urban areas. The objective of the project was to increase access to and use of modern contraceptives (Sanogo, 1993; Doucoure et al., 1993).

The preparatory phase of the project lasted for one year, from July 1990 to June 1991. During this phase, 54 widely scattered study villages were selected to participate in the project, and 108 male and female CBD agents who were inhabitants of the study villages were trained.

None of the villages had health centers or commercial sources of contraceptives. The CBD agents, none of whom were health workers, were responsible for community education and prescription and resupply of the contraceptive

Edited English summary translated and reprinted with the permission of the Population Council from *Rapport Final des Trois Etudes de Recherche Operationnelle Realisées dans le Cadre du Projet de Distribution Communautaire des Contraceptifs au Mali*, 1993.

methods. As remuneration for their efforts, CBD agents were allowed to keep 40 percent of the price of the contraceptives they sold. Originally, methods offered by the CBD program were limited to spermicides and condoms. Agents were supervised by community development technicians and nurses.

The implementation or demonstration phase of the project began in July 1991 and lasted for 18 months until December of 1992. During this period, the distribution of barrier methods was conducted and monitored, and distributor supervision and motivation activities for potential clients were conducted. During the implementation phase, in each of the 54 villages, a traveling drama troupe performed an original social drama that drew its themes from the baseline survey's results. This play was well attended and was important in publicizing the new program and the role of the local CBD workers. Villagers requesting services not available from local distributors were referred to health centers located outside the villages.

Once the program was established, the safety and feasibility of adding oral contraceptives to the CBD method mix was tested in a limited number of villages. The oral contraceptive experiment, or the expansion phase of the project, lasted for one year from January to December 1993.

Methodology

The operations research consisted of two studies. The first, the demonstration phase, evaluated changes in contraceptive knowledge, attitudes, and practice in the 54 study villages, before and after the introduction of the CBD program. The design was a before-and-after comparison without a control group. Information on contraceptive use was gathered in the participating villages through three surveys, each consisting of approximately 1,300 interviews. A baseline survey was conducted from May to June, 1991 at the end of the preparation phase of the project. A follow-up survey was conducted at the end of the implementation phase in February 1992 and at the end of the expansion phase in December 1993.

A quasi-experimental design was used to study the impact of introducing oral contraceptives during the expansion phase. Eighteen of the original 54 villages were selected for oral contraceptive distribution, and the remaining 36 served as a comparison group. Distribution of condoms and spermicides continued in both the intervention and comparison groups. The ability of CBD workers to provide oral contraceptives correctly was measured as the agreement between supervisors and workers' assessments of whether clients had contraindications to the use of oral contraceptives, and through a monitoring of the extent to which the workers discussed how to use the method, and described contraindications and side effects when counseling clients. The effect of CBD distribution of oral contraceptives was evaluated by comparing the change in contraceptive prevalence in the intervention and control groups between the first and second follow-up surveys.

Results

Demonstration phase: The CBD intervention had a positive effect on contraceptive use in the villages. Only 1 percent of women reported current practice of contraception prior to the project launch. Twelve months after the project launch, the first follow-up survey reported that contraceptive use had increased to 11.6 percent. The most frequently used method was the condom, and the reports of women surveyed were supported by the results of interviews with men. The number of men reporting ever use of condoms rose from about 50 percent to almost 85 percent.

Introduction of oral contraceptives: Prior to the introduction of oral contraceptives, contraceptive prevalence in both intervention and control villages was approximately 11.6 percent. Six months after the introduction of oral contraceptives, survey results from the 18 intervention villages indicated that contraceptive prevalence had increased to 31 percent, while prevalence in the 36 control villages where oral contraceptives were not introduced had increased by a lesser amount, to 21 percent.

Data collected during the study indicated a near-perfect correspondence between CBD agents and their nurse supervisors regarding the pill's suitability for selected new clients. The study findings also revealed that in 95 to 98 percent of cases, CBD agents talked to clients about how to use oral contraceptives and described their advantages, disadvantages, and side effects.

Discussion

The study demonstrates both the effectiveness of the CBD approach in rural Mali and the importance of including noncoitally-dependent methods among the contraceptives offered by the program. The impact of the intervention activities translated into important increases in modern contraceptive use in the study villages. The addition of the oral contraceptive to the original CBD method mix almost tripled contraceptive use within six months in the villages where it was introduced. The results of the introduction of oral contraceptives also demonstrated that Malian CBD agents were capable of prescribing pills safely.

This project represents a number of "firsts" for Mali. In terms of service delivery, the project was the first in the country to use the CBD approach, and the first to make contraceptive products available in rural areas. That the CBD agents were residents of the villages in which they carry out their activities, and that two agents per village (one man and one woman) were selected, are also innovations in the Malian context. Finally, for the first time in Francophone Africa, a national family planning program introduced the distribution of oral contraceptives in a pilot CBD project.

Over the life of the CBD project, three dissemination seminars, one at the end of each phase of the project, were organized to discuss results. The seminars were attended by local and central-level Ministry of Health officials and representatives of donor agencies. Findings from each important step were used to define strategies and improve program implementation. For instance, results from the demonstration phase led to the execution of a study of oral contraceptive distribution during the third and final phase of the project. The success of the OR project led to the initiation of a multimillion-dollar national CBD program funded by USAID/Bamako to expand contraceptive distribution in all regions of Mali.

References

Doucoure, Arkia Diallo et al. 1993. *Rapport Final des Trois Etudes de Recherche Operationnelle Realisées dans le Cadre du Projet de Distribution Communautaire des Contraceptifs au Mali.* Bamako: The Population Council.

Sonogo, Diouratie. 1993. *Les programs de distribution à base communautaire (DBC) comme mode de presentation de services de planning familial en milieu rural: Experience du Cameroun et du Mali,* Conference Proceedings, End of Project Conference, Africa Operations Research and Technical Assistance Project (4–7 October), The Population Council, Nairobi.

United Nations Development Program (UNDP). 1993. *Human Development Report.* New York and Oxford: Oxford University Press.

Acknowledgment

This project was financed by the United States Agency for International Development, Office of Population.

The Need for Quasi-Experimental Methodology to Evaluate Pricing Effects

Federico R. León and Agustín Cuesta

Programmatic issue: *What the impact of different prices is on clinic use.*

Programmatic processes/components: *The study examined the price-setting process and the effect of price increases. At the time of the study, price setting in APROFE was decentralized, and individual clinics were encouraged to raise prices to help compensate for reductions in funding from the organization's main donor, USAID. Clinic directors established their own prices, based on whatever criteria they perceived to be relevant.*

Research design: *APROFE wished the research to be as unobtrusive as possible, so a retrospective analysis was conducted to assess client price behavior. Clinics opted for a wide range of price increases (7 percent–61 percent, depending on the clinic) creating a natural experiment. The authors were able to take advantage of the natural experiment and compare groups of clinics that had instituted different price increases. As implied by its title, the report is also intended as a rebuttal to advocates of less rigorous research designs. The authors applied different designs to the data to learn if they would yield different results.*

Findings: *The study found that price increases greater than about 20 percent reduced demand for IUD insertions, but that price increases also increased clinic revenues, with the greatest price increase (61 percent) resulting in both the greatest revenue increase and greatest client loss. Also, more rigorous comparison-group designs resulted in radically different conclusions than did the less rigorous pretest-posttest approach.*

Program response to findings: *The retrospective analyses revealed that client loss resulted from price increases, a fact that had been obscured in earlier, routine management reviews of clinic performance data. As a result, APROFE recentralized some of the price-increase decisionmaking process and eventually attempted to replace the use of idiosyncratic (and usually anecdotal) information in price setting with standard quantitative indicators for all clinics that attempted to match prices with client ability to pay (APROFE, 1997). No information is available on what happened to* *users who could not afford the higher prices. However, a lower-cost option, the Ministry of Health was available to users.*

Discussion: *Although client loss did occur, revenues increased—suggesting that demand for IUD insertions in Ecuador is inelastic. The study also provides an example of the superiority of more rigorous comparison-group designs, compared with the less rigorous pretest-posttest design.*

Unlike the demonstration project in Mali (see Doucoure et al. in this volume), APROFE had been established for more than 30 years and utilization of its services was affected by competition, seasonality, and long-term trends in program growth. Such an environment requires a rigorous design to avoid drawing erroneous conclusions from the data. Although the designs used by the authors are more powerful than a simple before-and-after demonstration, they do not eliminate all sources of bias from the study. Each clinic decided whether to raise prices and the size of the price increase. Therefore, self-selection bias cannot be ruled out as contributing to the results: That bias can only be eliminated with random selection.

The Need for Quasi-Experimental Methodology to Evaluate Pricing Effects

Federico R. León and Agustín Cuesta

Mature family planning associations and national programs in less developed countries are placing increased emphasis on financial self-reliance. Increased cost-recovery through raising the price of services has been one of the strategies used to improve program sustainability (Jensen, 1991). Some experts, however, have questioned this strategy on the assumption that it will diminish the demand for services (Harvey, 1991). Research on the subject has produced mixed findings. Lewis (1986) cited studies conducted in Colombia, Jamaica, Sri Lanka, and Thailand that showed that demand was relatively inelastic; for example, it was reported that a doubling of the price of injectable contraceptives at public clinics in Thailand had no effect on the number of new or current users. On the other hand, Haws et al. (1992) found that the increase in sterilization fees at 17 clinics in Brazil, the Dominican Republic, and Mexico produced a decline in caseloads at 14 of them. Lande and Geller (1991) reported mixed findings from a review of other studies. In Ecuador, Bratt et al. (1991) found a reduced demand for IUDs immediately following a price increase, then a gradual movement back to original levels. In a recent review of five data sets from contraceptive social marketing programs, Harvey (1993) found that increased prices hurt demand.

There are two possible explanations for the diversity of findings. First, the elasticity of demand for family planning may be contingent on situational factors. Since the relative size of the price increases, the absolute amount of the payments per service, the user purchasing capacity, and so on, evidently varied across the studies, diverse results could be expected from them.[1] Here we would be dealing with a problem of *external validity* of the findings: The elasticity of demand demonstrated in a study would apply only to situations that are essentially similar to those of the study.

The second possible explanation concerns the *internal validity* of the studies, that is, the legitimacy of the attribution of cause or the possible spuriousness of the findings. For example, when demand decreases, was it the in-

Reprinted with the permission of the Population Council from *Studies in Family Planning* 1993. 24,6: 375–381.

creased price or an uncontrolled variable that produced the decrease? When the intrinsic weakness of the research designs used in some studies are into account, there are reasons to suspect that some effects may have been spurious. Thus, contradictory reports could be expected from pricing studies using different research designs, even though they shared the same situational characteristics.

One of the research designs employed in pricing studies has been the single-group pretest-posttest design, diagrammed below. In this type of pre-experiment, pretest observations (O_1) are

$$O_1 \ X \ O_2$$

recorded for one group of subjects—for example, the number of new sterilization acceptors in specified clinics during the three months preceding the intervention. The clinics later receive the treatment (X), for example, the introduction of a price increase for sterilization services. Then, posttest observations (O_2) are made for the same clinics, that is, the number of new sterilization acceptors in the specified clinics during the following quarter is recorded, and evaluators can assess the difference between pretest and posttest results in order to conclude whether the treatment had an impact: whether it increased demand, decreased it, or produced no effects.

The problem with this design is that it generally fails to rule out alternative interpretations of the results, such as those pertaining to seasonal trends, the continual expansion of family planning, or specific historic events (Campbell and Stanley, 1963; Cook and Campbell, 1979; Fisher et al., 1983). If evaluators choose to ignore the competing explanatory hypotheses, they may attribute the change in the number of acceptors (or lack of change) to the price increase, when in fact the change (or lack of change) was determined by other factors. In the end, program managers may be misled.

This report offers data from natural experiments conducted by the Asociación Pro-Bienestar de la Familia Ecuatoriana (APROFE) in 17 Ecuadorean clinics that (1) illustrate the erroneous conclusions that can be derived from the single-group pretest-posttest design and (2) demonstrate the practical advantage of using quasi-experimental designs that were invented to overcome the deficiencies of pre-experiments.

A Single-Group Pretest-Posttest Study

Between 1 August 1990 and 1 July 1991, APROFE kept constant the prices of services for reversible family planning methods in its clinics in 15 Ecuadorean cities. At a workshop attended by APROFE's central management unit and clinic

Table 1. Price charged per clinic for an IUD insertion and consultation on 1 August 1990 and 1 July 1991, and numer of new IUD clients in the three months preceding and three months following the July 1991 increase in price, four APROFE clinics, Ecuador

Clinics	Price in Sucres*		Number of new clients[†]	
	1 August 1990	1 July 1991	April–June	July–September
Portoviejo	3,100	5,000	273	354
Ambato	3,100	5,000	198	183
Chone	3,100	4,600	109	111
Manta	3,100	5,000	211	194

* The price corresponds to the Copper T IUD. The average exchange rate fluctuated between US$1=S/840 in mid-1990 and US$1=S/1,250 by the end of 1991.
† This is the number of women who (1) came for the first time to the APROFE clinic and requested an IUD insertion or (2) were already IUD users from other providers and came for the first time to the APROFE clinic for a control visit; the latter represent a small fraction of the total number. (This is not the official definition of new IUD users at APROFE, in its routine reports, APROFE uses the definition provided in Note 3 of the text.)

directors in May 1991, the participants examined several alternative ways to deal with price increases. As part of a move toward decentralized decisionmaking, decisions concerning whether or not to raise prices and the amount of the increases were left to the discretion of individual clinic directors.

In July 1991, three clinics raised the price of IUD services by 61 percent, and one clinic raised its price by 48 percent. All four clinics maintained the new prices throughout the second semester of 1991. Table 1 shows the price increases as well as the number of new IUD clients per clinic in the months immediately preceding and following the increases. A rise in the demand for IUD services can be observed from the second to the third quarter in two of the four clinics, and a decrease in demand occurred in the other two. In order to assess the relative magnitude of the changes, a percent change in the number of new IUD users was calculated as percent change = 100 (posttest–pretest)/pretest. Of the four clinics, Portoviejo was one where a substantial change in demand occurred, and the change was positive (30 percent); the percent changes at the other three clinics (–8, +2, –8) were small and could be attributed to random fluctuations.

In order to gain confidence in these data, the evaluators checked the number of new IUD users registered in the four clinics in the third quarter of 1990;[2] two clinics (Portoviejo and Manta) showed a greater demand in 1991 than in 1990, while the opposite occurred at the other two clinics (Ambato and Chone). Thus, whether compared with the prior quarter or the equivalent quarter of the prior year, the results of this single-group pretest-posttest study would suggest that, on the whole, the 48–61 percent price increases introduced at the beginning of the third quarter of 1991 did *not* reduce the demand for IUD services. Management would not be surprised, since the price increases only moderately surpassed the annual inflation rate of 45 percent.

Figure 1. Average number of new IUD clients in the second, third, and fourth quarters of 1987–90, APROFE

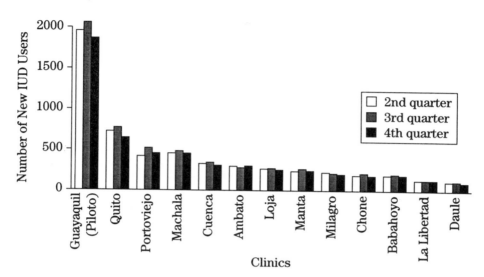

In actuality, however, the clinics lost potential clients because of the price increases, but this fact was concealed by a seasonal trend that was undetected by the single-group pretest-posttest design. Figure 1 shows that in the previous four years (1987–90), the number of new IUD clients increased from the second to the third quarter and fell in the fourth quarter in 10 of the 13 APROFE clinics offering reversible methods that were founded before 1987;[3] the demand increased from the second to the third quarter in 11 of the 13 clinics, a statistically significant finding.[4] Thus, gains in demand were likely to occur from pretest to posttest in the four clinics of the single-group pretest-posttest study in 1991 simply because the second and third quarters define the ascending portion of a seasonal trend. That only one clinic in the pretest-posttest study showed clear gains is probably indicative of the negative impact of price increases on demand, but the research design used was too weak to detect this effect and thus led to the spurious finding of a lack of negative effects.

A Nonequivalent Control Group Study

The more rigorous nonequivalent control group quasi-experiment with pretest and posttest diagrammed below is better able to capture the loss of potential demand. The first line

$$O_1 \ X \ O_2$$
$$O_1 \quad O_2$$

Figure 2. Pretest-posttest percent change in the number of new IUD clients at APROFE clinics, experimental and control groups, second and third quarters, 1991

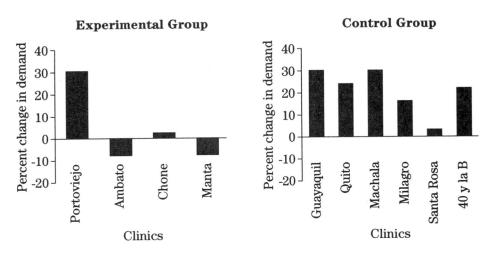

is similar in structure to the single-group pretest-posttest design; this is called the experimental group because it receives the treatment. The second line corresponds to the control group, which does not receive the treatment but receives pretest and posttest measurements. The design is known as a nonequivalent control group because the subjects (in the present case, clinics) are not randomly assigned to experimental and control groups and the groups may therefore display important differences (such as, the size of the clinic, the past history of prices, and the clients' purchasing capacity).

In the natural experiment of 1991, six APROFE clinics maintained the 1990 prices for IUDs, thus forming a control group for the clinics that raised their prices by 48 percent or 61 percent. Important information is obtained from a comparison of the demand gains and losses of the two groups. Figure 2 depicts the percent change in demand calculated for each clinic;[5] the average change was positive in the experimental group (mean percent change = +4 percent), but attained a higher value in the control group (mean percent change = +21 percent); furthermore, in the control group, the six clinics—large and small, based on the coast or the sierra—without exception showed increases in demand.[6] This comparison allows us to conclude that the clinics of the experimental group would have attained a larger number of IUD users in the third quarter of 1991 if they had not raised prices.

Two questions useful to the program may be asked at this point. First, what is the effect on demand of smaller price increases? Perhaps increases of 20 percent or less do not affect potential demand. Second, what happens to demand

Figure 3. Average percent change in IUD demand at three groups of APROFE clinics, according to change in price of IUDs, 1991

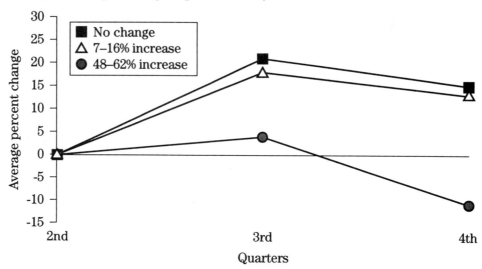

over time? Perhaps the losses of the experimental group were ephemeral. These questions can be readily answered since seven APROFE clinics (Cuenca, Babahoyo, Loja, La Libertad, Daule, La Troncal, and Mapasingue) raised prices by between 7 percent and 16 percent on 1 July 1991, and information on demand from the second through the fourth quarters was available for all clinics. Figure 3 shows the average percent change in demand for each group of clinics; the baseline is the second quarter of 1991.[7] The seasonal trend is clearly visible. The differences between the first two groups are small but systematic, while those between the first two and the third group are large from the beginning and widen further in the fourth quarter. Thus, the nonequivalent control group design allowed APROFE to detect some important practical consequences of raising prices by 48–61 percent versus raising them by 7–16 percent.

These consequences can be seen in more detail in Figure 4, which shows the distribution of the 17 APROFE clinics in the bivariate space defined by the increases in prices (horizontal axis) and the percent changes in demand from the second to the fourth quarters (vertical axis). The linear regression line gives information concerning the general trend: The greater the price increase, the smaller the gain or the larger the loss of potential clients.[8] But the figure also shows that the variability in demand change within the group of clinics that increased prices by 48–61 percent is smaller than the variability observed within the groups that established moderate increases or maintained the old prices. This finding suggests that price became an important determinant of demand change in the former group, pushing it down; in the other two groups, the wide

Figure 4. Changes in IUD demand at 17 APROFE clinics as a function of price increases, 1991

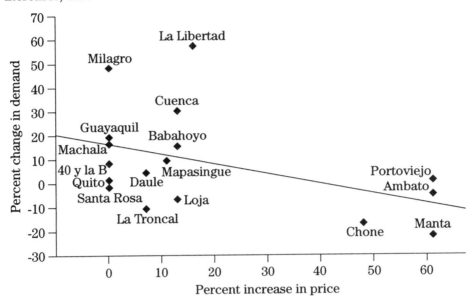

variability in demand change suggests the action of other determinants. The farthest outlier—the most distant point from the regression line—corresponds to the La Libertad clinic, where demand increased beyond any expectations derived from its level of service pricing (a 16 percent increase). Organizational psychologists who visited this clinic in August 1991 reported the existence of a commitment to expanding services (Boado et al., 1991), and a survey conducted in April 1992 found that APROFE led the market in long-acting contraceptives in this city (CEPAR, 1992). These and other analyses will allow APROFE to discover what it takes to succeed at raising or maintaining demand despite increased prices.

A Time-Series Study

Family planning associations or programs may not be able to establish different prices at different clinics. Under these circumstances, the nonequivalent control group design cannot be implemented and there may be a temptation to use the single-group pretest-posttest. There are, however, better alternatives for the analysis of single-group data. In the time-series design diagrammed below, several pretests (O_1, O_2, etc.) precede the treatment and several

$$O_1\ O_2\ O_3\ \ X\ \ O_4\ O_5\ O_6$$

Figure 5. Quarterly number of new IUD users at the Piloto clinic of APROFE in Guayaquil during periods of price constancy and price increases, 1987–92

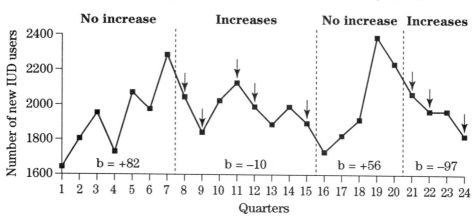

Note: b = rounded regression coefficients.

posttests (O_4, O_5, O_6) follow it. The basic structure of this design can be modified to fit diverse situations. For example, APROFE's Piloto clinic in Guayaquil raised prices a number of times between 1987 and 1992. Figure 5 shows the quarterly IUD demand curve at this clinic[9] from the first quarter of 1987 (1) through the fourth quarter of 1992 (24). Price increases for the IUD services in this period are indicated by the vertical arrows. The graph is segmented into four parts according to whether price increases occurred or did not occur within the period. The demand curve ascends when nominal prices are held constant (or, given inflation, when real prices diminish) and descends when prices are increased; the rounded regression coefficients provide information concerning the average number of new IUD users gained (+) or lost (–) per quarter. Thus, the evidence clearly indicates that IUD demand is negatively related to price at APROFE's Piloto clinic. Had we based our conclusion on a single-group pretest-posttest design around two points in time, the conclusion might have been the opposite; for example, the number of new IUD users in the quarter following the price increase of 1 July 1989 (third quarter = 2,119 clients) was greater than that registered in the quarter preceding it (second quarter = 2,018 clients).

The time-series results extend the external validity of the findings from the nonequivalent control group study, since they show that the negative impact of pricing on demand was not particular to a given group of clinics (Portoviejo, Ambato, Chone, and Manta) or to time interval (third and fourth quarters of 1991).

Time-series designs are useful tools that can be employed by program evaluators to monitor natural changes that take place over extended time periods. A minimum of one year must be considered in order to detect seasonal trends, though this is no guarantee of accuracy, because seasonal trends may be affected by program actions and other temporal factors. Consider the highly consistent inverted-U-shaped curve involving the second, third, and fourth quarters that appeared in each of 10 APROFE clinics in Figure 1; the curves were based on an average of the demand for IUD services observed during four years (1987–90). Such a strong seasonal trend, however, failed to show up in the data from the Guayaquil Piloto clinic in the year 1990 and again in 1992 (see quarters 14–16 and 22–24 in Figure 5), probably owing to the interfering effect of the price increases of 1989–90 and 1992. A time-series study limited to the years 1990–92 would have had problems detecting both the seasonal trend and the negative effects of price increases on demand.

Discussion

The challenge in operations research is to strike a good balance between overly simple research designs that may appear practical but that actually distort what is going on and overly complex ones that go too far to prove the obvious. Generally, the best alternative to these extremes is the nonequivalent control group quasi-experiment with pretest and posttest. Paradoxically, over the past decade a shift of emphasis has been observed from quasi-experimentation toward the single-group pretest-posttest design and other pre-experiments (Reynolds, 1991) believed to be more practical and to better fit most field conditions (for example, see Seltzer et al., 1993). The message from the present report is that while pre-experiments may be less costly and easier to implement, they cannot replace quasi-experiments. The analyses presented have shown that the results of pre-experiments may be misleading, and that the consequences of deceptive results from operations research are not just academic. Failure to detect a negative effect may lead program managers to make decisions that have undesired consequences for programs; by failing to detect positive effects, program managers may erroneously discard potentially useful solutions. Real programmatic disasters may follow when management decisions are based on illusions that have the appearance of scientific findings. It follows that, in the end, pre-experiments may be more costly than quasi-experiments and that their use must be avoided, particularly in the case of pricing studies, where many nuisance variables are beyond the control of evaluators.

Notes

1. Lande and Geller (1991) referred to the following situational factors as possible causes for the variability of findings across studies: type of contraceptive, initial price versus cumulative cost, the role of substitutes, nonmonetary costs, economic situation, and perception of value.

2. Comparable data were not available for the second quarter of 1990. APROFE began to register new users (defined in the note under Table 1) in the third quarter of 1990.

3. Information on demand for these years is based on a different definition of new IUD users. The new user could be either (1) a woman who came for the first time to the APROFE clinic and requested an IUD insertion, or was already an IUD user from another provider and came for a control visit, or (2) an IUD user, or former IUD user, from an APROFE clinic whose case had been closed by the clinic because the woman had decided to abandon family planning or had failed to show up at the clinic for four years and then returned to the clinic for a control visit or a reinsertion. The first group represents about 80 percent of the total number of new IUD users according to this definition.

4. The finding was statistically significant at $p < .03$, two-tailed, sign test. Actually, the averages represented in Figure 1 underestimate the extent of the seasonal trend observed in 1987, 1988, and 1989. The seasonal trend was weak or nonexistent in 1990, probably in response to the considerable and frequent price increases introduced the previous year in all clinics and the increase of 1990.

5. The definition of new clients is in the note to Table 1.

6. This finding is statistically significant at $p < .04$, two-tailed, sign test.

7. The definition of new clients is in the note to Table 1.

8. The product-moment correlation between percent price increase and percent change in demand was $r = -.44$ at $p < .07$, two-tailed. This may be an underestimate, however, since the line of best fit is perhaps curvilinear. Unfortunately, the distribution of data points does not lend itself to a finer analysis.

9. Here we employed the definition of new IUD user presented in Note 3 above in order to maintain consistency in the data from 1987 through 1992. Price increases before mid-1991 include those for the Lippes loop, while those after that time include the Copper T only.

References

Boado, Miguel, Oswaldo Otoya, and Gustavo Quiroz. 1991. "Diagnóstico de Personal en 14 Clínicas de APROFE, Ecuador." *Technical Report for APROFE and USAID/Ecuador.* Lima, Peru: The Population Council.

Bratt, John H., Barbara S. Janowitz, and Daniel B. Fried. 1991. "Impacts of a Price Increase in Eight Ecuadorean Family Planning Clinics." *Final Report.* Research Triangle Park, NC: Family Health International.

Campbell, Donald T. and Julian C. Stanley. 1963. "Experimental and Quasi-Experimental Designs for Research on Teaching." In *Handbook of Research on Teaching.* Ed. N.L. Gage. Chicago: Rand McNally.

CEPAR. 1992. "Encuesta de Planificación Familiar en Siete Ciudades del Ecuador: Informe sobre Mercado." Technical Report. Quito, Ecuador: Centro de Estudios de Paternidad Responsable.

Cook, Thomas D. and Donald T. Campbell. 1979. *Quasi-Experimentation: Design and Analysis Issues for Field Settings.* Chicago: Rand McNally.

Fisher, Andrew A., John E. Laing, and John E. Stoeckel. 1983. *Handbook for Family Planning Operations Research Design.* New York: The Population Council.

Harvey, Philip D. 1991. "In poor countries, 'self-sufficiency' can be dangerous to your health." *Studies in Family Planning* 22, 1: 52–54.

———. 1993. "To maximize contraceptive prevalence, keep prices low." *DKT International* 3: 1–5.

Haws, Jeanne, Lynn Bakamjian, Tim Williams, and Karen Johnson Lassner. 1992. "Impact of sustainability policies on sterilization services in Latin America." *Studies in Family Planning* 23, 2: 85–96.

Jensen, Eric E. 1991. "Cost-effectiveness and financial sustainability in family planning operations research." In *Operations Research: Helping Family Planning Programs Work Better.* Eds. Myrna Seidman and Marjorie Horn. New York: Wiley–Liss.

Lande, Robert E. and Judith S. Geller. 1991. "Paying for Family Planning." *Population Reports*, Series J, No. 39.

Lewis, Maureen A. 1986. "Do contraceptive prices affect demand?" *Studies in Family Planning* 17, 3: 126–135.

Reynolds, Jack. 1991. "A reconsideration of operations research experimental designs." In *Operations Research: Helping Family Planning Programs Work Better.* Eds. Myrna Seidman and Marjorie Horn. New York: Wiley–Liss.

Seltzer, Judith R., Robert C. Blomberg, Elba R. Mercado, and Marcia Townsend. 1993. "Evaluation of the Operations Research in Family Planning and Maternal-Child Health for Latin America and the Caribbean (INOPAL II) Project." Arlington, VA: Population Technical Assistance Project.

Acknowledgments

The data presented in this article were collected as part of a diagnostic study conducted by APROFE with technical and financial assistance from the INOPAL II Project of the Population Council, sponsored by the United States Agency for International Development (S&T/POP/R) through Contract No. DPE-3030-2-00-9019-00. USAID/Ecuador cosponsored a component of the diagnostic study. The authors are indebted to Anrudh Jain, Jim Foreit, and Susan Brems for their editorial suggestions.

PREFATORY REMARKS

Safe Provision of Oral Contraceptives: The Effectiveness of Systematic Laboratory Testing in Senegal

John Stanback, Jason B. Smith, Barbara Janowitz, and Fadel Diadhiou

Programmatic issue: *The study examines the effect of subjecting contraceptive pill users to mandatory laboratory testing in terms of the cost of the tests and frequency and accuracy of detection of contraindications to hormonal method use.*

Programmatic processes/components: *The research examined the health and use effects of a widely applied program norm requiring all prospective pill users to undergo a series of costly laboratory tests prior to method prescription*

Research design: *The authors conducted a diagnostic study, gathering data on the costs and accuracy of testing a cohort of women for pill contraindications. The contraindications included in the norm were also reviewed in the light of contemporary professional opinion. No intervention was involved.*

Findings: *The tests were judged largely irrelevant to hormonal contraceptive use. Many contraindications included by the program like Class III pap smears and high cholesterol levels are not considered by scientific sources to be contraindications to pill use. Only 3 percent of women tested showed one or more "contraindications." Very low test-retest reliability was found. Existence of the contraindication was not confirmed in eight of the nine women who could be retested. The cost of the tests to the client ranged from US $55 to more than $200. Such costs—as much as five times the monthly average salary in Senegal—were identified by the authors as a potential barrier to pill use.*

Program response to findings: *The study recommended elimination of routine laboratory screening for use of hormonal contraception. The recommendation was eventually accepted by the Ministry of Health in Senegal, but in a situation frequently encountered in OR, the study was not completely successful in changing provider behavior. Many individual physicians continued to demand laboratory screening of oral contraceptive clients.*

Discussion: *Unnecessary laboratory tests have been identified as a wide-spread barrier to contraceptive use in many settings for many years (see Huber and Huber, 1975). Even when tests are justified, low laboratory quality puts the reliability of test results in question. Large numbers of physicians in Senegal apparently did not accept the recommendation to eliminate laboratory tests as a prerequisite for pill use—a lifetime of practice and belief is unlikely to be overturned by the results of a single study. In dealing with medical barriers, OR needs to focus on the problem of training medical students in and informing physicians of advances in family planning, and of ways of obtaining provider compliance with new, scientifically sound, program norms.*

Reference

Huber, Douglas and Sallie Craig Huber. 1975. "Screening oral contraceptive candidates and inconsequential pelvic examinations." *Studies in Family Planning* 6,2: 49–51.

Safe Provision of Oral Contraceptives: The Effectiveness of Systematic Laboratory Testing in Senegal

John Stanback, Jason B. Smith,
Barbara Janowitz, and Fadel Diadhiou

Since oral contraceptives were introduced more than 30 years ago, more than 100 million women have used the convenient method of fertility control.[1] Today, the pill is still the most commonly used hormonal contraceptive method.[2] As formulations have changed and more has been learned about the safety of oral contraceptives, many early fears about the short-term and long-term side effects of the pill have diminished. However, physicians and policymakers in many countries still have deep-seated concerns about the safety of hormonal methods. These concerns manifest themselves in the form of medical policies that limit access to the pill and other hormonal contraceptive methods.

Some of the more restrictive policies exist in Francophone Africa, where de jure and de facto health regulations require women to undergo laboratory testing prior to receiving prescriptions for the pill. These policies, which assume that laboratory tests can effectively screen for underlying conditions such as diabetes, anemia and high cholesterol, are undoubtedly motivated by concern for contraceptive safety. However, excessive and inappropriate testing not only constitutes a medical barrier to family planning but may also fail to identify women at risk. For these reasons, systematic testing in Africa has recently been called into question.[3]

In 1988–1989, a study of laboratory testing prior to prescribing the pill in one Francophone country, Senegal, was conducted by the Department of Obstetrics and Gynecology at Aristide Le Dantec Hospital in collaboration with the Family Health and Population Project of the U.S. Agency for the International Development (U.S. AID), Family Health International , and the International Science and Technology Institute. This article describes the findings of the study and makes policy recommendations regarding the use of laboratory tests for ensuring contraceptive safety.

Reprinted with the permission of The Alan Guttmacher Institute from *International Family Planning Perspectives* 1994. 20,4: 147–149.

Methodology

From November 1988 to July 1989, researchers in Dakar, Senegal, conducted a prospective study of first-time oral contraceptive users to determine the percentage of women identified as poor risks for the pill by laboratory tests recommended in Senegal.

Study participants were recruited from three different centers: the maternity clinic at Le Dantec Hospital, the Dakar clinic of the Senegalese Family Planning Association, and the Centre de Protection Maternelle et Infantile de Medina, a government maternal and child health center. The study population consisted of the first 500 women who came to the clinics and requested the pill as first-time users. Because participation consisted initially of only a few questions and the women were offered free laboratory testing, all agreed to participate.

After admission to the study, the women received a routine physical examination and their medical history was taken. The participants received vouchers for free laboratory testing at the Pasteur Institute in Dakar. Ordinarily, women have such testing done at Le Dantec Hospital or a private laboratory; however, for this study, all women were sent to the Pasteur Institute, which is generally regarded as the best laboratory testing facility in the city. Study participants were also given bus fare for the trip to the Institute.

The study protocol required all participants to have the same laboratory tests that were recommended for first time oral contraceptive users in Senegal at the time. Pap smears were taken to determine cervical cancer risk, and urine was tested for glucose levels to detect diabetes. Fasting blood samples were tested for liver function (alkaline phosphotase, direct and indirect bilirubin, SGOT and SGPT), lipids (triglycerides, HDL, LDL and total cholesterol), glucose levels and sickling of erythrocytes. The study coordinator, an obstetrician-gynecologist from Le Dantec Hospital, used the laboratory test results to determine whether the pill was contraindicated for each participant. Contraindications to oral contraceptive use were based on U.S. Food and Drug Administration Physician Labeling Guidelines.[4] Clients with a contraindication were asked to come back for retesting as soon as possible to confirm the results.

The data collection instrument contained the results of the laboratory screening as well as background information about the study participants. The data were scanned, coded, entered and cleaned in Dakar. Analyses (tests of central tendency and correlation, univariate and bivariate analysis) began in Dakar and were completed at Family Health International in the United States

Results

Among the 500 women admitted into the study, 77 never obtained their initial laboratory examinations, 11 were ineligible because they were former pill users

Table 1. Laboratory contraindications to the pill among first-time acceptors in Dakar, by test round, 1989 (N = 410)

Acceptor	First round	Second Round
1	Class III Pap smear	Downgraded
2	Class III Pap smear	Downgraded
3	Class III Pap smear	Downgraded
4	Class III Pap smear	Downgraded
5	Class III Pap smear	Downgraded
6	Class III Pap smear	Downgraded
7	Class III Pap smear	Downgraded
8	High cholesterol	Normal
9	Hyperglycemia	No change
10	Class III Pap smear	Not retested
11	Class III Pap smear	Not retested
12	Class III Pap smear	Not retested
13	Class III Pap smear	Not retested
14	Sickle cell anemia	Not retested
15	Sickle cell anemia	Not retested
16	Liver function	Not retested
17	Liver function	Not retested
18	Liver function	Not retested
19	Elevated bilirubin	Not retested
20	Hyperglycemia	Not retested

at another center, and two clients from one center had not completed the questionnaire, leaving an analysis set of 410 women. Among these participants, 213 were clients at the Centre de Protection Maternalle et Infantile de Medina, 100 at the Family Planning Association clinic and 97 were clients at the maternity clinic of Le Dantec Hospital.

As Table 1 shows, the first round of laboratory tests identified 20 women with possible contraindications to using the pill; among them, only nine returned for a second, confirmatory test. Eight of nine participants who were retested had negative results, indicating one of three possibilities: changed health status, false positive on the first test, or false negative on the second test.

Seven of the nine confirmatory test were for Class III Pap smears (mild to moderate atypia consistent with dysplasia), which indicate potential risk of cervical cancer. In Senegal at that time, a Pap smears of Class III or higher was considered a contraindication for pill use. One test indicated high cholesterol levels, and one found hyperglycemia. Upon retesting all seven of the Pap smears were downgrade to Class I (benign) or Class II (inflammation) and the one case of high cholesterol was found to be within the normal range. The blood glucose level remained high in the one case of hyperglycemia, and, for this woman, oral contraceptive use was confirmed to be contraindicated.

Eleven women for whom the pill was contraindicated by their initial laboratory test results either could not be found or refused to have a second test. Four of these women had Class III Pap smears, two had results that indicated sickle cell disease (neither had ever been symptomatic), four indicated liver function problems (two had elevated SGOT and SGPT, one had elevated alkaline phosphotase, and one had slightly elevated direct bilirubin), and one indicated hyperglycemia. If we take the conservative position and assume that all 11 unconfirmed tests were confirmed as contraindications, then 3% of clients tested would have contraindications to the pill.

The cost to detect a contraindication was calculated. This calculation was restricted to the cost that would be paid by the client, exclusive of transportation and opportunity costs (cost of her time). Clients in Dakar have a choice of laboratories, ranging from the relatively expensive Pasteur Institute to other less expensive private and hospital laboratories. According to the calculations, laboratory tests recommended at the time of the study for new acceptors of the pill could cost a client US$55–$216. Laboratory testing for this study at the Pasteur Institute was done at a volume discount of $80 per client or $32,800 for all 410 study participants. Consequently, even if all 11 unconfirmed tests were true positives, the direct study cost per contraindication detected (12) would be more than $2,733.

Discussion

The prevalence of contraindications to pill use among the study sample was low (3%), even with the very conservative assumption that all unconfirmed tests actually reflected an underlying clinical condition that warranted denial of the pill. Low prevalence suggests that universal laboratory testing of all clients may not be the most efficient means of discovering these contraindications.

Low prevalence may also adversely affect the accuracy of testing because the predictive value of a test is a function of not only the sensitivity and specificity of the test, but also the prevalence of the condition being tested for. If the medical condition of interest is relatively rare in the population, as is the case with many contraindications to pill use, the results of massive testing may inflate the number of people incorrectly identified as having the condition.

The reversal in test results between the first and second rounds of laboratory testing may have been the result of changes in the clients' physical condition, but it also raises the question of test reliability. The reliability of a test is its ability to give consistent results when repeatedly applied to the same person under the same circumstances. The degree to which a test is reliable may vary considerably, depending on the proper implementation of the test—a multistage process involving a precise coordination of people, facilities and chemical agents.

In developing countries, a number of problems could arise. There may not be enough facilities to handle the number of tests required. Laboratories may be poorly equipped and chronically lacking in materials necessary for timely processing of specimens. The overall level of training and expertise among laboratory personnel may be low or may vary widely both within and between labs.

The cost of laboratory testing to detect a woman with contraindications is high, particularly in relation to per capita health expenditures: The estimated cost is almost 100 times the 1990 per capita health expenditures for Senegal.[5] During the study, testing was provided at no cost to the client; however, laboratory tests that cost 1–5 times the monthly per capita income in Senegal[6] could be a barrier to contraceptive use. Given the expense, it is unlikely that many women whose initial laboratory tests find a contraindication even opt for retesting. In most cases, the women would be encouraged to accept a nonhormonal method, such as the IUD.

Denial of oral contraceptives to these women may increase the risks of sickness and death from unwanted pregnancy and childbirth; these risks are much greater than those associated with the use of the pill. The maternal mortality ratio for Senagalese women was recently estimated to 850 deaths per 100,000 live births,[7] whereas the annual mortality related to use of the pill has been estimated at one death per 100,000 in Africa overall.[8]

The results of this study provide a strong argument for the elimination of systematic testing prior to prescribing oral contraceptives. At most, laboratory testing should be reserved as a confirmatory measure for those women identified as possible high-risk cases through simpler and less expensive mechanisms, such as medical histories or clinical exams.

After completion of this study, strong interest in the issue was shown by the Senagalese medical community and U.S. AID–Senegal, prompting a regional meeting to discuss the results. The International Symposium on Laboratory Testing Prior to Contraception was held in Dakar in February 1990 and was attended by representatives from Senegal, Côte d'Ivoire, Niger, Burkina Faso, Togo, Benin and Morocco. Presentations were made concerning the family planning programs in all of these countries. At the conclusion of the meeting, a 15-point resolution was approved whose first recommendation called for the elimination of routine laboratory screening for hormonal contraception.[9] The government of Senegal has since approved this recommendation and no longer requires systematic laboratory testing. However, many doctors and midwives have resisted the recommendation, and laboratory testing prior to prescription of the pill is still widespread in urban Senegal.

References

1. D. M. Potts and J. B. Smith, "The Future of Hormonal Contraception," *International Journal of Fertility*, Vol. 36, Supplement 3, 1991, pp.57–63.

2. Ibid.

3. P. Buekens et al., "Is Blood Testing Necessary Before OC Prescription in Africa?" *Studies in Family Planning*, 21:178–180, 1990.

4. U. S. Food and Drug Administration, "Labeling Guidance Text for Combination Oral Contraceptives Physician Labeling, Revised February 11, 1988," *Contraception*, 37:434, 1988.

5. The World Bank, *World Development Report*, Washington, D.C., 1993, p. 210.

6. Population Reference Bureau, *World Population Data Sheet*, Washington, D. C., 1990.

7. A Gueye et al., "Rapport de la Deuxième Mission d'Identification por la Réduction de la Mortalité Maternelle au Senegal," Goverment of Senegal. Dakar, 1989.

8. Centers for Disease Control, *Family Planning Methods and Practice: Africa*, Atlanta, 1983.

9. F. Diadhiou et al., "Rapport Final, Symposium International sur le Bilan Paraclinique Préliminaire à la Contraception," Université Cheikh Ant Diop, Dakar, Senegal, Feb. 1990.

The Impact of Mass Media Advertising on a Voluntary Sterilization Program in Brazil

Karen G. Foreit, Marcos Paulo P. de Castro, and Eliane F. Duarte Franco

Programmatic issue: *The Pro-Pater agency wished to increase, in a cost-effective manner, the number of vasectomies it performed.*

Programmatic processes/components: *Pro-Pater tried to increase client recruitment, by increasing information, education and communication activities. Because it islocated in São Paulo, a large city with a highly literate population, the agency decided to experiment with advertisements in mass-circulation magazines.*

Research design: *The magazine promotion study employed a simple time-series analysis using program service statistics for the baseline, intervention, and postintervention periods.*

Findings: *During a ten-week campaign, the number of new clients doubled and eventually stabilized at a daily rate that was more than 50 percent higher than precampaign levels. The study hypothesizes about the complementary roles of mass media and interpersonal promotion as they relate to the growth of a sterilization program, and touches on such programmatic issues as the up-front costs of a mass media campaign and its effects on program revenue.*

Program response to findings: *As a result of the study, Pro-Pater decided to continue to use the mass media for vasectomy promotion. The study was later replicated by Kincaid et al. who substituted television promotion for magazines. The two studies produced broadly similar findings, except that the number of vasectomies performed failed to reach a plateau at a higher level after the TV campaign as was the case after the magazine campaign, a finding that appears to have more to do with changing programmatic conditions than with differences between the two media.*

Discussion: *The effectivess and cost-effectiveness of using mass media to promote vasectomy is one of the generalizable findings in the OR literature. Relatively few operations research studies attempt to draw theoretical implications from their findings. The Pro-Pater study is notable for its* *attempt to describe the process of growth for sterilization services and to discuss the role of mass media promotion in stimulating the program growth process.*

Finally, once again, the study illustrates how OR design alternatives are limited by program conditions. The number of potential research designs available was limited because the agency operated only a single clinic, making the use of controls impossible. However, the time series is a relatively powerful design for the study of interventions in a one-facility setting. Unlike a demonstration project with a single pretest and a single posttest design, the time series controls for pretest time trends. By comparing the number of vasectomies performed before and after the campaign, the authors also controlled for possible seasonality in clinic performance by comparing the postintervention calendar months with the same preintervention calendar months of the year before.

Reference

Kincaid, D. Lawrence et al. 1996. "Impact of a mass media campaign in Brazil." *International Family Planning Perspectives* 22,4: 169–175.

The Impact of Mass Media Advertising on a Voluntary Sterilization Program in Brazil

Karen G. Foreit, Marcos Paulo P. de Castro, and Eliane F. Duarte Franco

Mass media advertising has been shown to be effective in promoting a wide range of health behavior, from smoking cessation (Cummings et al., 1997; Flay, 1987) to adopting family planning (Sweeney, 1977; Betrand et al., 1982). Advertising may create an awareness of a health problem, provide information on interventions or products to resolve the problem, and indicate where the product may be obtained.

Family planning advertising is characterized by two different traditions. The first, "generic," approach seeks to sensitize the audience to the issue of fertility regulation or to provide information on a wide range of contraceptive methods. The messages in this form of advertising tend to be general, often promoting such concepts as "responsible parenthood."

The second, "selective," approach resembles commercial, consumer products advertising campaigns. Specific brands of contraceptives and outlets are promoted. Contraceptive social marketing (CSM) is perhaps the best known example of this approach.

Generic campaigns may be responsible for the findings of stronger correlations between exposure to family planning messages and family planning use in areas with relatively lower contraceptive prevalence, than in areas of relatively higher prevalence (Bertrand et al., 1982). The consumer product approach has also been successful in low-prevalence settings. Selective promotion of vasectomy in Guatemala increased acceptance of that method (Bertrand et al., 1987).

Where contraceptive prevalence is already high, generic messages are unnecessary. Advertising in such areas should be more selective, promoting an underutilized method of underutilized source. The present study illustrates this selective approach and describes the effects of an advertising campaign to promote vasectomy in São Paulo, Brazil.

Reprinted with the permission of the Population Council from *Studies in Family Planning* 1989. 20,2: 107–116.

Program Setting and Background

São Paulo is the largest city in Brazil, and the nation's most important commercial and manufacturing center. The metropolitan area is estimated to contain between 15 and 17 million inhabitants. São Paulo state also displays some of Brazil's highest contraceptive prevalence rates. In 1986, 73 percent of women in union aged 15–44 reported using a family planning method; however, vasectomy accounted for only 2 percent of couples, versus 31 percent prevalence of female sterilization (Arruda et al., 1987).

The study described in this report was carried out at *Promocao de Paternidade Responsavel* (Pro-Pater), a private voluntary organization devoted to male reproductive health primarily vasectomy. The Pro-Pater is located in a commercial neighborhood near the city center. The clinic was opened in 1981 and by 1984 had become the largest single provider of voluntary sterilization in Brazil, performing 3,046 vasectomies in that year alone.

Initially, Pro-Pater relied on interpersonal promotion, primarily by word-of-mouth from satisfied clients. Approximately 73 percent of new clients surveyed in 1982 and 1983 (de Castro et al., 1984) had been referred by another client. In December 1983, a three-minute report on vasectomy and Pro-Pater wsa aired on a national television station to an estimated viewing audience of 40 million. In the month that followed, clinic attendance increased by 100 percent and 1984 performance remained 50 percent higher than 1983 levels. No further promotional efforts were undertaken, and clinic performance did not increase over the new plateau: performance during the first six months of 1985 was only marginally higher (10 percent) than in 1984.

Therefore, in mid-1985, Pro-Pater decided to undertake a formal advertising campaign, using full-page advertisements in local editions of "quality" national magazines. The advertisements appeared over a ten-week period, from mid-September to the end of November, 1985, and clinic performance was continuously monitored for 15 months. The remainder of this report describes the campaign and its effects.

Study Design

The 1985 campaign was Pro-Pater's first attempt at mass media advertising, and it involved a considerable financial investment; therefore, an operations research (OR) component was designed as an integral part of the process. The purpose of the OR was to closely monitor all phases of campaign implementation and impact on clinic operations to discover reasons for its success or failure. It was hoped that the lessons learned could be applied to vasectomy promotion in other regions of Brazil and perhaps in other countries as well.

As part of the OR process, three general objectives and two specific hypotheses were formulated. The first objective was to increase the awareness of vasectomy in the general population. This objective could not be measured directly, as the study design did not include a population survey. Therefore, it was measured indirectly, by comparing previous contact with vasectomized men among new clients referred by the campaign with those referred by traditional sources. A finding of fewer prior vasectomy contacts among the media-referred group was taken as affirmation of this objective.

The second objective was to increase the number of new clients and vasectomies performed. This objective could be measured directly, by comparing patient volume before, during, and after the campaign. Standard measures of statistical significance were used. As corollaries of this second objective, two operational hypotheses were formulated, both of which predicted negative side-effects of the campaign. The first hypothesis was that the number of new clients ineligible for vasectomy would increase. Pro-Pater provides full counseling and physical examinations as part of the routine intake procedure for all new clients, some of whom are subsequently judged to be ineligible for vasectomy. Eligibility criteria include maturity, completed family, and marital stability; patients exhibiting uncertainty, stress, or signs of coercion from their spouse are referred for further counseling before being accepted for vasectomy. While Pro-Pater does not view orientation of new clients ineligible for vasectomy as a program "failure," since only vasectomy acceptors pay a fee for services received, each ineligible new client represents a financial drain on clinic resources.

Because past outreach efforts had been highly selective, previous increases in new client volume had not been accompanied by relative increases in ineligibility (although the *number* of ineligible new clients had increased in absolute terms). Mass media advertising, by nature, is less selective than one-to-one interpersonal communication. The degree to which the *relative* percentage of ineligible new clients increased was taken as a failure to tailor the advertising message narrowly enough to appeal only to those men eligibile for vasectomy.

The second hypothesis was that mass media promotion would change the new client profile. This hypothesis has both positive and negative aspects. A downward change in demographic characteristics (younger age, fewer children) would be associated with increased ineligibility, as explained above. On the other hand, the campaign was also designed to attract a higher-income client who could afford to pay a higher fee, thus improving clinic self-sufficiency. In addition, it was hoped that the wide circulation of the magazines selected would attract new clients from neighborhood and geographical areas that Pro-Pater had not yet succeeded in entering. This hypothesis was evaluated by comparing client characteristics detailed in the intake interview before, during, and after the advertising campaign, and by comparing clients referred by various sources.

Finally, the third objective was to measure the costs and cost-effectiveness of mass media promotion. This was an ancillary objective of the study. Because the primary objective was to determine whether mass media advertising could be an effective tool for promoting vasectomy, the advertising director was charged with developing an optimum campaign within the stipulated budget, and not with comparing two approaches or media. Nevertheless, for the purpose of future applications, it was important to evaluate which advertisements or magazines were the most effective in attaining project goals. Standard market research techniques were used for this objective, including client recall of the advertisement and the magazine in which it appeared.

Methodology

The study design was a simply before-and-after time-series analysis utilizing the single Pro-Pater São Paulo clinic and a single intervention, the mass media promotional campaign. Service statistics for the years 1984–85 provided the baseline; clinic performance was continously monitored during the intervention and for a 12-month post-intervention period.

Mass Media Campaign

The advertising campaign was designed by a local advertising agency. Initially, all media outlets were explored, including television, radio, the printed media, and billboards. Television was rejected as being too expensive. Alternative campaigns using radio and magazines were developed. In the final analysis magazines were chosen on the grounds that more information could be transmitted in the printed media, that the printed advertisement constituted a more permanent record that could be passed on from reader to reader, and that magazines could reach a higher-income audience. Final layouts were pretested in the Pro-Pater waiting room. Figure 1 presents the four advertisements that were published.

Prior to publication, the advertising company orchestrated a pre-campaign promotion around an international conference on counseling for sterilization, sponsored by Pro-Pater and the Association for Voluntary Surgical Contraception (AVSC), and held in São Paulo two weeks before the appearance of the first advertisement. News reports and interviews appeared on radio, television, in daily newspapers, and advertising weeklies. A week before the campaign began, a taped television report, including interviews with patients in the waiting room and an actual vasectomy procedure, aired at midnight on a local television show. That single exposure resulted in 58 telephone calls to the clinic during the following week.

The formal campaign began on 16 September 1985, with advertisement 3 (see Figure 1) in *Veja*, a weekly news magazine, and ran until 27 November. A total of 27 insertions appeared, 18 in weekly magazines and 9 in monthly magazines, with an estimated target readership of 4.4 million men over 30 years of age.

Dependent Variables and Data Sources

Dependent variables included program performance and client characteristics. Program performance was measured by number of new clients admitted per month, number of vasectomies performed per month, and number of telephone calls received. Client characteristics included neighborhood of residence, age, spouse's age, education, type of employment, number of living children, age of youngest child, number of abortion, income, reason for not wanting more children, past and current contraceptive status, eligibility for vasectomy, and source of referral.

Clinic records furnished the primary data base, and new forms were implemented to register telephone calls. Patient records were updated as clients were vasectomized or dropped out of the program. Data collection ended on 30 November 1986, one year after the appearance of the last advertisement. By the end of the study, the patient file included 3,403 records for the baseline period, 1,475 records for the campaign, and 5,388 records for the post-campaign period. The telephone calls file contained 4,393 records, and the letters file 386 records.

Records were entered in dBase III on an IBM-compatible microcomputer, printed out in batch, and checked manually against the original forms. Editing and tabulations were carried out with SPSS (Statistical Package for the Social Sciences).

Figure 1. Advertisements used in the advertising campaign to promote voluntary sterilization, São Paulo, Brazil

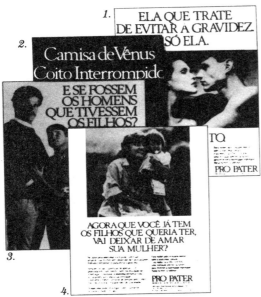

1. *It's up to her to avoid pregnancy, only her.*

2. *Condom—coitus interruptus*

3. *And if men had children?*

4. *Now that you have the children you want, are you going to stop loving your wife?*

Results

Telephone Calls and Letters

A clear impact of the advertising campaign was demonstrated, both in terms of total number of telephone calls received and in terms of source of referral. The volume
of calls increased in the first weeks of the campaign, peaking at 220 calls during the
second week, with lower and fluctuating totals during the remainder of the campaign and throughout the post-campaign period. The mean daily number of telephone
calls during the campaign was 30, declining to 20 in the post-campaign period.[1]

The increased volume can be attributed directly to the magazine advertisements. The ads generated 32 percent of all telephone calls received, 47 percent
of calls received during the campaign itself, and 9–10 percent of the calls received in the second half of the post-campaign year. As referrals by advertisements dropped off, they were partially replaced by increased referrals from traditional sources. Thus, it appears that we are seeing the first evidence of a
"multiplier effect." That is, telephone callers referred by the campaign became
new clients and vasectomy acceptors, who in turn referred new callers in the
post-campaign period. A stable residual effect of the campaign persisted throughout the study: even 12 months after the final advertisement appeared, some 10
percent of the telephone callers gave a magazine ad as their referral source.

Magazine referrals were significantly less likely to schedule an intake interview
than were callers referred by traditional sources (51 percent versus 78 percent; $\chi^2 =$
280, degrees of freedom = 1, p<.01). While this might suggest that mass media promotion is less effective than interpersonal communication, a more positive interpre-
tation would be that the mass media campaign had reached a previously un-
touched population, that of men who had had no opportunity or the initiative to
discuss vasectomy among their circle of friends. During the study, the clinic also
received 338 letters, of which almost 42 percent cited a magazine advertisement.
Although the campaign was restricted to the São Paulo inserts of the magazines,
only 54 percent of the letters came from São Paulo state; the remaining 46 percent represented nearly all the other states and territories in Brazil.

New Clients Admitted and Vasectomies Performed

Clinic performance, both in terms of new clients and vasectomies performed,
was positively and significantly affected by the advertising campaign. The mean
daily number of new clients doubled durihng the campaign as compared to the
baseline period, and remained 60 percent higher in the post-campaign period.
Similarly, the mean daily number of vasectomies performed rose 76 percent from
the baseline to the campaign period and stabilized at a level 54 percent higher than
baseline during the post-campaign period. Table 1 summarizes clinic performance
levels during the baseline, campaign, and post-campaign periods. Pre- and post-
campaign levels in vasectomies performed are graphically presented in Figure 2.

Examination of sources of referral demonstrated the direct effect of the advertising campaign on the increased client load. Eighteen percent of the new clients arriving during the campaign reported having seen a magazine ad, as opposed to 4 percent of the new clients in the post-campaign period (χ^2 = 338, degrees of freedom = 1, p<.01). Whereas 74 percent of the new clients during the campaign had spoken with a clinic patient, 88 percent of new clients in the post-campaign period had done so (χ^2 = 161, degrees of freedom = 1, p<.01). Finally, 36 percent of new clients arriving during the campaign reported having spoken with friends or relatives about va-

Table 1. Daily clinic performance, by period, September 1984 to November 1986

	Period		
	Baseline	Campaign	Post-campaign
Service	(3 Sept. '84– 30 Aug. '85)	(16 Sept. '85– 29 Nov. '85)	(2 Dec. '85– 28 Nov. '86)
Number of telephone calls			
Mean	—	30.1	20.1
Total[a]	—	1,788	2,430
Number of new clients admitted			
Mean	13.7	27.3	21.9
Total	3,403	1,475	5,388
Number of vasectomies performed			
Mean	11.2	19.7	17.2
Total	2,470	1,123	3,810

Note: Calls were not registered during the baseline period.
[a] An additional 175 telephone calls were registered in the two weeks prior to the campaign (2–13 September 1985).

Figure 2. Clinic performance before and after an advertising campaign to promote voluntary sterilization, São Paulo

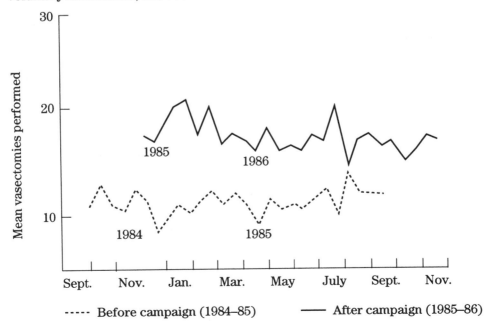

----- Before campaign (1984–85)   —— After campaign (1985–86)

sectomy, compared with 52 percent of new clients in the post-campaign period (χ^2 = 120, degrees of freedom = 1, p<.01). These trends in source of referral for new clients follow the same pattern observed for telephone callers, which is not surprising since virtually all intake interviews are previously scheduled by telephone. Moreover, since telephone callers referred by an advertisement were less likely to schedule an interview than those referred by traditional sources, fewer new clients than telephone callers reported contact with the campaign (18 percent of new clients versus 47 percent of telephone callers during the campaign).

Client Characteristics

To measure campaign impact on the profile of the potential vasectomy acceptor, a number of client characteristics were examined, including age, place of residence, age of spouse, number of living children, education, income, and current practice of contraception. Client profiles across the three time periods (baseline, campaign, and post-campaign) were compared, as well as profiles of clients referred by the campaign versus clients referred by traditional sources. Clients referred by the campaign were those who had seen a magazine advertisement and had not spoken with another clinic client prior to the intake interview. Clients referred by traditional sources were those who had spoken to another clinic client and had not seen a magazine advertisement.

The *age* variable was available for both telephone callers and new clients. The mean age of male telephone callers was 33 years and did not differ between those referred by a magazine ad and those referred by traditional sources. The mean age age of new clients arriving at the clinic was also 33 years and did not vary across time periods. However, new clients referred by the campaign were, on the average, one year older than those referred by traditional sources (33.9 years versus 33.0 years, t = 2.37, degrees of freedom = 5284, p<.02).

Number of living children did not vary by period; mean number of living children was 2.5 for new clients arriving before, during, and after the campaign. Clients referred by the campaign had slightly fewer children (2.3) than those referred by traditional sources (2.5).

Mean *educational level* rose slightly during the campaign, after which it returned to baseline levels. A similar and stronger effect was seen comparing clients referred by the campaign with those referred by traditional sources: median educational level among the campaign referrals was post-secondary, compared with a median of primary education among the traditional referrals.

Other client characteristics, including residence, spouse's age, contraceptive status, and so forth were examined. No consistent effects of period or source of referral were found for these other variables.

Cost-effectiveness Analysis

The present study was designed to test the effectiveness of mass media promotion of vasectomy, and as such did not attempt to determine which advertising approach would be most cost-effective. However, if the technique is to be used in the future or with other programs, cost-effectiveness should be an important issue. Therefore, the cost-effectiveness of the campaign as it was actually conducted was analyzed, and the effectiveness and cost-effectiveness of a cheaper campaign using fewer magazines was simulated.

In essence, the cost-effectiveness ratio is simply the ratio of program costs divided by program outputs. In the present study, program costs are those associated with the campaign: production costs (photography, layout, and so forth), publicist costs (for arranging press coverage), and publication costs. The production costs are one-time start-up costs that can be amortized over several campaigns. The publicist costs are also one-time start-up costs, but they would need to be repeated for each new campaign. Publication costs are recurrent costs and vary with the magazines used and the number of insertions.

Program outputs are the additional vasectomies performed as a result of the campaign. It was assumed that clinic performance would have remained stable in the absence of the intervention. Using the post-campaign plateau (which underestimates total impact), a 54 percent increase was calculated in mean daily vasectomies performed per year. Because new clients referred by the campaign refer other new clients (the multiplier effect), and because the new performance plateau appears stable, the time period of the analysis should be longer than the campaign. In the present analysis, one-year and three-year projections were used (1,500 and 4,500 additional vasectomies, respectively).

In order to simulate the effectiveness and cost-effectiveness of a cheaper campaign, it was necessary to calculate the relative returns of the two major publicity channels, radio/television and magazines. Within magazines, the relative returns of the two most successful magazines (*Veja* and *Isto É*) and of the other magazines were calculated. The calculations were based on the source of referral cited by new clients arriving during or after the campaign, and who went on to be vasectomized. It was assumed that once vasectomized, these clients would refer new clients in equal numbers, regardless of their original source of referral.

Table 2 presents final costs by cost category and their associated rates of return. Among those clients reporting a mass-media contact with the clinic, almost 12 percent had seen or heard a report on radio or television (the result of the press agent), and 88 percent had seen one or more magazine ads. Comparing these relative outputs to their relative costs, the press agent (radio/television coverage) proved to be the most cost-effective vehicle, followed by advertisements placed in *Veja* and *Isto É*. Advertisements placed in the narrow-audience magazines were the least cost-effective. However, before concluding that television might be a more cost-effective medium than magazines, it should be remembered that the television coverage was inserted into regular newscasts, daytime

Table 2. Costs and returns of components of the advertising campaign

Cost category	Total cost (US$)	Relative cost (%)	Relative return (%)	Cost-effectiveness
Production	2,960	5.1	—	—
Press agent[a]	3,590	6.1	11.6	1.9:1
Publication	51,740	88.8	88.4	.9:1[b]
Veja, Isto E	25,880	44.4	75.1	1.6:1[b]
Others	25,860	44.4	13.3	.3:1[b]
Total	58,290	100.0	100.0	na

[a] Radio and television coverage.   [b] Includes production costs.

interview shows, and so on, rather than as paid commercials.

If all promotion costs are included and a one-year return is allowed, each additional vasectomy performed costs approximately US$39; extending the return period to three years cuts the per-client costs by a factor of three, to US$13. At the same time, the extra return to Pro-Pater generated by patient fees was $45 per client, for a net return of $6 per client over a one-year period, and $32 per client over a three-year period.

As Table 2 indicates, publication in the less effective magazines cost 44 percent of the total advertising budget and generated only 13 percent of the return. Thus, if these magazines were eliminated, we could expect a return of approximately 1,300 additional vasectomies per year. In addition, the production costs (5 percent of the total) could be amortized over more than one campaign. Recalculating the cost-effectiveness ratio based on the costs of only the most effective magazines, 50 percent of the production costs, 100 of the publicist costs, and the reduced additional return, yields cost-effectiveness ratios of US$24 and US$8 per additional vasectomy performed for the one- and three-year return periods, for a net gain of $21 per client and $37 per client, respectively.

Discussion

The study formulated three objectives: to increase the awareness of vasectomy in the general population; to increase the number of new clients and vasectomies performed; and to measure the costs and cost-effectiveness of mass media promotion.

Indirect evidence suggests that the first objective of increasing awareness of vasectomy in the general population was attained. New clients recruited by the advertising campaign appeared less knowledgeable about vasectomy than new clients referred by traditional sources. Clients recruited by the ads were interested in receiving information about vasectomy but not as ready to schedule an intake interview; when they did arrive at the clinic, they were less likely to have spoken with a previous client or a family member or friend about vasectomy; and when accepted for vasectomy, they waited longer to schedule their surgery date. Thus, it appears that the campaign not only promoted the Pro-Pater clinic among men already interested in vasectomy, but also raised awareness of the procedure among men who were unfamiliar with it.

Regarding the second objective, the number of new clients admitted in the campaign period was double the observed 1984 plateau, and post-campaign admissions stabilized at a level 60 percent higher than baseline. The number of vasectomies performed rose 76 percent in the campaign period and stabilized at 54 percent higher.

The first hypothesis—that the number of clients ineligible for vasectomy would increase—was confirmed. The proportion of new clients not meeting the clinic's criteria for eligibility rose from 14 percent in the baseline period to 19 percent during the campaign. Post-campaign ineligibility rates returned to baseline levels. New clients recruited by the advertising campaign showed higher ineligibility rates than those referred by traditional sources.

The second hypothesis—that mass media promotion would change the new client profile, but have not effect on the characteristics of the vasectomy acceptor—was partially confirmed. No period effects were found among new clients in terms of age, age of spouse, number of living children, or current contraceptive use. New clients referred by magazine ads were somewhat older, better educated, and showed higher income levels than those referred by traditional sources. As predicted, the profile of the vasectomy acceptor did not change.

These results demonstrate the success of the campaign in reaching the targeted audience. The higher ineligibility rates produced by the campaign were not due to failure to match the desired demographic criteria, but rather reflected the fact that candidates recruited by the media campaign had had less previuos exposure to vasectomy information than candidates arriving through the traditional channels, and therefore were judged by clinic counselors to be less prepared to adopt permanent, surgical contraception.

The third objective was to measure costs and cost-effectiveness of mass media promotion. Allowing a three-year pay-back period, the campaign cost US$13 per additional vasectomy performed (which represents 28 percent of the clinic's operating costs per procedure). Eliminating the less productive magazines would reduce this cost to US$8 per additional vasectomy performed (18 percent of clinic costs). Either cost ($13 or $8) was more than compensated for by the additional revenue generated by the increase in vasectomies performed.

Conclusions

The results of the present study clearly demonstrate that mass media advertising was an effective and cost-effective vehicle for increasing the demand for vasectomy services in São Paulo, Brazil. Whether these findings would apply to other services and settings is a matter for further study, as is the question of the most cost-effective approach to mass media promotion. It is not clear, for example, to what extent Pro-Pater's existing client base influenced the results. It is possible that had the experiment been applied to a less well established clinic, the effect might have been different.

The success of the campaign in attracting the target audience without bringing in large numbers of vasectomy-seekers whose demographic and other characteristics would have made them ineligible for this family planning method deserves mention. The advertisments focused on a single contraceptive method, vasectomy, rather than promoting family planning in general. They clearly delineated the intended recipient of the message: men who already had all the children they wished to have, and who were potentially interested in a permanent method of contraception. Not only was this approach extremely successful in attracting positive attention, it also avoided negative reactions that might have been generated by a more diffuse message (fertility control, for example).

The present results also have implications for a larger operational question, namely, how family planning service delivery programs grow. Unlike programs offering temporary methods, programs that offer permanent methods (male and female sterilization) rely on essentially one-time patient contact. Once the patient has been successfully sterilized he or she does not return, whereas the user of a temporary method generates a continual need for follow-up or resupply services. Thus, for a sterilization program to remain active, each acceptor must be continously replaced by a new acceptor, and for the program to grow, each acceptor must be replaced by more than one new acceptor. Programs offering temporary methods, on the other hand, can show incremental growth by adding new acceptors on a one-to-one basis (each acceptor refers one more acceptor), providing that continuation rates are high enough.

It appears that, at least in the case of a well established sterilization program, as is Pro-Pater, two separate mechanisms are at work: one maintains equilibrium, and the other induces program expansion. Interpersonal communication, the promotional technique previously stresed by Pro-Pater, appears to be adequate to maintain program equilibrium. From year to year, each vasectomy acceptor, on the average, refers a new vasectomy acceptor, producing performance plateaus that remain stable over a year or more. However, in order to raise performance, to increase the client base that serves as the referral source for new clients, some kind of mass promotional event is necessary. Pro-Pater has experienced such an event twice, first with the unsolicited television coverage and second with the present advertising campaign. In both cases, clinic performance showed a sudden and sharp peak, which declined to a stable plateau higher than the previous equilibrium state. Direct evidence for the two-mechanism hypothesis is provided in Figure 3. Telephone calls referred by traditional sources were essentially stable in the

Figure 3. Weekly telephone calls to Pro-Pater before, during, and after an advertising campaign to promote voluntary sterilization, São Paulo, Brazil

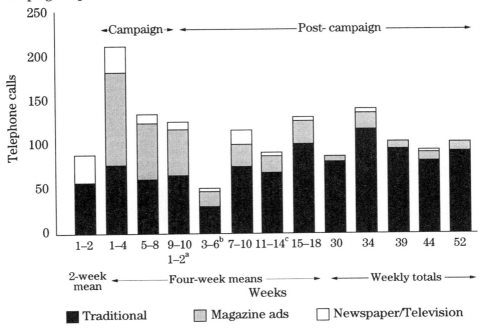

[a] Campaign weeks 9–10 and post-campaign weeks 1–2.
[b] Includes Christmas and New Year holidays.
[c] Includes Carnival holidays.

first months of the study (when the client base had not yet increased) and were matched in number of calls stimulated by the advertising campaign. When the campaign terminated, so did the majority of the inquiries it directly stimulated; however, the broadened client base began to result in an increasing number of telephone calls motivated by interpersonal communication.

Finally, we see that the impact of the campaign will extend far beyond the three months in which the advertisements were printed, or even beyond the 12 months given for the study. First, the campaign raised clinic performance to a new plateau, which can be maintained through interpersonal communication, or the "multiplier effect." Second, even 12 months after the last advertisement appeared, 10 percent of all telephone callers still referred to a magazine ad indicating that either the issues were still in circulation (for example, in a waiting room, or passed on from friend to friend) or that the advertisement itself had been clipped for future reference. For whatever reason, this suggests that the magazine vehicle may be ultimately more effective than other media, such as television, with larger immediate but no delayed impact. Third, it appears that the campaign successfully promoted vasectomy to a new population who had not previously realized that the option existed for them. While these "new recruits" may take longer to make the decision to adopt vasectomy than clients referred by interpersonal communication (see Mumford, 1983, for a decision-making model for vasectomy acceptance), they will ultimately make a major contribution to the ongoing success of the program.

Notes

This study was financed under contract DPE-3030-C-00-4074-00 between the Population Council and the Agency for International Development, and subcontract No. CI 85.13A between Pro-Pater and the INOPAL Project of the Population Council.

The authors would like to express their appreciation to James R. Foreit, Associate Director of INOPAL, for his comments and critical review.

1.   The normal work-week is five days. Some weeks were shorter due to holidays.

References

Arruda, José Maria, Naomi Rutenberg, Leo Morris, and Elisabth Anhel Ferras. 1987. *Pesquisa Naciónal Sobre Materno-Infantil e Planejamento Familiar: PNSMIPF-Brasil, 1986.* Rio de Janeiro: Sociedade Civil Bem-Estar Familiar no Brasil.

Bertrand, Jane T., Roberto Santiso G., Rosa Judith Cisneros, Felix Mascarin, and Leo Morris. 1982. "Family planning communications and contraceptive use in Guatemala, El Salvador, and Panama." *Studies in Family Planning* 13, 6/7: 190–199.

Bertrand, Jane T., Roberto Santiso G., Stephen H. Linder, and Maria Antonieta Piñeda. 1987. "Evaluation of a communications programs to increase adoption of vasectomy in Guatemala." *Studies in Family Planning* 18, 6: 361–370.

Cummings, K. Michael, Russell Sciandra, and Samuel Markello. 1987. "Impact of a newspaper-mediated quit-smoking program." *American Journal of Public Health* 77, 11: 1452–1453.

de Castro, Marcos Paulo P. Diogo A. Mastrorocco, Bernadete M. de Castro, and Stephen D. Mumford. 1984 "An innovative vasectomy program in São Paulo, Brazil." *International Family Planning Perspectives* 10, 4: 125–130.

Flay, Brian R. 1987. "Mass media and smoking cessation: A critical review." *American Journal of Public Health* 77, 2: 153–160.

Mumford, Stephen D. 1983. "The vasectomy decision-making process." *Studies in Family Planning* 14, 3: 83–88.

Sweeney, William O. 1977. "Media communications in population/family planning programs: A review." *Population Reports*, No. 16: J289–J320.

PREFATORY REMARKS

The Effect of Counseling on Sterilization Acceptance by High-Parity Women in Nigeria

Alexander E. Omu, Sharon S. Weir,
Barbara Janowitz, Deborah L. Covington,
Peter R. Lamptey, and Nadine N. Burton

Programmatic issue: *The program wished to increase low levels of post-partum sterilization and other contraceptive use among high-parity women who gave birth in Nigerian hospitals.*

Programmatic processes/components: *Little or no information on family planning and sterilization was given to women delivering in Nigerian hospitals. The study tested an intervention designed to provide women with family planning and sterilization counseling on four occasions during prenatal visits, hospitalization for childbirth, and at six weeks postpartum.*

Research design: *A true experiment was conducted. More than 1,000 women were randomly assigned to intervention and control groups. The intervention group received counseling and materials; the control group received only the family planning materials routinely provided to patients by the hospital. Dependent variables included contraceptive prevalence and patients' knowledge of family planning.*

Findings: *Women receiving counseling had greater knowledge of family planning, higher levels of sterilization (13 percent versus 3 percent) and higher modern method contraceptive prevalence in general (70 percent versus 51 percent) than did women who received only family planning materials.*

Program response to findings: *At the time the project was completed, key staff were transferred from the study hospital to a facility in another part of Nigeria. Participants believe that the disruption in staff continuity prevented full implementation of study findings.*

Discussion: *The study shows the importance of interpersonal communication in the adoption of family planning. However, the study did not examine an important operational issue—whether four contacts were needed to inform women adequately.*

Experiments are relatively easy to conduct in hospital settings. As in this study, true random assignment can often be accomplished, or other random-like assignment processes can be used to guard against the introduction of systematic bias. Nirapathpongporn et al. (1988) in a study comparing no-scalpel and standard incisional vasectomy techniques during the King's birthday vasectomy festival, assigned men on a first-come-first-served basis to operating tables, half of which were manned by physicians using the new technique. K. Foreit et al. (1993) in a study of postpartum IUD promotion in Peru, assigned women to experimental and control delivery wards on an available beds basis. In the Thai setting, true random assignment would have resulted in slowing down the rate at which vasectomies were performed, thus increasing provider costs and client inconvenience; while in the Peru study, true random assignment was impossible because it would have required women in labor to wait until a bed in the ward to which they had been randomly assigned became available.

References

Foreit, Karen et al. 1993. "Acceptability and cost-effectiveness of postpartum contraception in Lima, Peru." *International Family Planning Perspectives* 19, 1: 19–24.

Nirapathpongporn, Apichart et al. 1988. "No scalpel vasectomy at the King's Birthday vasectomy festival." *The Lancet* 335: 894–895.

The Effect of Counseling on Sterilization Acceptance by High-Parity Women in Nigeria

Alexander E. Omu, Sharon S. Weir,
Barbara Janowitz, Deborah L. Covington,
Peter R. Lamptey, and Nadine N. Burton

Background

During pregnancy, women older than 35 and women who have had four or more children are at increased risk of hemorrhage and high blood pressure, two of the most common causes of maternal death in developing countries.[1] Because women in the developing world often start to have children in their late teens or early twenties and do not practice family planning to space their pregnancies, women often achieve high parity at a comparatively young age and are thus exposed to the dangers of high-risk pregnancies for many years. As a result, most women in regions where the total fertility rate is high face an elevated risk of maternal morbidity and mortality during their later childbearing years. It is, therefore, important for high-parity women to have access to a troublefree, reliable method of contraception to protect them from potentially dangerous pregnancies.

Voluntary female sterilization is one of the most widely used methods of contraception, especially among women over the age of 35, in every region of the world except Sub-Saharan Africa. Among currently married women age 35–44 practicing contraception, 43 percent in Asia, 42 percent in Latin America and 25 percent in the Middle East rely on sterilization. In contrast, only eight percent of comparable women in Sub-Saharan African have undergone sterilization.[2]

Nigeria has one of the lowest rates of female sterilization in the region: Less than one percent of older women practicing contraception are sterilized.[3] In part, this is because Nigerian family planning programs are new. Until recently, there was little demand for family planning programs as a result of the widespread traditional desire for large families. A majority of Nigerian women want

Reprinted with the permission of The Alan Guttmacher Institute from *International Family Planning Perspectives* 1989. 15,2: 66–71.

another child immediately after or within a year of delivering their last baby.[4] The 1981–1982 Nigeria World Fertility Survey found that urban women aged 35–44 with four or more children wanted an average of two more children; the total fertility rate in Nigeria was 6.3.[5]

Extended breastfeeding and postpartum abstinence have traditional provided for birthspacing and protected Nigerian women from some high-risk pregnancies but rapid urbanization and other social changes are fast eroding these traditional practices. Yet, public knowledge and utilization of family planning methods, especially sterilization, are still very low. Only 32 percent of Nigerian women aged 15–44 know of any method of contraception modern or traditional. Furthermore, just seven percent have heard of voluntary surgical contraception.[6]

By contrast, in Kenya, Senegal and Zimbabwe—African countries with comparatively more exposure to family planning programs—at least 45 percent of women 15–44 know of female sterilization.[7] In those countries, family planning utilization is growing at a faster pace, reflecting the increased availability of services and of information and education programs.

According to a 1980 survey of women delivering at three hospitals in Benin, Nigeria, major reasons for not using contraception were spousal opposition, religious values and fear of side effects.[8] Another study, at the University of Benin Teaching Hospital, found that women who had had more than four deliveries represented 20 percent of maternity patients but accounted for 55 percent of maternal deaths at the hospital.[9] On the basis of these studies and his own research and clinical experience in obstetrics and gynecology, the senior author of this article decided to launch a project in collaboration with Family Health International that would implement and evaluate a family planning information and education program for high-parity women. The program would attempt to inform these women of the dangers associated with multiple pregnancies and of the availability, safety and effectiveness of all methods of contraception. It would also stress the appropriateness of voluntary surgical contraception for high-parity women.

The setting for the project was University of Benin Teaching Hospital, a 450-bed referral hospital that serves a catchment area of approximately four million inhabitants. About 4,000 deliveries per year occur at the hospital; a 1981 obstetric surveillance study found that one-third of the deliveries were for a fourth-order birth or higher.[10]

The project's goal was to demonstrate that taking the time to educate and inform women at risk of pregnancy complications because of high parity would increase the acceptability of postpartum family planning in a population otherwise reluctant to accept any method of contraception, especially surgical methods. Guidelines for the program were based on the premise that counseling must elicit an informed and free choice. The counselor's responsibility was threefold: They were to assess the readiness of the woman to end her fertility, provide complete information to the patient about the risk associated with surgical contraception and inform her of the availability of reversible methods. Women included in the study received no inducement to participate. Those who selected sterilization went through a careful informed-consent procedure that included information about the permanence of the method, ample time to reflect on their decision without external pressures and a witnessed signature.

The objectives of the evaluation component were to determine whether the program affected the demand for voluntary surgical contraception among high-parity women delivering at the University of Benin Teaching Hospital, whether counseling improved the understanding of and attitudes toward of sterilization among these women, and whether the information and education increased the postpartum demand for all family planning methods by high-risk women.

Methods

In this study, a high-parity woman was defined as one who had had four or more previous deliveries and was at or beyond the 28th week of gestation. All high-parity women who were scheduled to deliver at the hospital and who had attended its prenatal clinic during a 19-month period were included in the study, except women for whom a physician had recommended sterilization for medical reasons. The study ran from September 1984 through March 1986.

By a random allocation process, high-parity women were assigned to one of two groups at the time of their initial visit to prenatal clinic. One group became the treatment group and was exposed to an information and education program that included individualized counseling on family planning and the health risks associated with high parity. The second group became the control group.

Women in the treatment group were to receive information four times: at admission to the study (during the 29th to 35th weeks of gestation), during a prenatal visit after the 36th week of pregnancy, during hospitalization for delivery and at six weeks postpartum. Nurses conducted the first and third counseling sessions; physicians did the second and fourth. They were trained for the counseling by staff members from Family Health International according to a protocol developed with the Association for Voluntary Surgical Contraception and using materials provided by that organization.

The protocol called for the treatment group to receive information on the health effects of high parity and the benefits of family planning at the first, third and fourth sessions. Education regarding all methods of contraception was scheduled for the second and third sessions. Voluntary surgical contraception was presented in some detail, and the advantages and limitations of the method were discussed in the context of high-risk pregnancies. Those who expressed interest in sterilization received more in-depth counseling at the second, third and fourth sessions to ensure that they fully understood the permanence of the method and potential complications associated with surgical procedure.

The control group received only the standard family planning information usually provided at the clinic. Although all the methods of contraception available at the hospital were discussed, the information did not stress the increased risks associated with high parity. The staff providing this counseling had received no special training in information and education procedures and did not follow a standard protocol. The information they provided on surgical contraception was incomplete and did not address the major fear of women in the Benin region: that sterilization in this lifetime would make them infertile in subsequent reincarnations.

At the time of their enrollment in the study, women in both the treatment and the control groups were interviewed to obtain information on their social and demographic characteristics, as well as on their knowledge of contraceptive methods, contraceptive use and desire for additional children. Sterilizations were performed at delivery or immediately postpartum. Women from both groups were also interviewed at six weeks postpartum to obtain information on delivery outcomes, contraceptive plans and attitudes toward sterilization. Hospital records were checked to identify sterilized women who failed to return for their postpartum visit. Women who were not interviewed at six weeks and who did not have a sterilization record were assumed not to have been sterilized.

More than 99 percent of those admitted to the study were interviewed at admission. Almost 90 percent of the women in the treatment group received counseling all four times; only two did not attend any sessions. In addition, more than 90 percent of the women were interviewed at six weeks postpartum. A patient's failure to return for prenatal visits and at six week postpartum was the primary reason that patients missed counseling sessions or did not have a follow-up interview.

Patient Characteristics

More than 1,000 high-parity women were admitted for prenatal care during the study period. Baseline social, demographic and reproductive health characteristics are presented in Table 1. There were no significant differences between the treatment and control groups with regard to any of the characteristics surveyed. Neither were any differences found between women who returned at six weeks postpartum and those who failed to return. Since the random allocation suc-

Table 1. Percentage distribution of high-parity women at the University of Benin Teaching Hospital, by study group, according to various characteristics, Nigeria, 1984-1986

Characteristics	All women (N=1,012)	Treatment group (N=509)	Control group (N=503)
Age			
20–24	4.5	5.7	3.4
25–29	30.3	28.3	32.4
30–34	37.8	39.9	35.8
35–39	21.3	21.6	21.1
>40	5.0	4.1	6.0
Unknown	0.9	0.4	1.4
Ethnicity			
Edo	53.3	51.9	54.7
Ibo	14.6	14.3	14.9
Ishan	10.4	11.2	9.5
Other	21.5	22.2	20.9
Unknown	0.2	0.4	0.0
Education			
None	16.4	17.3	15.5
Primary	52.4	49.9	54.9
Secondary	17.0	17.5	16.5
Post Secondary	14.1	15.1	13.1
Unknown	0.1	0.2	0.0
Religion			
Protestant	42.5	45.0	40.0
Catholic	27.2	26.9	27.4
Traditional	24.5	22.4	26.6
Other	5.2	5.1	5.4
Unknown	0.6	0.6	0.6
Previous deliveries			
4	26.3	26.9	25.6
5	30.3	28.9	31.8
6	21.9	24.8	19.1
≥ 7	21.3	19.3	23.5
Unknown	0.1	0.2	0.0
Living children			
0–3	9.6	9.2	9.9
4	32.9	34.0	31.8
5	30.3	29.3	31.4
6	16.1	17.9	14.3
≥ 7	11.0	9.4	12.5
Unknown	0.1	0.2	0.0
Infant deaths			
0	70.3	70.5	70.0
1	22.5	23.2	21.9
≥ 2	7.1	6.1	8.2
Unknown	0.1	0.2	0.0
Cesarean sections			
None	92.6	92.1	93.0
1	6.1	6.3	6.0
≥ 2	1.1	1.2	1.0
Unknown	0.1	2.0	0.0
Planned method			
Sterilization	8.2	9.4	7.0
Pills/injectables	45.8	45.2	46.3
IUD	16.4	17.1	15.7
Other*	16.8	18.3	15.5
None	11.9	9.0	14.7
Unknown	0.9	1.0	0.8
Total	**100.0**	**100.0**	**100.0**

* Includes condoms, contraceptive foams and jellies, abstinence, breastfeeding, rhythm and withdrawal.

ceeded in creating similar treatment and control groups, and since the women who did not complete follow-up were similar to those who did, we feel confident in attributing any differences in sterilization rates to the information and education program.

Women in the study had a mean age of 31, and 90 percent were aged 25–30. However, five percent of the women pregnant with their fifth-order birth or higher were age 20–24, and five percent were 40 or older. More than half came from one ethnic group, the Edo; 15 percent were Ibo, 10 percent Ishan and the remaining 22 percent came from at least 10 other smaller ethnic groups. The high-parity women who deliver at the teaching hospital in Benin are urbanized and better educated than are most Nigerian women. Almost 85 percent of the women had had at least a primary education, and 14 percent had had some postsecondary schooling. Forty-three percent of the high-parity women were Protestant, 27 percent were Catholic and 25 percent followed a traditional religion.

As for reproductive health characteristics, 43 percent of the women had six or more previous deliveries, and 21 percent had seven or more. Only seven percent of the women, however, had ever had a cesarean section. In spite of the high parity, 10 percent of the women currently had fewer than four living children and only half of those who had borne seven or more children had that many living children. Overall, 30 percent of the women had experienced the loss of at least one child in its first year of life, and seven percent had seen two or more children die as infants.

The women in the study were more knowledgeable about family planning than are most Nigerian women. Forty-five percent of them knew about female sterilization, and more than 85 percent knew about injectables, IUDs and oral contraceptives (not shown). In addition, 32 percent had used oral contraceptives at some point, 11 percent had used IUDs and seven percent had used injectables. As Table 1 shows, 87 percent planned to use a contraceptive method after delivery, including eight percent who said at their first prenatal visit that they planned to be sterilized.

Table 2 contains information on the women's attitudes toward their current pregnancy and whether they desired more children. Fifty-five percent of the women said they wanted their current pregnancy as well as more children, 30 percent said they wanted the current pregnancy but no more children and 11 percent said they wanted neither the current pregnancy nor more children. The latter proportion increased with the number of living children, so that slightly more than one-third of the women with seven or more children said that they did not want the current pregnancy. Only among women expecting at least their seventh child did more than half report that they did not want any more children.

Table 2. Percentage distribution of high-parity women, by study group and number of living children, according to desire to limit family size

Group and no. of living children	N	Wanted current pregnancy and more children	Wanted current pregnancy but no more children	Didn't want current pregnancy or more children	Not sure	Total
Total						
All	1,011*	54.7	30.0	11.3	4.0	100.0
0–3	97	82.5	15.5	0.0	2.0	100.0
4	333	70.3	21.9	2.7	5.1	100.0
5	307	55.7	32.6	8.8	2.9	100.0
6	163	33.1	39.9	22.7	4.3	100.0
≥ 7	111	13.5	45.9	36.9	3.7	100.0
Treatment						
All	508*	57.0	30.3	9.6	3.1	100.0
0–3	47	91.5	6.4	0.0	2.1	100.0
4	173	69.9	24.9	1.7	3.5	100.0
5	149	60.4	30.9	5.4	3.3	100.0
6	91	30.8	41.8	24.2	3.2	100.0
≥ 7	48	16.7	50.0	33.3	0.0	100.0
Control						
All	503	52.5	29.8	12.9	4.8	100.0
0–3	50	74.0	24.0	0.0	2.0	100.0
4	160	70.6	18.8	3.8	6.8	100.0
5	158	51.3	34.2	12.0	2.5	100.0
6	72	36.1	37.5	20.8	5.6	100.0
≥ 7	63	11.1	42.9	39.7	6.3	100.0

* Excludes one woman who refused to be interviewed.

Unless women were to change their minds, these data indicate that only 40 percent would be candidates for female sterilization, and fewer than 25 percent of women with four living children might be interested. Among those who did not want any more children, almost half (48 percent) said they could not afford more children, and 14 percent gave health reasons.

Data collected at six weeks postpartum indicate that most women in the study delivered vaginally; only three percent had a cesarean section. Among 97 percent of the women, the baby was still alive at the time of the interview; among two percent, the child had died after a live birth. The remainder of the women experienced a miscarriage or a stillbirth. One woman was known to have died, and 84 did not return at six weeks.

Counseling Results

Women in the treatment group were more likely to choose sterilization than were women who received no special information—13 percent, compared with three percent. The difference was statistically significant (p<0.001). The proportion of women sterilized is presented in Table 3, according to various social,

Table 3. Percentage of women who underwent sterilization, by various characteristics, according to study group

Characteristic	Treatment		Control	
	%	N	%	N
Total	**13.0**	**509**	**3.4**	**503**
Age				
<30	3.5	173	1.7	180
30–34	11.8	203	1.1	180
35	27.5	131	8.8	136
Unknown	0.0	2	0.0	7
Ethnicity				
Edo	12.9	264	3.3	275
Ibo	12.3	73	4.0	75
Ishan	10.5	57	4.2	48
Other	14.8	115	2.9	105
Education				
None	15.9	88	2.6	78
Primary	11.8	254	2.5	276
Secondary	14.6	89	6.0	83
Post secondary	11.7	77	4.5	66
Unknown	0.0	1	0.0	0
Religion				
Catholic	13.1	137	3.6	138
Protestant	14.8	229	2.5	201
Traditional	11.4	114	4.5	134
Other/unknown	3.4	29	3.3	30
Living children				
0–3	4.3	47	4.0	50
4	5.8	173	0.0	160
5	8.7	149	5.7	158
6	20.9	91	4.2	72
≥ 7	45.8	48	4.8	63
Unknown	0.0	1	0.0	0
Type of delivery				
Vaginal	12.2	460	2.8	436
Cesarean	50.0	12	26.7	15
Miscarriage	0.0	2	0.0	0
Unknown	11.4	35	1.9	52
Contraceptive plan at admission				
Sterilization	79.2	48	42.9	35
Pill, injectables, IUD	4.1	317	0.3	312
Other/unknown	14.3	98	0.0	82
None	2.2	46	1.4	74
Family limitation desires				
Didn't want pregnancy/didn't want more	38.8	49	10.8	65
Wanted pregnancy/didn't want more	23.4	154	6.0	150
Wanted pregnancy/wanted more	3.1	290	0.4	264
Unknown	12.5	16	0.0	24

demographic and reproductive characteristics. In every category, women in the treatment group were more likely than women in the control group to undergo sterilization. This was especially true among counseled women in the 30–34 age-group and those with seven or more living children, both of whom were about 10 times more likely than controls to choose sterilization.

Within the treatment group, the older a woman was and the more children she had, the more likely she was to choose sterilization. This association probably reflects the counseling on increased health risks among high-parity and older women. Among women in the control group, only those 35 or older were significantly more likely to be sterilized; parity had no effect. Regardless of study group, the proportions choosing sterilization were small among women who had four or fewer children, not counting the current delivery.

In both groups, there was little variation by ethnicity, education and religion in the proportion of women who chose to be sterilized. Women who delivered by cesarean section, however, were more likely to obtain a sterilization than were women who delivered vaginally: Half of the women in the treatment group and a quarter of those in the control group who delivered by cesarean sections obtained sterilizations, compared with 12 percent and three percent, respectively, of those who delivered vaginally. Two of the six women in the treatment group who had cesareans and opted for sterilization had had three prior cesarean deliveries and would have been strongly advised by their obstetrician to select a permanent method of contraception. According to the protocol, they should not have been included in the study. If they are excluded from the analysis, the overall sterilization rate declines slightly (to 12.6 percent), but the difference between the groups remains significant.

Almost 80 percent of the women in the treatment group who said that they planned to be sterilized went through with the operation. This was true for only 43 percent of the control group. Unless they have a solid understanding of sterilization, women who express interest in the procedure may not feel strongly enough to follow through on their desire. The proportion of women in the treatment group who were sterilized was lower among those who had planned to use a clinical method than among those who had planned to use other methods. Perhaps women who are knowledgeable about other effective methods are less likely to choose sterilization.

In both groups, women who wanted neither the current pregnancy nor more children were the most likely to choose sterilization, with 39 percent of the treatment group and 11 percent of the control group doing so. Among women who wanted the current pregnancy but no more children 23 percent of the treatment group chose sterilization, as did six percent of the control women. A few women (nine in the treatment group and one in the control group) who said at admission to the program that they wanted more children also decided to be sterilized; three of these women had indicated at admission that they planned to be sterilized. Three other women had cesarean sections for this delivery and had medically indicated sterilizations; the remaining four may have changed their minds about having more children.

Sixty-six women in the treatment group underwent sterilization following childbirth. Although 63 women reported at the end of the first counseling session that they wanted to be sterilized, only 45 of those women carried through with their decision. An additional 24 women selected sterilization at later counseling sessions, and 21 of them actually had the operation. Although 68 percent of the women who chose sterilization made their decision in the first counseling session, the later sessions may have been of greater benefit than implied by these data: More women might have changed their minds if there had been only one counseling session early in the prenatal period. The later sessions may have provided additional information to reinforce the original decision and helped some women who were unsure to make a decision.

After six weeks postpartum, women in the treatment group who had decided against sterilization were asked why. Thirty-three percent said they wanted more children, and 28 percent said they had done so because of fear of the operation or its complications. Another 16 percent said they did not want the operation because they believed sterilization might persist through reincarnation, six percent said their husband objected to sterilization and three percent said they preferred a reversible method. The remaining women gave a variety of reasons.

Understanding Sterilization

Counseling improved the understanding of female sterilization. At admission, only 45 percent of the women in the study had heard of the operation. Most of those who had heard of it did not understand the procedure, and they described it as an operation where the womb is tied or the womb is turned. Only seven percent understood sterilization to be having the fallopian tubes tied.

At six weeks postpartum, however, all of the treatment patients said they had heard of sterilization, and these women, especially those who had chosen sterilization, were the most well-informed about the operation. At six week postpartum, 61 of the 62 women in the treatment group who underwent sterilization and returned for the checkup correctly described the operation; almost 90 percent of counseled women who were not sterilized all gave a correct description. In comparison, 90 percent of women in the control group said they had heard of sterilization, either during their admission interview or by talking with counseled women at the hospital. They still had a limited understanding of the surgery, however, with almost 90 percent describing it as tying or turning the womb.

Women who said they had heard of sterilization were asked about their attitudes toward it, and the results are shown in Table 4. At admission, between half and three-quarters of the women had no opinion or held an unfavorable opinion about whether the operation was safe, weakened women, changed women's sex drive or changed their status. By six weeks postpartum, attitudes

Table 4. Percentage distribution of women who had heard of sterilization, by attitude toward the operation, according to when questioned and treatment group

Attitude	At admission	Six weeks postpartum		Control group
		Treatment group		
	All patients	Sterilized	Not sterilized	
N	456	66	414	383
Operation is safe				
Agree	30.9	100.0	61.1	20.4
Disagree	17.8	0.0	31.4	30.0
No opinion	51.3	0.0	7.0	49.6
Unknown	0.0	0.0	0.5	0.0
Women are as strong as before				
Agree	22.4	98.4	62.1	19.8
Disagree	20.8	0.0	13.3	14.4
No opinion	56.8	1.6	24.2	65.8
Unknown	0.0	0.0	0.5	0.0
No change in sex drive				
Agree	30.5	91.9	64.0	18.3
Disagree	6.4	3.2	4.1	8.8
No opinion	63.1	4.8	31.4	74.9
Unknown	0.0	0.0	0.5	0.0
Woman's status does not change				
Agree	38.8	96.8	66.9	23.8
Disagree	8.1	1.6	18.8	6.8
No opinion	51.1	1.6	13.8	69.5
Unknown	2.0	0.0	.5	0.0
Total	**100.0**	**100.0**	**100.0**	**100.0**

Note: Women who did not complete the baseline interview or who did not return at six weeks postpartum are excluded. The 17 women in the control group who were sterilized are also excluded.

toward the operation had improved among all counseled women. This improvement was especially great among those who were sterilized, but women in the treatment group who did not undergo the operation also had much more positive attitudes toward it than did those who were not counseled. For example, slightly more than 60 percent of those in the treatment group who were not sterilized said they believed the operation was safe, compared with 20 percent of women in the control group. Nonetheless, they were not as convinced as women who had the operation that there would be no ill effects. Women in the control group were just as uncertain about the operation at six weeks postpartum as they were at admission.

The program also had an important effect on contraceptive use after delivery. At admission, half of the women had never used a contraceptive method, but almost 90 percent said they planned to use a method after delivery. At six weeks postpartum, counseled women were significantly more likely than those in the control group to have followed through on their intentions ($p < 0.001$), as is shown in Table 5. Seventy-one percent of the counseled women were using a medical or

Table 5. Percentage distribution of women using a contraceptive method at six weeks postpartum, by method, according to study group

Method	Treatment group (N=480)	Control group (N=453)
Clinical	70.5	50.8
Sterilization	13.8	3.8
Pills/injectable	35.2	27.8
IUD	19.6	17.0
Barrier	1.9	2.2
Traditional	14.5	18.6
None	14.1	28.9
Unknown	0.9	1.7
Total	100.0	100.0

Note: This table excludes women who were not sterilized and who did not return for the sixth week interview, because their contraceptive use is unknown.

barrier method of contraception. In contrast, 51 percent of control women were using one of these methods.

Conclusions

The information and education program had a significant impact on a woman's decision to utilize a contraceptive method postpartum. In addition, counseled women of every ethnic and religious group were more likely to request sterilization. The study suggests that the current low rates of voluntary female sterilization may be due, in part, to a lack of knowledge and understanding of sterilization, since half of the women admitted to the program had never heard of the operation, and most of those who had did not understand what it entailed.

A sterilization rate of 13 percent among high-parity women counseled four times about the health impact of multiple birth and benefits of family planning may not seem impressive when compared to the worldwide prevalence of voluntary female sterilization. However, it is notable among Nigerian women for several reasons. First, the rate is almost twice as high as the seven percent sterilization rate among high-parity women at the same hospital in 1981.[11] Second, there is a strong preference for large families in Nigeria where childbearing is of great social importance. Women may, therefore, be reluctant to choose a permanent method despite the risk to their health of further childbearing. Finally, one-fourth of the women in this study had experienced the death of a child during infancy, and 10 percent of them had experienced infant death following their most immediate previous pregnancy.

In this setting, consideration needs to be given to the cost-effectiveness of counseling women with less than a minimum number of children. Sixty-two percent of women in the treatment group who chose sterilization had six or more children, not including the current pregnancy, and 82 percent had five or more living children. If women with fewer than five children had been counseled only once, the number of counseling sessions would have decreased by a third, and the number of sterilizations would have decreased by no more than 10 percent, assuming rates similar to those in control group.

Even women with five or more children may not need to have as many as four counseling sessions. Women who decide to be sterilized on their first visit may need only one additional session to be provided with more detailed information. Sessions should be conducted as early as possible after the 20th week of gestation to enable the couple to think through this important decision.

Another way to decrease the costs of the program could be to see only once those women who say at admission that they want more children, since this was the most common reason for not having the operation. If such women had had only one session, the number of sterilizations in the treatment group would have decreased by a maximum of 14 percent, and the number of counseling sessions would have declined by 44 percent.

While either strategy to limit the number of sessions would decrease program costs, it might also decrease the number of women who choose some other method of contraception. Some postpartum counseling on contraception is undoubtedly needed for all women.

One-fourth of women said they chose not to undergo sterilization because of fear or dislike of surgery. Therefore, the program obviously needs to emphasize the safety of the operation in order to allay these fears. Overall, the program had an impressive impact on women's knowledge and attitudes toward female sterilization. Improvement in these areas may translate into an increased demand for sterilization services later, either among those exposed to the program or among those with whom they share information.

A good counseling program, however, must be designed to help women understand all methods of family planning. This will enable them to make well-informed, well-considered decisions about their fertility. The process should not attempt to persuade a couple to select a particular method, such as sterilization. If the process has been respectful of individual preferences, the chances that the couple will regret the sterilization decision will be minimized. Satisfied clients can then become advocates for family planning, and their support will increase demand for services and help to reduce maternal mortality.

References

1. W. Rinehart, A. Kols and S. Moore, "Healthier Mothers and Children Through Family Planning," *Population Reports*, Series J, No, 27, May–June 1984.
2. K. London et. al., "Fertility and Family Planning Surveys: An Update," *Population Reports*, Series M, No. 8, Sept–Oct. 1985.

3. National Population Bureau, *Nigeria Fertility Survey, 1981–1982: Principal Report*, Vols I & II, Lagos, 1984.

4. K. London et al., 1985, op. cit. (see reference 2), Table 7.

5. National Population Bureau, 1984, op, cit. (see reference 3).

6. Ibid., Table 4.2.1–1

7. K. London et al., 1985, op. cit. (see reference 2), Table 3.

8. A. E. Omu and J. A. Unuigbe, "Acceptance of Contraception Practice by Grand-multipara in Benin City, Nigeria," *International Journal of Gynaecology and Obstetrics*, 24:145, 1986.

9. S. Okojie, "Maternal Mortality at the University of Benin Teaching Hospital," in D. A. Ojo et al., eds., *Obstetrics and Gynaecology in Developing Countries*, 1977, p. 280–286.

10. Family Health International, "A Report on Obstetric Deliveries at the University of Benin Teaching Hospital in Benin City, Nigeria," Research Triangle Park, N. C., July, 1983.

11. Ibid.

A Comparison of the Performance of Male and Female CDB Distributors in Peru

James R. Foreit, Maria Rosa Garate, Alfredo Brazzoduro, Felix Guillen, Maria del Carmen Herrera, and Flor Cardosa Suarez

Programmatic issue: *The programs wished to determine if the use of male CBD distributors would increase distribution of condoms and increases the number of male CBD users.*

Programmatic processes/components: *Meeting the objective of increased male involvement resulted in having to change CBD distributor recruitment tactics and introduced problems into supervisor–supervisee relations.*

Research design: *The design was a quasiexperiment with post-test comparisons of intervention and comparison group results. Dependent variables included number of clients recruited, clients' gender, and methods distributed. Opinions of supervisors and other program staff about using men as CBD distributors was obtained through in-depth interviews, a qualitative technique.*

Findings: *The study found that men recruited more male clients and distributed more condoms, whereas women distributors recruited more female clients and distributed more oral contraceptives. Men also recruited as many or more new clients than women, and distributed as many couple years of protection (CYP) as did their female counterparts. In-depth interviews with program supervisors, who were women, revealed a reluctance to allow men to become distributors.*

Program response to findings: *In one of the programs, the female supervisory staff and CBD director never accepted the idea of using men as CBD distributors, and the number of male distributors rapidly diminished through attrition. In the other program, the idea of using men as CBD distributors was better accepted, and men continued to be recruited for a period of two to three years after the study. In the mid-1990s, international donor assistance to the agencies was withdrawn and both ceased to exist.*

Discussion: *The study shows that programs can overcome psychosocial barriers produced by client–provider gender differences, and increase condom distribution and male involvement by using men as CBD distributors.*

This study again demonstrates how the program situation determines methodological options. The independent variable, distributor gender, is an organismic variable that cannot be randomly assigned.

A Comparison of the Performance of Male and Female CBD Distributors in Peru

James R. Foreit, Maria Rosa Garate, Alfredo Brazzoduro, Felix Guillen, Maria del Carmen Herrera, and Flor Cardoso Suarez

In 1981, the International Conference on Family Planning in the 1980s, held in Jakarta, Indonesia, affirmed that men had the same reproductive rights as women, noted that existing services did not reflect those rights, and recommended that priorities for the coming decade include establishing more programs for men. Extending reproductive rights and services to men has important implications for women and for the demographic effectiveness of family planning programs. The increased use of male contraceptives strengthens the rights of women by permitting couples to share the burden of responsibility for family planning. Making male methods available may also raise contraceptive prevalence, because each additional method attracts new family planning users (Jain, 1989).

The condom is the only available male method that can be used for birth spacing. It is also the only method that offers protection against sexually transmitted diseases (STDs), including AIDS. Nevertheless, few agencies target men, and condoms are among the least popular contraceptive methods. In Peru, for example, fewer than 0.7 percent of couples of reproductive age (15–49) used the method in 1986 (Instituto Nacional de Estadistica, 1987).

Community-based distribution (CBD) of contraceptives is an important source of temporary family planning methods in Latin America, but most CBD progams distribute far fewer condoms than oral contraceptives. One limitation to serving men may be that CBD distributors are almost always women. Evidence suggests that the most successful distributors are those who share the same characteristics as their target populations, while the least successful are those who differ greatly from the target group (Rogers, 1973; Repetto, 1977; Azcona et al., 1980). Thus, gender differences between distributors and potential users may limit the sale of condoms. To overcome this barrier, some programs have attempted to recruit male CBD workers, but little has been reported about their effectiveness as distributors (Gallen, 1986).

Specifically, family planning organizations need to know if it is feasible to recruit and supervise both men and women, if men and women distribute the

Reprinted with the permission of the Population Council from *Studies in Family Planning* 1992. 23,1:58–62.

same or different method mixes, if they will distribute the same volume of contraceptives, and if they serve the same or different user groups. This report presents the results of an operations research experiment to determine the effectiveness of male CBD distributors in two regions of Peru.

Two private, nonprofit family planning agencies, Promoción de Labores Educativas y Asistenciales en Favor de la Salud (PROFAMILIA) and the Centro Nor-Peruano de Capacitación y Promoción Familiar (CENPROF), participated in the study. Although their CBD programs were administratively similar, they displayed important differences in size, target population, method mix, and distributor characteristics.

PROFAMILIA is located in Lima, Peru's capital and largest city. The CBD program functions in low-income urban areas in the southern part of the city, where the population numbers about 850,000. According to program staff, many clients are from traditional rural backgrounds and are members of non-Spanish-speaking indigenous groups. Distributors are mostly housewives operating out of their own homes. Prospective clients are attracted to the CBD posts by signs on the homes of distributors and through family planning talks in the community.

Prior to the study, the PROFAMILIA CBD program was composed of 185 female and 15 male distributors. Approximately 67 percent of the men and 82 percent of the women had not completed a secondary education. In the 12 months prior to the study, oral contraceptives made up over 75 percent of all couple-years of protection (CYP) distributed, while condoms made up 22 percent, and spermicidal foam and tablets, 3 percent.

CENPROF is located in Trujillo, a coastal city 420 km. north of Lima, with a population of approximately 565,000. Its CBD program is also located in low-income areas inhabited by immigrants from rural areas. Unlike PROFAMILIA, the target population is largely Spanish speaking. CBD distributors include community leaders and students. Prior to the study, the program had 40 female and 8 male distributors, who were generally better educated than their PROFAMILIA counterparts: 67 percent of the men and 44 percent of the women had more than a secondary education. During the 12 months prior to the study, condoms made up almost 63 percent of all CYP distributed, while orals accounted for 22 percent, and foam and tablets, 15 percent.

Methodology

Hypotheses

The study tested three hypotheses: (1) male distributors would sell more condoms and female distributors would sell more oral contraceptives; (2) male distributors would serve more male clients and female distributors would serve more female clients; and (3) male distributors would sell less contraceptive protection than would female distributors. (The last hypothesis was added by administrators and supervisors who felt that men would be less effective than women as CBD distributors.)

Design

An experimental design with one independent variable, distributor gender, was utilized. Dependent variables included quantities sold of condoms, pills, and spermicides, total CYP for all methods combined, number of new clients, and client gender.

Both agencies recruited additional male and female CBD distributors during the period from November 1987 to January 1988. Only these new distributors were included in the study. Men and women were trained together, received the same client information materials and contraceptives to distribute, and were assigned to the same supervisors. Distributors received an 80 percent commission on all sales of oral contraceptives, condoms, foam, and vaginal tablets. Field observation lasted 10 months, from April 1988 through January 1989. Data on the dependent variables were obtained from the distributors' service statistics forms. Both CENPROF and PROFAMILIA used the same definition of new acceptors and CYP.[1]

Information on the sociodemographic characteristics of distributors was obtained from agency personnel records. Additional information was gathered from structured interviews with supervisors and from forms designed to record information on recruitment activities.

Results

Recruitment of Male Distributors

The agencies first tried to recruit distributors through group lectures in factories, union halls, and clubs; when doing so proved unsuccessful, they shifted to a strategy of individual recruitment. Virtually all of the PROFAMILIA distributors and 87 percent of the CENPROF distributors were recruited individually by supervisors. Men were more difficult to recruit than were women, especially in Lima. PROFAMILIA enrolled 38 men and 171 women, and CENPROF recruited 52 men and 94 women. Both agencies found it necessary to hold distributor training on weekends to accommodate the schedules of male recruits.

Supervisor Attitudes

With only one exception, the supervisors in both agencies were women. Further, most supervisors were reluctant to include men as family planning distributors, saying that the activity was "women's work." The attitudes of the 19 PROFAMILIA and six CENPROF supervisors are summarized in the remarks quoted below:

"Men only want to sell contraceptives. They don't want to keep records and give talks."

"Men are very hard to contact. They don't work in the community."

"Men don't want to do this kind of work. Many are too embarrassed."

"Men don't think the work is important."

"You can't even talk about the subject [family planning] with older men."

"It is easier for women to talk to women."

"Men have less free time to do the work."

"Men have trouble talking about family planning with women."

"Women have more users."

"Men produce less."

Distributor Compliance

Supervisors in both agencies were concerned that men would be less likely than women to keep records and turn in monthly reports. (Lack of reporting usually indicates lack of contraceptive distribution and inattention to other program activities, and is often used as a proxy for distributor dropout.) We found no statistically reliable reporting differences by gender. Reporting differences between programs were greater than gender differences within the same program. In CENPROF, both men and women turned in 60 percent of their monthly reports. In PROFAMILIA, men turned in 80 percent of the required reports, and women turned in 90 percent of them.[2]

Contraceptive Sales

The distributions of contraceptive sales were highly skewed: A few distributors sold large quantities, while the remainder were clustered around a much lower sales level. Means were always larger than medians (see Appendix A). In PROFAMILIA, the standard deviations for most indicators were approximately equal to 1.6 times the value of the means, while in CENPROF the standard deviations for most indicators were approximately 1.5–3.3 times greater than the means. Therefore, we selected the median as the most appropriate measure of central tendency.

Differences between male and female distributors were evaluated with a nonparametric statistic, median test by chi-square. Like all nonparametric tests, this measure is highly conservative.[3]

Table 1 compares monthly median contraceptive sales and total CYP sold by male and female distributors affiliated with CENPROF and PROFAMILIA. All distributors contributed 10 months of observation. Months when no sales were reported were coded as zero.

Table 1. Monthly median sales of contraceptives per distributor, according to the distributor's gender and program affiliation (PROFAMILIA or CENPROF), Peru

	Distributor	
Program and method	Male	Female
PROFAMILIA	(n = 38)	(n = 171)
Pills (cycle)	3.0	6.5**
Condoms (units)	48.9	23.9**
Vaginal tablets (units)	2.0	3.0
Foam (can)	0.3	0.2
Total CYP (all methods)	1.1	1.0
CENPROF	(n = 52)	(n = 94)
Pills (cycle)	1.8	2.9
Condoms (units)	162.1	87.7**
Vaginal tablets (units)	27.7	25.5
Foam (can)	0.2	0.7
Total CYP (all methods)	2.8	1.8 *

*p <.05   **p <.01
Note: A unit of condoms = 1 condom; a unit of tablets = 1 tablet.

In both PROFAMILIA and CENPROF, men sold two times more condoms than did women. Women sold more pills than did men in both programs, but the difference was statistically reliable only for PROFAMILIA. The results for PROFAMILIA distributors confirm the hypothesis that men sell more condoms and women sell more pills; for CENPROF, this hypothesis was partially confirmed. It is interesting to note that there were no significant differences between men and women in sales of female barrier methods, perhaps because sales levels were so low. Men and women distributed equal amounts of CYP than did women in PROFAMILIA, while men distributed more total CYP than did women in CENPROF.

New Clients

Male distributors in PROFAMILIA served a median of 3.2 new clients per month, and women, 2.8. The difference was not statistically reliable. In CENPROF, men recruited significantly more new clients per month than did women, a median of 6.2 compared with 4.2, respectively.[4] These results, together with the findings on total CYP, fail to support the hypothesis that male distributors would sell less contraceptive protection than would female distributors.

User Characteristics

Hypothesis 2 predicted that male distributors would serve more male clients, and female distributors, more female clients. This was confirmed in CENPROF: Male clients accounted for 74 percent of sales by male distributors, while 71 percent of sales by female distributors were made to women. In PROFAMILIA, both male and female distributors served a largely female clientele. However, men accounted for 39 percent of sales by male distributors but only 13 percent of sales by female distributors. Both differences are statistically reliable.[5]

Distributor Gender vs. Sociodemographic Differences

Male and female distributors also differed on several sociodemographic factors other than gender. Male distributors were younger, better educated, less likely to be married, and had fewer living children than female distributors. Therefore, it is possible that any one of these differences rather than gender *per se* was responsible for the observed differences in performance. We reasoned that if a factor other than gender were responsible for the differences observed between men and women, it should also have the same systematic influence on within-gender performance differences.

None of the variables examined (age, education, marital status, or living children) produced statistically reliable differences in male distributor performance. Similarly, none of the variables influenced female distributor performance in PROFAMILIA. Among female CENPROF distributors only one factor, education, had a significant impact on one performance indicator, total CYP.

Discussion

The results have important implications for programs that seek to increase male involvement in family planning. In two different settings in Peru, male distributors were more likely to serve male clients, and female distributors were more likely to serve female clients. There were no gender differences in distributor compliance with program norms, and gender was found to exert an impact on method mix independent of other factors. Contrary to expectations, men sold as much or more total CYP than did women, and they recruited as many or more new clients.

These findings indicate that men can be effective CBD distributors. The study suggests that CBD programs can influence method and client mix by recruiting more men as distributors. Finally, the results also demonstrate that successful programs for males can be incorporated within existing CBD structures and do not require special training or client materials.

However, we also found that men were more difficult than women to recruit as CBD distributors, and that female supervisors were less comfortable working with male distributors than with other females. Males may be more difficult to recruit than females because they are more likely to be employed and have less time to volunteer, or because the small commissions available from selling contraceptives do not attract them. It is also possible that the female staff and women's health orientation of CBD programs discourage male participation. The use of male supervisors might make men easier to recruit as distributors and make supervisor-distributor relations less difficult. Future operations research should focus on discovering successful strategies for recruiting men as CBD distributors and for supervising them once recruited.

Appendix

Appendix A. Male and female distributors: Monthly means and standard deviations per distributor

Distributor and method	Male		Female	
	Mean	SD	Mean	SD
PROFAMILIA				
Pills	4.2	4.8	8.2	7.2
Condoms	66.7	59.6	36.9	52.5
Vaginal tablets	8.9	14.2	5.5	7.1
Foam	0.6	0.8	0.7	1.1
Total CYP	3.3	0.8	2.0	0.9
CENPROF				
Pills	2.2	4.0	4.4	14.4
Condoms	237.0	511.4	111.1	262.5
Vaginal tablets	70.7	143.9	38.5	59.7
Foam	1.0	1.7	1.2	1.3
Total CYP	3.3	5.8	2.0	3.1

References

Azcona, Sergio Correu et al. 1980. "Agent characteristics and productivity in the Mexican rural health program." *Studies in Family Planning* 11, 7/8: 247–254.

Gallen, Moira E. et al. 1986. "Men—new focus for family planning programs." *Population Reports*, J 33.

Instituto Nacional de Estadistica. 1987. *Encuesta Demográfica y de Salud Familiar.*

Jain, Anrudh K. 1989. "Fertility reduction and the quality of family planning services." *Studies in Family Planning* 20, 1: 1–6.

Peatmen, John G. 1963. *Introduction to Applied Statistics.* New York: Harper & Row.

Repetto, Robert. 1977. "Correlatives of field-worker performance in the Indonesian family planning program: A test of the homophily heterophily hypothesis." *Studies in Family Planning* 8, 1: 19–21.

Rogers, Everett. 1973. *Communications Strategies for Family Planning.* New York: Free Press.

Notes

1. A new acceptor is a person who takes a method from the program for the first time. Thirteen cycles of oral contraceptives = 1 CYP: 100 condoms or 100 vaginal tablets = 1 CYP; 5 cans of foam = 1 CYP.

2. To determine if men were less likely than women to report, we divided the number of reports of each promoter by the number of months he/she was elegible to report.

3. The median test by chi-square is a distribution-free method of testing for statistical significance. It determines whether the median of a variable is the same in different independent samples defined by a grouping variable. Measurables are ordered into two intervals, above or below the median of the combined samples. The significance of the difference is tested by chi-square. (See Peatmen, 1963.)

4. $\chi^2 = 4.1$; df = 1; p<.05

5. PROFAMILIA: $\chi^2 = 16.5$; df = 1; p<.01
   CENPROF: $\chi^2 = 39.4$; df = 1; p<.01

Acknowledgments

The authors wish to acknowledge the participation of Maria del Pilar Fortunic, who conducted interviews with CENPROF and PROFAMILIA supervisors, and Demetrio Elgueta, who programmed the project data bases and helped both institutions computerize their service statistics systems. The project was conducted with funding from the USAID Office of Population under the INOPAL Operations Research in Latin America and the Caribbean project.

RESOURCES

Introduction

James R. Foreit

Considerable resources are required to provide family planning and reproductive health services. Some of these resources include money to pay salaries, to purchase materials and contraceptives, and to construct and maintain facilities. Other resources, such as volunteer time, may not be paid for in monetary terms. The value of all the resources needed to provide a given service to a client is known as the production cost of that service. Typically, programs provide family planning and other reproductive health services to their clients at less than the cost of production. Family planning programs have been heavily subsidized by governments of developing countries, as well as by bilateral and international donors, because of their assumed positive effects on health status and socioeconomic development.

In the mid-1990s, subsidized family planning programs faced three challenges. First, demand for services was growing. Between 1992 and 2000, the number of married women of reproductive age, 15–49, was projected to increase by approximately 20 to 40 percent, depending on the country being considered. At the same time, the proportion of women using contraceptives is also growing. The combination of increasing population size and increasing contraceptive prevalence led many health and development authorities to forecast that the number of contraceptive users in their countries would double or even triple in the same decade, implying higher program costs and an increased need for funds (Haaga and Tsui, 1995).

A second challenge was presented by the United Nations International Conference on Population and Development (ICPD) held in Cairo in 1994, which called for the expansion of programs that had been narrowly focused on family planning to include a wider array of other reproductive health services. The cost of implementing the action program recommended by the conference in developing countries was estimated at more than $17 billion in the year 2000. Implementation of the family planning component of ICPD is estimated to reach $10 billion in the year 2000, or about twice the amount spent in 1990 (Alcala, 1994).

Financial sustainability is the third challenge faced by programs at the turn of the millennium. In the mid-1990s, funds for family planning from some major international donors, notably USAID, reached a plateau or began to decline. Sustainable programs are those that are able to cover their operating costs after the withdrawal of international funding, and continue to maintain earlier output levels. Sustainability has become an especially serious problem for private, non-profit family planning programs in many parts of the developing world.

Increases in the number, types, and costs of services, and the need to become more sustainable, underline the need for operations research to focus on the problems of *resource allocation* (which refers to the effective use of available resources) and *resource mobilization* (which refers to the capture of additional resources).

In the area of resource allocation, operations research has been used to reduce waste and to discover new and less costly ways of operating programs. Many potential sources of waste exist: loss of purchased supplies, employment of more expensive procedures when less expensive alternatives would work equally well, requirement of unnecessary tests and visits, and maintenance of underused staff and facilities. More effective and less costly alternatives to existing practices have also been developed as part of operations research projects. OR has demonstrated that CBD programs that routinely summon distributors to costly retraining courses could produce greater improvements in provider knowledge more cheaply with on-the-job retraining. OR has also helped programs replace outdated norms and eliminate needless medical procedures and excessive administrative requirements.

Requiring patients to undergo unnecessary and unreliable laboratory tests prior to prescription of oral contraceptives (Stanback et al., in this volume) has already been discussed as a medical barrier to the practice of family planning. However, when these tests are also subsidized, they become a resource-allocation problem, wasting money that could be used for activities that have a positive effect on user health and fertility outcomes. Finally, building more capacity than is commensurate with need leads to underuse of staff, infrastructure, and materials and incurs unnecessary costs. The money invested in excess capacity has no effect on health and could be better used for other purposes.

This section presents three papers on resource allocation. The first (Foreit et al.) deals with the problem of eliminating unnecessary visits to family planning clinics operating at capacity, and the other two deal with the problem of underuse of staff and infrastructure. In the Bangladesh program (Janowitz et al.), a diagnostic study found that staff was underused because they did not show up for work. In the second instance in Peru (Foreit et al.), managers knew that staff was underutilized because of limited demand in the areas surrounding the sites where services were provided, and conducted an experiment to increase use by manipulating the frequency with which services were provided.

To obtain the funds necessary to provide more services to more users, programs must do more than eliminate waste and find new ways to provide services. They must also mobilize additional resources. OR can help programs mobilize resources in two ways, first by demonstrating the impact and efficiency of programs to high level-administrators and political leaders, as in the case of the Taichung and Mali studies discussed in earlier sections of this book, and second, by helping lower-level program managers to set prices and offer new, for-profit services.

As a way of mobilizing more resources for family planning, governments are starting to encourage more for-profit involvement in reproductive health and family planning programs. Increased involvement of the commercial sector, health insurance schemes, and private practitioners are assumed to be able to move users from subsidized to unsubsidized services. To date, however, very little OR has been carried out to help for-profit sector programs increase their effectiveness, efficiency, quality, and revenues. In the future, however, the private sector may become an important new client for family planning OR.

Evidence suggests that users with greater income reap the greatest benefit from subsidized services, and that users of most methods are willing to pay more than the prices currently charged for contraceptives (Haaga and Tsui, 1995; de Vargas et al., 1998). However, the paper by León and Cuesta in the previous section reminds us that demand is not insensitive to price, and that many price increases are associated with at least some client loss. Testing mechanisms for reducing client loss, such as sliding-fee scales and other means-testing schemes, should be a high priority for future operations research on resource mobilization.

In addition, or as an alternative to raising user fees, programs can also begin to sell new services in high demand at a profit and use the money earned to cross-subsidize other services for which a lesser demand exists. Although adding for-profit services is less common in other regions, in Latin America, many new services such as ultrasound and laboratory tests are being marketed profitably by private, not-for-profit family planning organizations (Bratt et al., 1998). One paper, León et al., on generating revenues by adding services is included in this section. It describes an attempt by a family planning program in Peru to increase revenues by promoting other underused reproductive health services.

References

Alcala, Maria José. 1994. *Action for the 21st Century, Reproductive Health and Rights for All.* New York: Family Care International.

Bratt, John H., James Foreit, and Teresa de Vargas. 1998. "Three strategies to promote sustainability of CEMOPLAF clinics in Ecuador." *Studies in Family Planning* 29, 1: 58–68.

Haaga, John and Amy O. Tsui (eds). 1995. *Resource Allocation for Family Planning in Developing Countries: Report of a Meeting.* Washington, DC: National Academy Press.

de Vargas, Teresa et al. 1998. "Estimating consumer response to price changes in family planning and reproductive health services." Paper presented at the annual meeting of the Population Association of America, Chicago, 2–4 April.

Cost Control, Access, and Quality of Care: The Impact of IUD Revisit Norms in Ecuador

James R. Foreit, John Bratt, Karen Foreit, and Teresa de Vargas

Programmatic issue: *How to serve more clients in fully utilized clinics without increasing costs or reducing service quality.*

Programmatic processes/components: *IUD revisit norms were studied. IUD revisits accounted for most of the revisits in fully utilized clinics. The program wanted to know the effect of changing their IUD revisit norm on program and user costs, clinic attendance, and probability of detecting IUD-related medical problems.*

Research design: *The study simulated changes in the norm of four IUD revisits to one required revisit or an all-revisit-optional norm (clients would be asked to return if they had a problem or question). The simulation was based on estimates of the probabilities of revisiting under different norms, and on estimates of the number of medical problems that would go undetected if asymptomatic clients did not make routine visits. Client interviews and medical examinations provided information on the likelihood of making a revisit under different norms, and on medical problem rates.*

Personnel, materials, equipment, infrastructure, and overhead costs were estimated for the program. Travel and opportunity costs of time involved in clinic visits were estimated for clients. The simulation was partially validated by an examination of service statistics one year after the agency changed IUD revisit norms.

Findings: *Reducing the number of required revisits from four to one would eliminate about 8,000 clinic visits, save the program $10,000 and clients $23,000 per year. Changing the norm from four required revisits to an all-revisit-optional approach would eliminate about 15,000 clinic visits, save the program about $18,000 and clients about $41,000. However, going from a four-revisit to a one-revisit norm would reduce the number of problems detected from 582 to 527, and replacing the four-revisit norm with an all-revisit-optional norm would lower the number of problems detected from 582 to 423.*

Program response to findings: *CEMOPLAF replaced the four-revisit norm with the one-revisit norm, resulting in a 29 percent decline in IUD revisits. The subsidized IUD revisits were largely replaced by unsubsidized gynecology visits.*

Discussion: *This paper used relatively unintrusive diagnostic techniques to estimate changes in output and costs that would result from specified actions. Simulation models have much to recommend them from the point of view of cost and rapid availability of results, but because models often have heavy data requirements, the technique cannot be used often. Most important, because simulations are seldom subjected to empirical proof, little is known about the inaccuracy. Thus, program managers should attempt to validate the accuracy of their simulation predictions to verify that expected results are indeed being obtained.*

Cost Control, Access, and Quality of Care: The Impact of IUD Revisit Norms in Ecuador

James R. Foreit, John Bratt, Karen Foreit, and Teresa de Vargas

Introduction

Quality of care, costs, and access are dominant issues for family planning programs in Latin America. While the topic of quality of care is fairly new to family planning (see Bruce, 1990), its application in medicine goes back 80 years (see Brook, 1988). Historically, most approaches to assessing quality focused on the *process* of providing care (see Donobedian, 1969). The process approach still characterizes the family planning field.[1] However, in medicine, the assessment of *outcome* has become equally important, and increasingly, health care analysts are insisting that quality of care be linked to measurable outcomes. Seen in this way, *quality of care consists of program interventions or elements which increase the probability of positive client outcomes.*

Subsidized resources are growing more slowly than demand for family planning goods and services (Janowitz et al., 1990). As a result, family planning programs have been forced to pay closer attention to costs. At the same time, they are under pressure to improve quality of care, which may involve investment of resources in new interventions or in correcting program deficiencies. Managers are concerned that quality improvement will increase service costs at the same time that programs are attempting to become more cost efficient.

Access to family planning is also affected by costs. Increasing costs to clients, such as prices charged, time and transportation, may put family planning out of the reach of many potential users. In addition, if program resources are limited and costs per service increase as a result of quality improvement, programs will be able to serve fewer clients, and access will suffer.

In summary, quality of care, costs, and access are integrally related to one another. Any change in one will necessarily affect the other two (see Chelminsky, 1993). However, it is not inevitable that this interaction be negative. The challenge to program managers is to identify those operational parameters which can be manipulated to maintain or improve quality and access while eliminating unnecessary costs.

Reprinted with permission from *The Journal of Health & Population in Developing Countries* 1998. 1,2.

This paper reports the results of an operations research study to balance the costs, quality of care, and access to the Centro Medico de Planificacion Familiar (CEMOPLAF) of Quito, Ecuador. Client follow-up is considered an essential element of quality of care (Bruce, 1990). CEMOPLAF schedules routine revisits for new IUD acceptors (a program process) to detect and resolve medical problems arising from IUD use (a program outcome). These revisits represent real and opportunity costs for providers and clients, and revisits by users who have no problems add to clinic overcrowding and reduce access for new acceptors. Management felt the number of required revisits exceeded the optimal needed for a quality service. They wanted to reduce the number of revisits while avoiding an unacceptable number of undetected and untreated contraceptive use-related problems.

Program setting. CEMOPLAF provides family planning and other reproductive and child health services. Throughout Ecuador the agency operates 20 clinics. CEMOPLAF's goals are to be 87 percent self-sufficient by 1997, to increase new family planning clients by 10 percent per year, and to expand prenatal services. To meet these goals, the organization will have to increase productivity and efficiency. Eleven of its clinics are operating at or above capacity, and six more will reach capacity within the next two years.

IUD revisits are the most pressing clinic utilization problem. In 1991, they accounted for 74 percent of all visits and 68 percent of all costs. Despite the recommendations of international groups, norms requiring frequent IUD revisits remain commonplace throughout Latin America. The CEMOPLAF norm specified four revisits during the first year of use: the first at 8 days postinsertion, the second thirty-five days later, the third three months after the second, and a final revisit nine months after insertion. At each visit, the client is weighed, has her blood pressure taken, receives a pelvic exam and is asked if she has any questions or problems with her method.

The study compared the current norm of four required revisits with two simulations: (1) a norm of one required revisit with other revisits optional for clients with problems or questions, as recommended by international organizations such as WHO and IPPF (Adrian et al., 1992); and (2) an all revisits optional norm, which maximizes cost-control. To determine the most clinically-acceptable and cost-effective norm, the study modeled detection of medical problems, cost savings, and increased new client capacity.

Methodology

Theoretical framework. Routine revisits would be unnecessary if all family planning clients knew when they had problems and returned for consultation. However, some problems are unnoticed by the user or are not seen as important enough to warrant a clinic visit. The ideal revisit norm would capture all users with problems while avoiding revisits by clients without problems or questions. Signal detection theory (Coombs et al., 1970) demonstrates that such an ideal is impossible to attain.

Signal detection predicts the probability of identifying a weak stimulus (signal) in the midst of noise. In the typical experiment, an observer is presented segments of noise alone or noise plus a signal and responds whenever she believes the signal is present. If the observer waits to respond until she is *absolutely sure* that she hears the signal, she will fail to detect the weaker signals. If she reacts every time she thinks she *might* have heard the signal, she will detect all the signals but will also raise many false alarms. Inevitably, the observer will make errors no matter what strategy she adopts. The observer's strategy will be based on her judgment as to whether it is worse to miss a signal or raise a false alarm (Coombs et al., 1970; Marx and Hillix, 1979).

In the context of IUD services, the presence of a method-related medical problem is analogous to a signal and a revisit the response. Counseling at time of insertion should instruct the client to recognize problems. The probability of making a revisit is conditioned by the "payoffs" (perceived costs and benefits to both the client and the institution) of the four logically possible outcomes: (1) The client has a problem and makes a revisit to the clinic; (2) she has a problem and does not make a revisit; (3) she does not have a problem and makes a revisit; (4) she does not have a problem and does not make a revisit. In signal detection terminology, the first outcome is a "hit," the second a "miss," the third a "false alarm" and the fourth a "correct rejection," as shown in Figure 1.

Clients and services benefit when clients revisit when they have problems $(Y|y)$ and stay away when they do not have problems $(N|n)$. Clients and services incur unnecessary costs when clients revisit when they do not have problems $(Y|n)$. Finally, clients suffer when they have problems and do not revisit $(N|y)$. The probability of a problem is independent of the revisiting norm, but programs can raise or lower the probability of revisiting by setting different norms. Increasing routine revisits will increase both detection of problems and false alarms. Eliminating routine revisits will reduce false alarms and increase missed problems. The optimal schedule depends on the probabilities and costs and benefits of the four outcomes.[2]

Filling in the pay-off matrix requires independent estimates of the probability of making a revisit and the incidence of medical problems. We directly observed the frequency of revisiting, but were unable to observe directly the likelihood of a problem because we did not have access to clients who did not return to the clinic. Therefore, we measured problem rates among clients who did return and asked them if they would have revisited without a routinely scheduled appointment. We used this information to infer underlying method-related

Figure 1. Pay-off matrix for problems and revisits

Revisit

	Yes (Y)	No (N)
Problem — yes (y)	Hit (Y|y)	Miss (N|y)
Problem — no (n)	False Alarm (Y|n)	Correct Rejection (N|n)

problem rates and to model the impact of different norms on the probability of making revisits and on rates of hits, misses, and false alarms.

Design. Ten clinics were randomly selected for study, including four in Quito and six in other locations. A record search of IUD acceptors who had completed one year after insertion provided information on first year revisit rates. The search included the medical histories of all 3356 clients who had received an IUD in the study clinics between January 1–May 31, 1991. The number of revisits made in the twelve months following insertion was recorded for each client.

Client interviews and medical examinations provided information on problem rates among IUD users revisiting in the first year. The likelihood of returning without a routine appointment was obtained from the client interview. All clients making IUD revisits in the study clinics between January 1–May 31, 1992, and who had received their IUD within 12 months of the revisit date were interviewed. A total of 4985 interviews were conducted. Clients were asked if they had any questions to discuss with the service provider, if they had side-effects or problems, the reason for revisiting, and in the case of routine appointments, if they would have revisited without having been told to do so. Attending physicians and nurse-midwives recorded the presence of IUD related problems on clinical trial forms.

Estimation of costs. The study also examined client and agency revisit costs. Client costs included payments for transportation (including persons accompanying the client), clinic fees, and the opportunity cost of time spent traveling and in the facility itself. Clients were asked how much they had spent on transportation, and how much time they spent traveling. Patient flow analysis (PFA) measured time spent in clinic. Opportunity costs were calculated for the client only.

Agency costs included staff time, materials, furniture and equipment, infrastructure, and overhead. Net cost was the average agency cost of an IUD revisit, less the price paid by the client. Costs were estimated at six of the study clinics. PFA estimated staff time. Use of materials and equipment was observed directly. Overhead was assigned on a pro-rated basis.

Results

Current Patterns of Revisits and Problems Detected

Revisits. According to the record search, under the four revisit norm, IUD acceptors made an average of 2.31 revisits during the twelve months following insertion. Approximately 19 percent made no revisits, 16 percent made exactly four revisits, and 14 percent exceeded the norm and made five or more revisits. According to the client interviews, 66 percent of all revisits were made because of a previously-scheduled appointment; the remaining third were made because the client had a problem or wished to talk with a service provider.

Timing of revisits was obtained from the client interview. Revisits were classified by whether or not they were within an acceptable range of the time specified by the norm: visit #1 at 8 days (1–15 days after insertion); visit #2 at 43 days (30–59); visit #3 at 133 days (120–150); and visit #4 at 270 days (240–364 days). Clients who said they were returning for a problem were defined as returning if the revisit were optional. Clients keeping a routine appointment who said that they would have returned even if they had not been told to do so were also defined as returning if the revisit were optional. Clients with routine revisits who answered that they would not have returned or expressed weak motivations for returning were defined as not returning for an optional revisit.[3]

Table 1 combines the results of the record search and client interviews. It shows the percent of revisiting acceptors, revisits made at the time specified by the norm, and the percent of clients who stated that they would have made the revisit without a routine appointment.

Compliance with the norm was limited. Most clients made a first revisit at about the time indicated but subsequent revisits declined rapidly after the first appointment, as did the probability of returning at the time specified by the

Table 1. Four-revisit norm, percent of clients making revisits, and percent of revisits made at time specified by norm

Revisit	Record Search % Acceptors Making Revisit	Client Interviews % Revisits Made at Specified Time	% Would Return Without Appointment
1	81.3	69.6	31.3
2	61.6	33.4	63.9
3	44.5	23.7	63.7
4	29.6	16.8	61.1
No. cases	3356		

Table 2. Proportion of revisits with medical problems by number and timing of revisit

Revisit	Timing Conforming to Norm	Outside Norm
1	.022	.045
2	.054	.061
3	.072	.061
4	.037	.068

norm. The large proportion of revisits outside of prescribed periods appears due to lack of provider knowledge as well as lack of patient compliance. Approximately 66 percent of all revisits were made in response to a routine appointment, and about 81 percent of these were kept at the scheduled time. Discussions with providers revealed that many were not aware of the correct timing of revisits and that they gave routine appointments at times not prescribed by the norm.

Client questions. The interview found that in approximately 35 percent of revisits clients had questions they wished to discuss with providers. CEMOPLAF medical staff reviewed the questions and concluded that approximately 70 percent could have been avoided by better client education at insertion (for example, "Does the IUD cause cancer?" or "Can I get pregnant if my IUD is in place?").

Medical problems. Three IUD-related medical problems were studied: expulsion, suspected pelvic inflammatory disease (PID), and suspected pregnancy. Expulsions were found at 4.3 percent of revisits, suspected pregnancies at 2.5 percent, and suspected PID at 3.1 percent.

Table 2 shows the proportion of revisits with diagnosed medical problems at each of the first four revisits, both within and outside of the prescribed interval. First revisits made less than 15 days after insertion diagnosed the fewest problems. This is probably because the period since insertion was not long enough for most problems to develop. First revisits made after 15 days had diagnosis rates over twice as great as those made earlier, suggesting that a change in the timing of the first revisit would improve the effectiveness of the norm.[4]

Three fourths of returning clients with diagnosed medical problems reported they would have returned without a routine appointment. Probability of

Table 3. Probability that a client with a medical problem would have returned without an appointment by interval since insertion

Problem	Probability of Revisit		
	0–3 Months	4–12 Months	First 12 Months
Expulsion	0.500	0.786	0.646
Suspected pregnancy	0.786	0.727	0.750
Suspected PID	0.882	0.893	0.889

Table 4. Revisit patterns for three different norms

Frequency of Revisiting	Norm		
	Observed	Projected	
	4 Required Revisits	1 Required Revisit	All Revisits Optional
1	19.7% (M)	42.0% (M)	23.8% (O)
2	17.1% (M)	21.2% (O)	12.0% (O)
3	14.9% (M)	10.8% (O)	7.1% (O)
4	15.6% (M)	5.0% (O)	2.2% (O)
5+	14.0% (O)	2.3% (O)	1.0% (O)
Mean Revisits	2.31	1.48	0.83

M = Mandatory revisit; O = Optional revisit.

returning varied by type of problem, with suspected PID showing the highest probability and expulsion the lowest. Table 3 shows the probability that women with diagnosed problems would have returned without an appointment.

Modeling Revisits and Problems Detected Under Alternative Norms

One required revisit. When four revisits were required, 81 percent of new IUD clients returned at least once. We would expect the same to obtain if only one revisit were required. However, second and subsequent revisits would no longer be routinely scheduled, and the overall frequency of revisiting should decline. We calculated transitional probabilities of making optional higher-order revisits from the observed transitional probabilities under the four revisit norm and client reports as to whether or not they would have returned without an appointment. This allowed us to project the frequency distribution of total revisits and the expected mean.

All revisits optional. Modeling this norm follows the same logic as the one required revisit norm. However, since all revisits are now optional, we must calculate the probability of making a first revisit. Once the first revisit is made, we can use the same higher order transitional probabilities from the one revisit norm. Thus, the probability of making the first revisit was calculated as the sum of the probabilities of making exactly one (or two, or three, etc.) revisits under the old norm multiplied by the probability that at least one of these revisits would have been made without a routine appointment.

Table 4 presents projected frequencies of revisiting for the three norms. Requiring one revisit with others optional would produce an average of 1.48 revisits in the first year (a 36 percent reduction from current levels), and making all revisits optional would result in 0.83 revisits (a 64 percent reduction).

Problem detection. To estimate the rate of detection of method-related problems (hits) under the alternative norms, we need to know the problem rate among all new acceptors, whether or not they returned for a revisit. The client interview and medical examination provided information on problems for clients who returned for a revisit. We assumed that the problem rate among clients who did not return was greater than zero but less than that observed at the clinics. As an estimate, we used the problem rate among clients making a first revisit within three months of insertion who stated they would *not* have returned if they had not been given a routine appointment.

Probabilities of making at least one revisit (Y) and not making any revisit (N) were taken from the record search. The probabilities of hits (Y|y) and false alarms (Y|n) correspond to the proportions of revisits with and without diagnosed problems, multiplied by the probability of making at least one revisit. The probabilities of misses (N|y) and correct rejections (N|n) were estimated from the diagnosis rates among those clients who would not have returned for a revisit, multiplied by the probability of not making any revisit. The estimated underlying problem rate is the sum of hits and misses. The underlying rate for all problems was slightly less than 8 percent during the year after insertion. Estimated annual expulsion was 3.7 percent, and suspected pregnancy and PID 2.1 percent each. There was little variation in rates by time since insertion.[5]

Effectiveness of problem detection was calculated by dividing the probability of a hit by the underlying problem rate. We estimated that the current norm detects approximately 71 percent of expulsions, 67 percent of suspected pregnancies, and 83 percent of suspected PID.[6] Projected hit rates under the alternative norms are lower, reflecting the lower probabilities of making a revisit 0–3 months after insertion (all visits optional) and 4–12 months after insertion (one revisit required; all others optional). Table 5 shows underlying problem rates and detection levels for all norms.

The lower the frequency of revisiting, the greater the decline in percentage of medical problems detected. Therefore, the four revisit norm detects the most problems and the optional revisit norm the least. However, most clients with these problems reported that they would have returned without a routine appointment. Therefore, reducing the number of required revisits from four to one would capture only 7 percent fewer problems, or 55/10,000 insertions (roughly the CEMOPLAF annual caseload); while making all revisits optional would capture 20 percent fewer problems, or 159/10,000 insertions. Since clients appear to be better able to detect some problems than others and/or are more likely to seek treatment, changing the norms would have different impacts on the detec-

Table 5. Estimated annual problem and detection rate under three different norms

Indicator	Expulsion	Suspected Pregnancy	Suspected PID	Total
		Problem		
Annual problem rate	.0372	.0213	.0213	.0798
Problem detection Norm				
4 revisits	71%	67%	83%	73%
1 revisit	65%	57%	78%	66%
All optional	43%	50%	74%	53%

Table 6. Costs to the client for an IUD revisit

Type of Cost	Amount
Monetary costs	
Fee paid to CEMOPLAF	$0.76
Fares for transportation	$0.34
Total money costs	$1.10
Opportunity costs	
Transit time	$1.26
Clinic waiting time	$0.42
Total opportunity costs	
Total client cost	$2.78

tion of different problems. Detection of expulsions and suspected pregnancy would be most affected and detection of suspected PID least affected.

Client and program costs. Client costs included cash payments for transportation and clinic fees, and opportunity costs included time spent traveling and in the clinic. Opportunity costs were monetized by multiplying time by the official minimum wage (US $0.56 per hour). Travel time averaged two hours and fifteen minutes, and waiting time forty-five minutes. Almost half of clients were accompanied which contributed to transportation costs and clinic crowding. Transportation costs averaged US $0.34 for clients and their companions, and fees paid to CEMOPLAF averaged US $0.76. Table 6 presents the breakdown of client costs.

Opportunity costs comprise about 60 percent of costs, and cash payments the remaining 40 percent. The total estimated client cost of an IUD revisit is $2.78, the equivalent of five hours' pay at the minimum wage. Multiplying this by 2.31 visits a year yields US $6.39 in client costs under the current norm, or almost 13 working hours. The one revisit norm would have an estimated yearly cost per client of $4.11 (or about seven working hours), and the all revisits optional norm would reduce annual per client costs to $2.30 (or about four working hours).

The net cost of an IUD revisit to CEMOPLAF ranged from a low of $1.11 to a high of $2.25 over the six clinics studied. When the average client payment of $0.76 was subtracted, the net cost to CEMOPLAF ranged from $0.35–$1.49, with an average net cost in all clinics of $1.21.

Table 7. Comparison of three norms: Revisits, problems detected, and costs per 10,000 IUD insertions

			Outcomes		
				Annual Costs	
Norm	Revisits	Problems Detected	Agency	Client	Total
4 required revisits	23,100	582	$28,000	$64,000	$92,000
1 required revisit	14,800	527	$18,000	$41,000	$59,000
All revisits optional	8,300	423	$10,000	$23,000	$33,000

We also calculated total annual client and program costs for each norm. Table 7 shows estimated problems detected in the first year, revisits, and costs per 10,000 insertions.[7] Besides producing financial savings for both program and users, the alternative norms would also improve access. Requiring only one revisit could save 8,300 first year revisits (36 percent) a year at current levels of attention. This reduction in revisits would create openings for the equivalent of 3,000 new IUD clients without expanding clinic infrastructure. Making all revisits optional could save 14,800 first year (64 percent) revisits and create room for 8,000 additional new clients.[8]

The impact of changing the norm on *total* IUD revisits should be less than that shown in Table 7, for two reasons: First, some women make revisits during their second, third, and subsequent years of IUD use. They would be unaffected by the change in the first year norms. Second, some women who reported that they would not have made the revisit were it not for the norm, could be expected to make a revisit anyway (the reverse is less likely, that women who were not revisiting despite the norm, would begin to make additional visits if the norm were changed). We did not collect information on volume of IUD revisits made by women who had used the method for more than one year, and we have no way of assessing propensity to revisit beyond the clients' declared intentions in the interview.

Program impact. CEMOPLAF adopted a new norm of one required IUD revisit to be made no sooner than fifteen days after insertion. The new norm was implemented in all CEMOPLAF clinics during the first quarter of 1993. We evaluated the impact on total volume of revisits by comparing service statistics for the four quarters of 1992 with the four quarters of 1993. IUD consultations were classified as insertions or revisits.

The impact on the volume of revisits was almost immediate. Mean insertions per quarter remained the same between 1992 and 1993 (F < 1.0). Mean quarterly IUD revisits declined by 29 percent from 778 per clinic to 553 per clinic after changing the norm (F= 13.41, df 1,18, p < .01). Data on motivation for client revisits post-intervention (i.e., problems vs. routine check-ups) were not collected. Since revisits included women in their second and higher years of IUD use, the percent decline in IUD revisiting was less than predicted for women in their first year of use alone.

Discussion

As the present study illustrates, quality, cost, and access are interrelated. We have defined quality by outcomes to clients (i.e., detection of IUD-related medical problems), costs in terms of costs to both providers and clients (i.e., unnecessary visits), and access as provider capacity to serve and client capacity to pay in time and money. Program decisions necessarily involve tradeoffs, so that when administrators seek to improve one aspect, they must also consider potential impacts on the other two. This study was motivated by cost and access concerns. We found that changing the norm would result in a small decrease in quality (problems detected), but major cost savings and improvement in access.

Any norm specifying a routine revisit for all new acceptors will necessarily require clients who have no medical problems to come back. Regardless of their rarity, expulsion, PID, and pregnancy require prompt medical attention. Since most clients with these problems would return without a routine appointment, reducing the number of required revisits from four to one would capture only 7 percent fewer problems but reduce first year revisits by 36 percent.

Quality of care depends not only on the validity of the norm, but also on client compliance. Client compliance is conditioned both by anticipated benefits of detecting and resolving problems and by the costs incurred by unnecessary revisits. Thus, the original four revisit norm was fairly successful in ensuring compliance in making the first revisit, but was less successful in motivating subsequent revisits. Therefore, reducing routine revisits to a minimum and improving their timing not only improves program efficiency, it may also enhance client compliance.

This study suggests some methodological refinements for research on quality, costs, and access in family planning programs. While CEMOPLAF focused on IUD revisit norms, other factors may be equally important for cost containment, access, and quality. Programs should examine all operational procedures, beginning by asking why they were adopted in the first place. Some may be based on outmoded technology or reasons other than ensuring quality. The four revisit norm examined in this study, for example, was originally designed to gather data for clinical trials rather than to optimize client care.

Both managers and service providers must participate in identifying dysfunctional procedures and suggesting solutions. Preference should be given to data collection techniques that minimize program disruption. Research variables should include cost, access, and quality, and should not be limited to only one of the three factors as is usually the case in current family planning program research. Finally, in the study of quality, program processes need to be linked to client outcomes such as detection of medical problems, contraceptive acceptance and continuation, prevalence, and fertility impact.

This study relied on modeling, record review, and the collection of a small amount of interview data. It meets the criteria of staff involvement and unobtrusive design. It produced savings for program and users with minimal impact on problem detection, and created room for new users. More important, CEMOPLAF demonstrated that cost-control is compatible with quality, and that improvements in efficiency can improve rather than sacrifice access.

References

Adrian, L. K. et al. 1992. "Catalogue of Family Planning Service Delivery Guidelines. An Inventory of Policies and Procedures. Family Health International, Research Triangle Park, N.C. Unpublished Manuscript.

Brook, R.H. "Quality Assessment and Technology Assessment: Critical Linkages. 1988. in Lohr, K.N. and Rettig, R.A. *Quality of Care and Technology Assessment. Report of a Forum of the Council on Health Care Technology.* National Academy Press, Washington, D.C. pp. 29–38.

Bruce, J. 1990. "Fundamental Elements of the Quality of Care: A Simple Framework." *Studies in Family Planning* 21(2): pp. 61–69.

Chelminsky, E. 1993. "The Political Debate About Health Care: Are We Losing Sight of Quality?" *Science* Vol. 262 (22 October) pp. 525–528.

Coombs, C.H. et al. 1970. *Mathematical Psychology: An Elementary Introduction.* Prentice Hall, Englewood Cliffs, New Jersey.

Donebedian, A. 1969. *A Guide to Medical Care Administration. Volume II: Medical Care Appraisal-Quality & Utilization.* American Public Health Assoc., Washington, D.C.

Janowitz, B. et al. 1990. "Investing in the Future, A Report on the Cost of Family Planning in the Year 2000." Family Health International, Research Triangle Park, N.C.

Marx, M.H. and Hillix, W.A. 1979. *Systems and Theories in Psychology.* McGraw Hill, NY.

Tremaine, K. and Liskin, L. 1988. "IUDs—A New Look." *Population Reports* Series B, No. 5.

World Health Organization. 1987. "Mechanism of Action, Safety, and Efficacy of Interuterine Devices." Technical Report Series 756. Switzerland.

Notes

1. Two typical recent examples of family planning quality of care research are Miller et al, 1991, and Simmons, R. and Elias, C., 1993.

2. Cell probabilities are obtained by cross multiplying the probability of a problem with the probability of a revisit. Cell probabilities are multiplied by their relative benefits or costs to obtain the overall pay-off.

3. Clients who stated they had returned for a "check-up" were classified as weakly motivated.

4. Some clinical trials have found differential rates of problems by time since insertion (WHO, 1987). The constant rate found in the present study may reflect client self-

selection, with women experiencing problems more likely to return than women not experiencing problems.

5. Problem rates were estimated for two periods, 0–3 and 4–12 months after insertion to control for the possibility that problems, like revisits, varied over time. The probability of returning within three months of insertion was .732, and the probability of returning at least once between 4–12 months was .478. Detection of medical problems was cross tabulated by period and by whether or not the woman would have returned without a routine appointment.

We assumed that problem rates among clients who did not return were equal to the problem rates among clients who did return but who said they would not have returned if they had not had an appointment. Cross-multiplying probabilities of having or not having a problem provides cell estimates in the matrix. The estimated total expulsion rate is the sum of the rates in the first row of Table 1N.

Table 1N. Observed revisit rates and estimated expulsion rates, three months post-insertion

Problem	Revisit Yes	Revisit No	Total
Yes	(.732 * .023) = .0168	(.268 * .017) = .0046	.0214
No	(.732 * .977) = .7064	(.268 * .983) = .2634	.9786
Total	.732	.268	1.000

The TCU 380A was used by approximately 90 percent of the women interviewed. Estimated problem rates are within the range of published reports for 12 months of copper-bearing IUDs (see Tremaine and Liskin, 1988, Table 1, pp. 4–5). Table 2N presents problem detection rates and estimated underlying problem rates by period.

Table 2N. Probability of a problem in the first year after insertion

Problem	Detected 0–3 Months	Detected 4–12 Months	Detected Total	Estimated 0–3 Months	Estimated 4–12 Months	Estimated Total
Expulsion	.0168	.0096	.0264	.0214	.0158	.0372
Suspected pregnancy	.0066	.0076	.0142	.0074	.0139	.0213
Suspected PID	.0081	.0096	.0177	.0086	.0127	.0213
Total problems	.0315	.0268	.0583	.0374	.0424	.0798

6. The hit rate when all revisits are optional is the probability of detecting a given problem under the four revisit norm (Table 2N) × the probability that women with the problem would revisit without a routine appointment (Table 3). The hit rate under the norm of one required revisit is estimated as the sum of the hit rate at 0–3 months under the current norm plus the estimated hit rate at 4–12 months when all revisits are optional.

7. We calculated neither client or social costs resulting from misses nor client or social benefits resulting from greater access.

8. Capacity for additional users is calculated by dividing revisits saved by the estimated total visits per new acceptor (insertion visit + revisits) under the new norm.

Acknowledgments

The authors wish to thank Barbara Janowitz of Family Health International (FHI) for suggesting the research topic. The Office of Population, U.S. Agency for International Development, supported the study under contracts AID/DPE-3030-Z-00-9019-00, Operations Research and Technical Assistance in Latin America (Population Council) and DPE-3041-A-00-00-0043-00 (FHI).

Can the Bangladeshi Family Planning Program Meet Rising Needs Without Raising Costs?

Barbara Janowitz, Matthew Holtman,
David Hubacher, and Kanta Jamil

Programmatic issue: *How to provide more services without increasing program expenditures. Projections indicate that the number of couples of reproductive age will increase by about 40 percent (from 22 to 31 million) between 1994 and 2004.*

Programmatic process/components: *Outreach. Home visits by more than 23,000 field-workers are a basic component of the Bangladesh National Family Planning Program. Managers suspected that field-worker productivity (in this case, hours worked as a proportion of hours paid) was low, implying an important inefficiency in the service-delivery system. Reduction of the inefficiency would allow more clients to be served without hiring more field-workers and increasing personnel costs.*

Research design: *The project was a diagnostic study aimed at determining how field-workers spent their time, and at assigning costs to the activities they carried out. Data on field-workers' time use was collected through observation and record reviews. Salary costs were distributed by activity (for example, home visits, unauthorized leave, and meetings).*

Findings: *Only 59 percent of field-workers' paid time was spent on job-related activities. Unauthorized leave accounted for most of the time spent on non-job-related activities. According to estimates, elimination of unauthorized leave would increase the number of home visits from 219 to 293 per month, and the cost per couple year of protection among field-workers' clients would decline from $5.80 to $5.26. By the year 2004, population growth would require an increase in numbers of field-workers from 23,000 to almost 33,000, and would increase personnel costs from about $24 million to about $33 million, annually. In contrast, if unauthorized leave were eliminated, only 24,000 field-workers would be needed in 2004, and personnel costs would increase by less than $1 million.*

Program response to findings: *The study did not result in reforms to increase field-workers' productivity. A single study is seldom sufficient to rally the bureaucratic and political support needed to make fundamental changes in* *a government program employing thousands of workers. Research continues on changing the field-worker program in the public sector, including expanding the services package promoted by the worker.*

Discussion: *The authors increased the usefulness of their analysis by modeling three scenarios for increasing productivity by the year 2004. The scenarios included eliminating unauthorized leave, eliminating late arrivals and early departures and other wasted time to add one additional hour to the effective work day, and a combined approach that would eliminate both unauthorized leave and tardiness.*

The scenarios provide the manager with information on the results of different courses of action. A logical next step would be to determine which scenario would be possible to implement by conducting operations research to determine how best to reduce unauthorized leave and tardiness.

Can the Bangladeshi Family Planning Program Meet Rising Needs Without Raising Costs?

Barbara Janowitz, Matthew Holtman,
David Hubacher, and Kanta Jamil

Bangladesh is an emerging success story in family planning. In 1975, when the first national survey was conducted, 8% of married women of reproductive age were practicing contraception.[1] By 1983, the proportion had risen to 19%,[2] and in the subsequent 10 years, it more than doubled, reaching 45% in 1993–1994.[3]

Use of modern methods has grown steadily from 14% in 1983 to 36% in 1993–1994. Resupply methods (condoms, injectables and oral contraceptives) have accounted for most of this growth. For example, between 1983 and 1993–1994, the proportion of women using the pill rose from 3% to 17%, and the proportion relying on injectables grew from less than 1% to 5%. By contrast, over the same time period, the prevalence of IUD use increased only from 1% to 2%, and the prevalence of female sterilization grew from 6% to 8%.

Contraceptive methods are available through a variety of sources. Government and nongovernmental home service delivery programs provide resupply methods. Small fixed health facilities, known as family welfare centers, provide resupply methods and IUDs; satellite (mobile) clinics, which are scheduled once a month in existing facilities in different communities, also offer these methods. Family planning clinics located in *thana* (district) health complexes provide both temporary methods and sterilization. Two categories of workers provide services: family welfare assistants (fieldworkers) in the home service delivery program, and family welfare visitors (clinic workers) in the family welfare centers and thana health complexes. Both types of workers participate in service provision at the satellite clinics.

As the method mix has changed, so has the source of supply. Home service delivery programs provided 42% of resupply methods in 1989, but this share had increased to 70% by 1993–1994. Clinics accounted for a slightly smaller share of the source mix in 1993–1994 than in 1991, while the share of satellite clinics increased slightly.[4]

Despite the family planning program's great success, there are concerns that its expansion to meet the needs of a growing population and to raise contra-

Reprinted with the permission of The Alan Guttmacher Institute from *International Family Planning Perspectives* 1997. 23,5: 116–121, 145.

ceptive prevalence may entail unacceptably high costs. Cost increases could be most dramatic in the government home service delivery program. This program employs approximately 4,500 supervisors and 23,500 fieldworkers, who are assigned a geographic area and a specific number of couples whom they are expected to visit every two months, regardless of the couples' choice of contraceptive and method source. Yearly salaries and benefits for personnel in this program total $23 million. (The government hired 10,000 new fieldworkers between 1987 and 1991 in order to reduce the number of eligible couples for whom each worker was responsible. This increase undoubtedly contributed to the changes in both the method and the source mixes.[5])

In the clinic-based program, which encompasses approximately 3,000 family welfare centers and 350 clinics in thana health complexes, salaries and benefits for service delivery personnel and support staff total more than $7 million annually. Ensuring that all facilities and personnel are used as productively as possible is important to prevent unnecessary construction of new facilities or addition of staff at existing sites, which could raise costs. (Since the satellite clinics operate out of existing facilities, such as local schools or homes, and are staffed by fieldworkers and clinic workers earning their regular salaries, these clinics involve no added costs to the program.)

In this article, we synthesize findings on the costs and productivity of both the home service delivery and the clinic programs in order to suggest ways that resources may be used most efficiently. The two service delivery systems cannot be analyzed separately because women are supposed to receive home visits from a fieldworker regardless of their choice of contraceptive method and source. Moreover, important functions of the family welfare assistant include motivating clients to use clinical methods and counseling them about side effects; therefore, the costs of providing clinical methods include costs associated with the home service delivery program.

Previous studies have provided valuable information about the costs of the family planning program in Bangladesh.[6] These have taken a "top-down" approach, using primarily macro-level data to develop a broad picture of the costs of the program. This approach has the disadvantage of providing too little information about operations at the service delivery level to identify opportunities for improving the system's efficiency. Other studies have collected micro-level observational data (a "bottom-up" perspective) addressing the productivity of service providers.[7] These studies have been useful in documenting work activities, but they do not provide information on costs or on the potential savings that could be realized through changes in work strategies.

Our analyses address both the relationship between provider-level productivity and costs and the effect on costs of having overlapping delivery systems. The impact of increasing provider productivity is examined both at the level of the basic unit of service (i.e., the costs per couple-year of protection if home service delivery and clinic staff increased their work effort) and at the aggregate level (i.e., the costs of modifying the home service delivery program and clinic program to meet increased demand). Overlap is examined by estimating the portion of clinic methods' cost per couple-years of protection that is attributable to the home-visit program.

Methods

Between October 1993 and February 1994, data were obtained on service personnel at different types of government clinics in rural areas. Facilities and employees were chosen randomly, in the following manner.[8] Within each of the country's four "old" divisions (Dhaka, Chittagong, Khulna and Rajshahi), we constructed a sampling frame consisting of thanas with a health complex and at least four family welfare centers. The thanas were listed according to their proximity to each other, and two from each division were selected using a systematic sampling procedure (random selection of a starting thana and application of an appropriate sampling interval). Once a thana was selected, its health complex was included in the study. The family welfare centers in the selected thanas were numbered, and a random sample of four from each was chosen. The inclusion of satellite clinics was dependent on the selection of thana health complexes and family welfare centers and the work schedules of the family welfare visitors. For each of the eight thanas selected for the clinic portion of the study, two neighboring thanas were chosen for the home service delivery portion. By using the original eight thanas as "anchors," we concentrated the work in one geographic location in each division, thereby reducing field costs. The selection of family welfare visitors and supervisors in each thana was done using a simple random sampling procedure.

An observational study was carried out to determine how clinic personnel and fieldworkers spent their time, and this information formed the basis of the calculation of the cost of services per visit. While this measure is easy to compute and to understand, it is not a very useful way of comparing the costs of different methods or delivery systems. Therefore, we examine the costs per couple-year of protection. This measure is based on information about the costs of different types of family planning visits that took place either at a woman's home or at a clinic, the numbers of visits made by fieldworkers and method continuation rates.

Calculating Family Planning Visit Costs

The total cost of a visit includes the costs of contraceptives, supplies, capital and labor. Contraceptive costs were obtained from the U.S. Agency for International Development and UNFPA. Costs of capital items, supplies and construction costs were obtained from government purchase orders.

To determine how workers allocated their time, we began by abstracting information from workers' logbooks to construct a monthly work pattern. The logbooks for 64 fieldworkers and 48 clinic workers were used to calculate the number of days spent in different activities (e.g., home visits, satellite clinic work, meetings and training, authorized annual leave, and services related to aspects of health care other than family planning, such as immunization camps).

Second, surveillance of 32 family welfare assistants and 16 supervisors was conducted to determine the amount of unauthorized leave they take in a typical month.[a] Workers and supervisors selected for surveillance worked in different areas from each other and from those whose logbooks had been reviewed. (This was to ensure that no worker contributed information to more than one data collection instrument.) Observers recorded whether or not workers left their homes; both those who left their homes and those who did not were asked what kind of work they had done or why they had not worked.

We also conducted surveillance of 36 family welfare visitors (32 at family welfare centers and four at thana health complexes). Observers stationed at the clinics noted whether these workers arrived there and how long they stayed; if workers did not arrive on a day they were scheduled to be at the clinic, observers spoke with other clinic staff to see if the reason for the absence was known.

Third, with the workers' knowledge, an observational study was conducted to determine what types of activities were carried out during the workday. Again, the family welfare assistants and supervisors chosen worked in different areas from each other, as well as from workers included in the surveillance study. Trained female observers accompanied 64 family welfare assistants to the field, for an average of three days each, and recorded their travel time to and from the field and between households, the number of women they contacted, the duration of contact time with clients and whether they provided contraceptives or information about family planning or maternal and child health. Observers also accompanied 16 supervisors to the field for two days each and noted how much time they spent on field visits and on administrative activities, and how much time they spent unoccupied.

Observers spent six days noting the activities carried out by 32 clinic workers (16 at family welfare centers and 16 at thana health complexes), including various types of family planning and maternal and child health services and all other health services. They also obtained information on activities not specifically connected with client visits, such as administrative tasks, time spent on tea and bathroom breaks, and time spent unoccupied (idle time, time with friends or family, and absence for brief periods for personal reasons). Neither the observational study nor the surveillance component included clinic workers' supervisors, since they do not work at the clinics and their role is the focus of less attention among policymakers.

Finally, information was obtained from selected government facilities on the salaries and benefits of fieldworkers and clinic personnel.

Calculating Costs of Method Use

To calculate the cost per couple-year of protection, we added the costs of all home and clinic visits associated with the acceptance and use of a method. For example, a woman may receive a home visit during which the family welfare assistant motivates her to use oral contraceptives, another visit at which she accepts pills and subsequent visits for resupply or follow-up information. Or a woman may be motivated by a fieldworker, but receive her pills from a clinic and obtain resupply from the fieldworker. All of these costs are included.

We then determined the median number of months for which a woman using each method was protected against the risk of pregnancy, to standardize the costs of method use to units of one year. For temporary methods, we calculated the median number of months by applying life-table techniques to 12-month continuation rates; for female sterilization, we used the difference between age 45 and the average age at acceptance from the 1993–1994 Demographic and Health Survey (DHS).[9]

Results

Costs of Home Visits

On days on which the surveillance was carried out, one-quarter of family welfare assistants and more than one-half of supervisors did not work but were not on authorized leave; among the 24 family welfare assistants who left their homes in order to work, the mean length of time spent working or away from home was 3.25 hours. Our findings from the observational component of our study show that on days that fieldworkers went to the field, they spent an average of 3.75 hours working. Thus, it seems that fieldworkers worked longer hours when they knew they were being observed. (While the family welfare assistants' working days are stipulated, their hours per day are not; however, 5–6 hours per day is a reasonable maximum for women working in rural areas.[10]) The workers spent about two-thirds of their time traveling and about one-third with clients. Similar results have been reported in smaller studies.[11]

In all, $52 (78%) of each fieldworker's monthly salary covers the provision of family planning–related costs (Table 1). Of this total, 48% supports time spent making home visits, 11% covers time spent in meetings or making reports, and the remaining 41% is equally divided between authorized and unauthorized leave. For supervisors, whose work is entirely in support of family planning services, monthly costs total $68. Supervisors spent only one-third of their days working; about 44% of their salary covers unauthorized leave.

Family welfare assistants' cost per unit time for home visits was calculated by dividing each of the cost categories listed in Table 1 by the number of minutes the fieldworkers spent per month making home visits. Visits averaged about four minutes in length;[b] adding travel time increased labor input to 12 minutes per visit. The costs of visits vary from about 25 cents to about 40 cents (not shown).

Costs of Clinic Visits

One in five family welfare visitors who were to be observed did not report to work. On days that they worked, these personnel spent about 4.5 hours at the clinic; of this time, 1.8 hours was spent with clients, including 38 minutes with family planning clients. Family welfare visitors spent about 1.5 hours on support-ing tasks and were unoccupied an average of 1.3 hours per day. As with fieldworkers, the number of hours to be worked daily is not specified in clinic workers' job descriptions, but 5.5 hours seems a reasonable minimum;[12] there-fore, another hour is classified as "not at [clinic]."

About $16 (25%) of family welfare visitors' salaries and benefits cover family planning activities. Of this amount, a little more than one-third covers time the work-ers are unoccupied (13%), not at the clinic because they have arrived late or gone home early (10%) or on unauthorized leave (13%); only 18% covers time spent deliv-ering family planning services to clients, and the rest is accounted for by costs of overhead, meetings and training, and authorized leave (Table 2).

Clinic visits for family planning averaged about seven minutes in length. The labor cost of these visits ranges from about 37 cents to $1.69. The full cost (including labor, contraceptives, supplies and capital) ranges from $1.15 to $3.42.

Costs per Couple-Year of Protection

Although clients are supposed to receive six annual visits from family welfare assistants, they actually receive, on average, 3.6 visits.[c] Our data do not show how the number of visits varies by method. However, using information on the visit patterns shown in the DHS, we estimate that the annual number of visits ranges from two for acceptors of female sterilization to seven for for women ac-cepting oral contraceptives.[d]

Table 1. Monthly labor costs and percentage distribution of costs associated with the provision of family planning services, by activity, according to type of worker, home service delivery program, Bangladesh, 1993–1994

Activity	Fieldworker			Supervisor	
	Cost	%		Cost	%
Total	**$52.11**	**100.0**		**$68.03**	**100.0**
Work time	**30.78**	**59.1**		**24.30**	**35.7**
Home visit	25.15	48.3		0.00	0.0
Meetings, reporting	5.63	10.8		0.00	0.0
Administration	0.00	0.0		24.30	35.7
Leave time	**21.33**	**40.9**		**43.73**	**64.3**
Authorized	10.75	20.6		14.00	20.6
Unauthorized	10.58	20.3		29.73	43.7

Table 2. Monthly labor costs and percentage distribution of costs associated with the provision of family planning services by clinic workers, by activity

Activity	Cost	%
Total	$15.80	100.0
Days at clinic	8.92	56.3
Providing services	2.87	18.2
Meetings, training	2.09	13.2
Personal overhead*	0.32	2.1
Unoccupied†	2.02	12.8
Arriving late, leaving early‡	1.62	10.3
Days not at clinic	6.88	43.6
Meetings, training	1.29	8.2
Authorized leave	3.62	22.9
Unauthorized leave	1.97	12.5

*Includes lunch, tea and bathroom breaks. †Includes idle time, absence for short periods for personal reasons and time with friends or family. ‡Difference between 5.5 hours and the time actually spent at the clinic.

Effect of delivery system overlap. Women who use clinical methods or who get resupply methods from a source other than a fieldworker probably do not require six home visits a year. Therefore, one way to reduce costs is to reduce the number of home visits to these women.

Table 3 illustrates how costs of home delivery and clinic provision overlap. The costs per couple-year of protection for the pill total $5.80 if the method is initially provided by a fieldworker and $6.39 if it is initially provided at a clinic. Most of the higher cost is attributable to the inclusion of the clinic acceptance visit, since all pill users receive the same number of home visits, regardless of where they obtain the method. Thus, overlap increases costs.

Effect of increasing productivity. The analysis for family welfare assistants addressed the question of what would happen to costs and to the number of visits if fieldworkers increased their number of workdays by eliminating unauthorized leave or if they increased the time they worked by one hour per home-visit day.[e]

The elimination of unauthorized leave would add 6.2 workdays to each fieldworker's month, allocated equally across monthly activities. This change alone would increase the number of visits per month from 219 per fieldworker to 293 and would lower the labor cost per couple-year of protection for oral contraceptives by 17%, from $3.05 to $2.51 (Table 4). Alternatively, an extra hour of fieldwork per day would increase the monthly number of visits to 312 and would bring the labor cost down to $2.35. The combination of eliminating unauthorized leave and adding an hour of work would almost double the number of monthly visits (to 417) and decrease the labor cost per couple-year of protection by approximately one-third (to $1.97).

For clinics, we chose for illustrative purposes to assess the impact of an increase in demand for services supported by an increase of 50% of working time

Table 3. Costs per couple-year of protection for oral contraceptives, by type of cost, according to where method was initially provided

Type of cost	Home		Family welfare center	
	Cost	%	Cost	%
Total	$5.80	100.0	$6.39	100.0
Clinic acceptance visit	na	na	0.70	11.0
Home visit	3.05	52.6	2.94	46.0
Motivation	0.40	6.9	0.40	6.3
Acceptance	0.45	7.8	na	na
Resupply	2.20	37.9	2.54*	39.7
Contraceptives	2.75	47.4	2.75	43.0

Note: na=not applicable.

at family welfare centers. Table 5 shows that the cost per couple-year of protection of clinic visits for IUDs would decrease by about one-third, from $1.94 to $1.32. This is because labor and capital costs would produce a higher volume of visits, thereby lowering the average labor and capital costs per visit.

The total reduction in the costs per couple-year of protection would be only 14% (from $4.54 to $3.92), largely because an important component of the cost, home visits, would remain unchanged. (The cost of contraceptives would also remain the same.) Labor costs are higher for visits made to the homes of IUD acceptors than for visits made by acceptors to clinics. Follow-up visits made to the woman's home account for 39% of the cost per couple-year of protection in the baseline calculation. Since some IUD users will obtain follow-up services from clinics, this demonstates the effect of system overlap.

Projecting Costs to the Year 2004

An important concern for the government of Bangladesh and for donors is how to meet the projected costs of the home service delivery program, and how to modify the program so that it effectively meets the country's needs. We examined a range of scenarios, making various assumptions concerning improvements in efficiency, to project costs to the year 2004.

Table 4. Number of visits a fieldworker makes per month and cost per couple-year of protection for oral contraceptives provided by fieldworkers, assuming various changes to increase productivity

Type of cost	No change	No unauthorized leave	Extra hour of fieldwork per day	Extra hour and no unauthorized leave
Visits per month	219	293	312	417
Total costs	$5.80	$5.26	$5.10	$4.72
Labor	3.05	2.51	2.35	1.97
Fieldworker	2.41	1.97	1.86	1.55
Supervisor	0.64	0.54	0.49	0.42
Contraceptives	2.75	2.75	2.75	2.75

Table 5. Cost per couple-year of protection for IUDs and projected cost if clinic workers' time spent providing services increased by 50%, by type of cost

Type of cost	Current	Projected
Total	**$4.54**	**$3.92**
Clinic	**1.94**	**1.32**
Labor	1.02	0.68
Acceptance	0.59	0.39
Follow-up	0.16	0.11
Removal	0.27*	0.18
Supplies	0.08	0.08
Capital	0.84	0.56
Home visit	**2.02**	**2.02**
Motivation	0.24	0.24
Follow-up	1.78	1.78
Contraceptives	**0.58**	**0.58**

* Calculated from mean time for removal observed at thana health center.

All of the scenarios assume that between 1994 and 2004, the number of couples of reproductive age will grow by about 40%, from 22 million to 31 million, and that the government program will continue to reach 77% of couples. They also assume that the method mix and, therefore, the number of visits per couple per year remain constant.[f] Results of these various assumptions are shown in Table 6.

Under the first scenario, we assumed that the program will grow proportionately with the number of eligible couples. The result would be a staff of 32,861 family welfare assistants and 6,295 supervisors (compared with 23,500 and 4,500, respectively, in 1994), with annual salaries and benefits totaling $33 million (up from $23 million).

The next scenario examines the effects of eliminating unauthorized leave. Assuming that the amount of contact time spent per client remains constant, this change would lead to an increase in the annual number of home visits made by each family welfare assistant from 2,599 to 3,511. The number of visits made per year to each couple is assumed to be the same; consequently, the numbers of family welfare assistants and supervisors would increase only slightly, and the change in costs would be small. However, the number of eligible couples for whom each family welfare assistant is responsible would be 973 (compared with 719 in 1994).

Another scenario assumes that family welfare assistants increase the number of hours that they work per day from four to five, but that they do not increase the number of days that they work. The results are similar to those of the previous scenario, in that the projected total costs of salaries and benefits would be almost identical to what they were in 1994.

Finally, we examined the impact of both eliminating unauthorized leave and increasing the number of hours worked per day. Under this scenario, costs

Table 6. Characteristics of the home service delivery program, 1994, and projections of characteristics in 2004, assuming various changes to increase productivity

Characteristic	1994	2004			
		No change	No unauthorized leave	Extra hour of fieldwork per day	Extra hour and no unauthorized leave
No. of home visit days per month per fieldworker	11.4	11.4	15.4	11.4	15.4
No. of home visits per day per fieldworker	19	19	19	27	27
No. of home visits per year per fieldworker	2,599	2,599	3,511	3,694	4,990
No. of home visits for all fieldworkers (in millions)	61.1	85.4	85.4	85.4	85.4
No. of couples (in millions)*	16.9	23.7	23.7	23.7	23.7
No. of visits per couple per year	3.61	3.61	3.61	3.61	3.61
No. of couples per fieldworker	719	720	973	1,023	1,382
No. of fieldworkers	23,500	32,861	24,326	23,124	17,118
No. of supervisors	4,500	6,295	4,660	4,430	3,279
Total salaries and benefits (in millions of $)	23.5	32.9	24.3	23.1	17.1

*Scenarios assume that the number of couples will grow from 22 million in 1994 to 31 million in the year 2004 and that the government program will continue to reach 77% of couples.

of salaries and benefits ($17 million) would be considerably lower in the year 2004 than they were in 1994. However, the number of eligible couples per family welfare assistant would roughly double, to 1,382.

Another concern is whether to increase the number of clinics serving women in rural areas. To address this issue, we analyzed the extent to which existing excess clinic capacity could be used to expand services without building new facilities.[8] The monthly number of visits per clinic was calculated for current levels of productivity and then projected under the assumption of increased working hours. We assumed that some of the observed work time now spent either unoccupied or away from the clinic would be used to provide services to clients.

We estimate that the current number of visits per month is 29.8 at family welfare centers, 18.8 at thana health complexes and 43.3 at satellite clinics. Using information from the clinic observations of how workers' time is distributed among different activities, we project that with the assumed increase in efficiency, these numbers would rise to 57.1, 23.7 and 65.8, respectively.

Table 7 shows the estimated and projected number of aggregate visits per month for all rural clinics.[h] More than 1.6 million visits are currently conducted by family welfare visitors who work at rural clinics; the potential number of visits would increase to 2.9 million if unused time were used to provide services to clients, assuming that contact time per client remained constant. Thus, the number of additional visits produced per month depends solely on the amount of unused time at each type of clinic.

Assuming an unchanged contraceptive prevalence rate, the total demand projected for the year 2004 would be 2.3 million visits, or about 80% of the projected number of visits if productivity increased. However, if we assume an increase in the contraceptive prevalence rate, the projected demand rises slightly above the projected number of visits to 3.1 million. Nevertheless, given that fairly conservative assumptions were made regarding the increase in productivity (no decrease in unauthorized leave, no decrease in time spent on administrative tasks and only 50% of unoccupied time used for visits), even with an increase in contraceptive prevalence, the existing number of clinics should be able to accommodate the increase in demand.

Discussion

Before discussing the implications of our results, we should point out some of the study's limitations. Our productivity estimates depended upon secret observations of both clinic providers and fieldworkers. Although the sample for these observations was selected randomly, the sample size is relatively small. Some of the workers who were secretly observed realized that they were being observed and may have altered their behavior; for example, some fieldworkers

Table 7. Number of clinic visits conducted in 1994 and number that would be conducted if unused time were reduced; and projected number of visits required in 2004, by trend in contraceptive prevalence rate; all according to type of clinic

	Conducted in 1994		Required in 2004	
Type of clinic	Actual	Reduce unused time	Constant prevalence	Increased prevalence*
Total	1,641,740	2,912,052	2,298,436	3,146,548
Family welfare center	1,110,364	2,125,673	1,554,509	2,128,116
Thana health complex	81,806	103,065	114,528	156,789
Satellite clinic	449,570	683,315	629,398	861,643

*We assumed that prevalence will increase from 46% to 63% (see: A. Barkat et al., *Strategic Directions for the Bangladesh National Family Planning Program, 1995–2005*, Ministry of Health and Family Welfare, Dhaka, 1996), that the demand for services other than family planning will increase in proportion to the demand for family planning services and that the method mix will remain unchanged.

may have left the house and gone to work even though they otherwise might not have done so.

Similarly, when workers were accompanied to the field or observed in clinics, their performance levels may have been higher if they wanted to impress the observer. Consequently, our results probably present a more optimistic picture of productivity and costs than is the norm. However, as we have pointed out, the findings for observations in which family welfare assistants were accompanied to the field are similar to those of other studies.

Another potential limitation is that the projected costs of the home service delivery program depend on the assumption that the method mix remains constant. However, even if the method mix shifts, contraceptive costs would change, but labor costs would remain the same as long as additional workers were not hired.

The increase in the contraceptive prevalence rate over the last few years is due in large part to the growth of the home service delivery program. At the same time, that growth has undoubtedly also contributed to the proportionate decline in the use of long-acting and permanent methods and to the lack of use of clinics. Now that the program is maturing, ways that it might be improved need to be considered, including changes in both the clinic and the home service delivery programs.

Although the increase in contraceptive use has led to a fall in the total fertility rate from 6.3 births per woman in the mid-1970s to 4.2 in 1990,[13] the population will continue to grow substantially over the next decade. If the current program structure is maintained, 32,861 family welfare assistants and 6,295 supervisors will be needed by the year 2004. Given that donor resources are unlikely to keep pace with costs, decisions will need to be made as to how to cut costs while maintaining the quality of care. Thus, the government of Bangladesh needs to consider how to strengthen management in order to increase performance levels of fieldworkers and supervisors.

Our calculations show that if fieldworkers were to increase the number of days and hours worked, the costs of the program could remain at the current level (or even fall) over the next 10 years. An important question is whether these changes are realistic, in that they assume an increased work effort on the part of fieldworkers. One way of answering this question is to compare government fieldworkers with fieldworkers from nongovernmental organizations who have similar salaries. Fieldworkers employed by nongovernmental organizations are less likely to take unauthorized leave and therefore spend more days making home visits than government workers;[14] this suggests that it is not unreasonable to expect fieldworkers to work additional days. Moreover, family welfare assistants can increase the number of eligible couples for whom they are responsible by visiting more couples per day.

Not only must management be strengthened, but technical issues concerning the appropriate job of the family welfare assistant also need attention. For example, given that family welfare assistants spend a high proportion of their workdays traveling, alternative service delivery strategies should be considered that can reduce travel time and increase client contact time.

One such strategy would be a cluster visitation system. Another strategy would be for family welfare assistants to reorganize their work plans to target specific subgroups of clients who are most in need of their services. For example, women who get their pills or condoms from a source other than the family welfare assistant and clients who are established users of resupply methods might be contacted less frequently. Women who use clinical methods, especially those who have been sterilized, do not need to be visited frequently.

A reduction in time spent on visits to women requiring less attention will allow more time to be spent with nonusers, new users, and users having side effects and other problems. The government should consider revising visit guidelines to reduce the number of required visits for users of particular methods.

In the last several years, the number of family welfare centers has expanded and the use of long-acting methods has stagnated. As a consequence, there is underutilized capacity in the clinic program. Existing facilities can therefore continue to accommodate client demand as the population of women of childbearing age grows, provided that women have reasonable access to these facilities. Decisions regarding clinic expansion should take into consideration that in the short run, these facilities are underutilized. Moreover, provision of long-acting methods can be expanded at low cost by using the unoccupied time of family welfare visitors. An important concern for the program, therefore, is how to encourage the acceptance and continued use of long-acting methods.

The existence of two overlapping systems of service delivery has important implications for the costs of family planning service delivery. Efforts to reduce costs per couple-year of protection must take this into consideration. For example, acceptors of methods at clinics also receive visits at home, and the home visit costs constitute a significant part of the total costs per couple-year of protection. If the number of home visits for clinic method acceptors were reduced, then the costs per couple-year of protection would decrease. However, this reduction of overlap will not lead to any reduction in overall costs per couple-year of protection for the home-visit program unless the time that the family welfare assistants save is redirected in ways that can increase contraceptive use and continuation rates, or the number of family welfare assistants is reduced.

The current structure of the family planning program has had remarkable success. The program has significantly increased awareness and use of family planning services. Moreover, the expansion of the home service delivery program has led to significant improvements in contraceptive use. However, challenges lie ahead, especially with regard to serving a growing number of married women of reproductive age under conditions of diminishing resources. This article points to areas that can be improved and to strategies that can be used to reduce costs. Changes in strategies and program structure should enable Bangladesh to make gains in contraceptive use while increasing use of long-acting methods without incurring significant increases in program costs.

Notes

a.   All data collection strategies for this study were approved by a steering/revision committee, headed by and composed largely of officials of the government of Bangladesh, which was a major sponsor of the study. Names of observed workers were never used on data collection forms in order to protect the workers' identities.

b.   More than three-quarters of visits lasted less than five minutes. More than half of visits to method acceptors were longer than four minutes, compared with fewer than one-third of visits to nonusers or continuing users.

c.   In 1993–1994, there were approximately 22 million couples of reproductive age in Bangladesh. There were about 30,000 outreach workers, of whom 77% were government family welfare assistants and 23% were employed by nongovernmental organizations. Assuming that the government fieldworkers covered 77% of eligible couples, or 17 million couples, then 101 million visits were made 4,409 per family welfare assistant. Field workers' logbooks indicated that they spent 15.4 days in the field each month; thus, they would need to make an average of about 24 visits per day to see each client every two months. Our data show that they made about 19 visits per day and spent about 11.4 days per month in the field. Therefore, they likely visit the average client 3.6 times per year, or once every 3.5 months.

d.   Calculations based on data from the DHS suggest that the annual number of visits averaged 2.5 (ranging from fewer than two among sterilization acceptors to about five for users of injectables or oral contraceptives). We inflated the method-specific estimates so that they averaged out to 3.6, the estimated annual number based on our findings, and used the adjusted method-specific averages to calculate the cost of follow-up visits associated with each method.

e.   Alternatively, fieldworkers could spend more time with each client.

f.   We have made this assumption in order to simplify the cost calculations. However, as the population grows and contraceptive prevalence increases, the method mix may continue to change in favor of resupply methods. Such a shift would likely have little, if any, impact on the number of visits; even if fieldworkers increased the number of visits they make to users of resupply methods, costs would change only if the number of workers increased.

g.   Our analysis is meant to be illustrative. The example ignores differences in the distribution of unproductive time by clinic and by time of day, and does not address whether clinics are easily accessible. Our data show that the average user of a rural clinic spends about an hour in transit to and from the clinic. However, we have no information on whether travel time constituted a barrier for women who did not use clinics. (See: S. Kabir, "Client Costs for Family Planning Services Delivered at Fixed Clinic Facilities in Bangladesh," in Population Council, *Key Issues in Family Planning Service Delivery in Bangladesh*, Dhaka, 1997.)

h.   While the estimated number of visits per day is highest at satellite clinics, the monthly total is highest at family welfare centers, as family welfare visitors spend more time at these facilities than they do at satellite clinics. The projected increase in the monthly total of visits is greatest for family welfare centers because time available to increase visits is highest at this clinic type.

References

1. M.N. Islam and M.M. Islam, *Bangladesh Fertility Survey, 1989: Secondary Analysis*, National Institute of Population Research and Training, Dhaka, 1993, pp. 29–72.

2. S.N. Mitra and G.M. Kamal, *Bangladesh Contraceptive Prevalence Survey, 1983: Final Report*, Mitra and Associates, Dhaka, 1985.

3. S.N. Mitra et al., *Bangladesh Demographic and Health Survey, 1993–1994*, National Institute of Population Research and Training (NIPORT), Mitra and Associates, and Macro International, Calverton, Md., USA, 1994.

4. Ibid.

5. S. Hussain et al., "Recruiting Appropriate Female Field Workers: Experiences from a National Recruitment Process in Bangladesh," paper presented at the International Centre for Diarrhoeal Disease Research, Bangladesh (ICDDR,B) annual scientific conference, Dhaka, Oct. 26–28, 1991.

6. G.B. Simmons, U. Rob and S. Bernstein, "An Economic Analysis of Family Planning in Bangladesh," Department of Population Planning and International Health, University of Michigan, Ann Arbor, Mich., USA, 1986; and G.B. Simmons, D. Balk and K.K. Faiz, "Cost-Effectiveness Analysis of Family Planning Programs in Rural Bangladesh: Evidence from Matlab," *Studies in Family Planning*, 22:83–101, 1991.

7. M.A. Koblinsky et al., "Helping Managers to Manage: Work Schedules of Field-Workers in Rural Bangladesh," *Studies in Family Planning*, 20:225–234, 1989; S.J.G. Brechin and M.A. Koblinsky, "Quality of Care in Community-Based MCH-FP Programs: The Field Worker's Perspective," ICDDR,B Working Paper No. 56, Dhaka, 1990; Y. Hasan and M.A. Koblinsky, "Work Routine of Female Family Planning Field Workers (FWA) in Rural Bangladesh," paper presented at the ICDDR,B annual scientific conference, Dhaka, Oct. 26–28, 1991; and M.A. Rashid et al., "Determinants of Utilization of Satellite Clinics," NIPORT, Dhaka, 1992.

8. B. Janowitz et al., "Productivity and Costs for Family Planning Service Delivery in Bangladesh: The GOB Program," Family Health International, Research Triangle Park, N.C., USA, 1996.

9. A. Larson, S. Islam and S.N. Mitra, *Pill Use in Bangladesh: Compliance, Continuation and Unintentional Pregnancies. Report of the 1990 Pill Use Study*, Mitra and Associates, Dhaka, 1991; M.B. Hossain, J.F. Phillips and J.G. Haaga, "The Impact of Fieldworker Visits on Contraceptive Discontinuation in Two Rural Areas of Bangladesh," paper presented at the annual meeting of the Population Association of America, Miami, Fla., USA, May 5–7, 1994; and S.N. Mitra et al., 1994, op. cit. (see reference 3).

10. Y. Hasan and M. Koblinsky, 1991, op. cit. (see reference 7).

11. M.A. Koblinsky et al., 1989, op. cit. (see reference 7); and S.J.G. Brechin and M.A. Koblinsky, 1990, op. cit. (see reference 7).

12. M.B. Rahman, director, Population, Development and Evaluation Unit, Ministry of Planning, Dhaka, personal communication, June 1994.

13. S.N. Mitra et al., 1994, op. cit. (see reference 3).

14. B. Janowitz et al., 1996, op. cit. (see reference 8); and——, "Productivity and Costs for Family Planning Service Delivery in Bangladesh: The NGO Program," Family Health International, Research Triangle Park, N.C., USA, 1996.

The Impact of Service Delivery Frequency on Family Planning Program Output and Efficiency

James R. Foreit, James E. Rosen, Miguel Ramos, Eduardo Mostajo, and Rosa Monge

Programmatic issue: *To determine the most cost-effective frequency for mobile clinic visits.*

Programmatic process/components: *Provision of services by mobile clinics has been a feature of many different family planning programs. Frequency of visiting by mobile clinics is a major determinant of the costs and outcomes of this program component. INPPARES, the Peruvian IPPF affiliate, wished to know the most cost-effective frequency for mobile clinic visits.*

Research design: *An experimental design known as a randomized block design was employed. Communities were matched by population size and other characteristics and randomly assigned to one of three interventions: once-per-week mobile clinic visits, twice-monthly visits and once-per-month visits. Dependent variables included total visits, family planning visits, IUD insertions, and costs.*

Findings: *Depending on the indicator, twice-monthly visits produced 1.5–2.1 times the output per session produced by once-per-month sessions, and 1.3–1.6 times the output per session produced by weekly sessions. The twice-per-month frequency was also 7–38 percent more cost effective than were monthly visits, and 6–28 percent more cost-effective than were weekly visits.*

Program response to findings: *INPPARES switched all mobile clinics to a twice-per-month visit schedule. Other NGOs in Peru also adopted the twice-per-month frequency for their mobile clinics.*

Discussion: *In this case, the use of an experimental design was neither intrusive nor overly costly. Little or no motive existed for reliance on a less powerful research technique. The design featured random assignment of matched study units. Matching is an common technique used to ensure the comparability of groups. It reduces the probability that outliers in the study population will end up in only some of the experimental groups and not in others. The technique is especially useful when the sample size is* *small. (In the case of the INPPARES study, each group had only 14 mobile clinic sites.) The need for matching declines as sample size increases, because a large sample size ensures comparability.*

The Impact of Service Delivery Frequency on Family Planning Program Output and Efficiency

James R. Foreit, James E. Rosen, Miguel Ramos,
Eduardo Mostajo, and Rosa Monge

Operations research (OR) can be distinguished from other social science research by its emphasis on the study of factors that can be manipulated by program administrators. The major limitation of OR as a family planning management tool is that it is usually situation-specific, with results limited to a single program at a particular point in time.

While family planning programs differ in size, approach, and contraceptive methods offered, they do share some operational features. One common but often overlooked factor controllable by managers is the frequency of performing program activities. For example, if output is sensitive to the frequency of supervisory visits, the manager can choose between the frequency that produces the most output or the most cost-effective output. If performance is insensitive to changes in frequency, supervisory visits can be reduced and resources assigned to more productive activities.

Foreit and Foreit (1984) examined the effect of varying frequency of supervision on a community-based distribution (CBD) program in Brazil. They found that reducing the frequency of supervisory visits from once a month to once every three months did not have an impact on program output. This finding allowed managers of one program to increase the number of distributors without increasing the number of supervisors. In other areas, the number of supervisors was reduced, producing large cost savings.

The present report extends the study of frequency from program support activities to service delivery. The operational variable was frequency of holding clinical sessions in medical back-up posts in a CBD program in Lima, Peru.

Program Setting

The Instituto Peruano de Paternidad Responsable (INPPARES) operates family planning clinics, community posts, and CBD programs throughout Peru. In mar-

Reprinted with the permission of the Population Council from *Studies in Family Planning* 1990.
21,4: 209–215.

ginal urban areas of Lima, CBD distributors sell pills, condoms, and spermicides and keep a proportion of the modest payment. Medical back-up for the distributors is provided at community posts by physicians who are brought into the community in an INPPARES van. Services are provided in space donated by the community. Physicians perform IUD insertions and follow-up, and check oral contraceptive users for contraindications and side-effects. (The program is voluntary. Women who wish to receive the pill from CBD workers are not required to see a post physician.) They also provide general reproductive health services. Physicians are assisted by CBD workers who also sell all oral contraceptives, condoms and spermicides to patients. All routine resupply visits are made to the distributors, making it unnecessary for the clients to return to the posts to just obtain a cycle of pills or a supply of condoms.

The community post component was developed in response to the legal requirement for medical supervision of family planning activities, to make the IUD readily available to the CBD program target population, and to provide an adequate quality of care for CBD acceptors.

During its first year (1984) the medical back-up component produced modest results. In 321 sessions, two physicians provided 1,221 family planning services and inserted only 125 IUDs. Probable causes for under-utilization were low visibility (posts functioned irregularly and their location often varied from session to session) and a reluctance by distributors to make IUD referrals.

To overcome these difficulties, INPPARES trained distributors in IUD counseling and began to pay them a small fee(US$0.29) for IUD referrals. Distributors brought women to the posts for insertions, and were paid the referral fee at the end of the session. Post sessions were held at fixed locations and on a fixed schedule. Finally, an OR study was conducted to determine the most effective, efficient, and cost-effective frequency of post sessions per month.

Methodology

The study included 42 posts in urban marginal areas of Lima. Three frequencies of post functioning were compared: once a month, twice a month, and weekly.

The experiment used a randomized block design. The 42 posts were matched in 14 blocks of 3 posts each, which were matched for prior performance, number of CBD workers, and district population size. Equal numbers of family planning talks were scheduled for each post, and physicians were randomly assigned to all three frequencies. The experiment lasted 12 months, from August 1985 through July 1986.

Three output indicators were constructed: effectiveness, efficiency, and cost-effectiveness. *Effectiveness* was operationally defined as the total number of services performed during the year of the experiment. *Efficiency* was defined as the mean number of services performed per session.

Services included family planning visits and non-family planning visits. A family planning visit was defined as any visit where a family planning service (including IUD insertion) was provided. A non-family planning visit was any visit where the client did not receive a family planning service. Non-family planning visits included gynecological and obstetric examinations, pap tests, and pregnancy tests. Women returning for the results of a test were counted as post visits. Women wishing just family planning information, or those who came only to purchase a method from a CBD worker, were not counted as post visits. Total visits were the sum of family planning and non-family planning visits. IUD insertions are also included as an output, as increasing the availability of this method was a major objective of the back-up component. The number of program acceptors (women making a first visit to a post for a family planning service) was also included as an indicator of the number of different persons receiving family planning services. Acceptors included active CBD users who came for an IUD insertion or to consult with a physician about pill side-effects, for example, as well as women who were new either to INPPARES or to family planning.

Cost-effectiveness was the ratio of total net costs associated with operating a post (net costs equal total program costs minus total program income) to total outputs produced by that post. Outputs include sessions, family planning visits, total visits, IUD insertions, and program acceptors.

Four cost components were identified. *Post start-up costs* are the one-time fixed costs of establishing posts and included CBD worker training and post equipment. *Session costs* included physician salaries, supervision, and transportation. *Patient costs* consisted of contraceptives, patient records, and consumable medical supplies. *Administrative costs* included the salaries of the CBD coordinator and secretary, and the indirect costs of salaries, services, and equipment. Costs were calculated in constant *intis*, using December 1986 as a base, and converted to dollars at the December 1986 financial market exchange rate (I/17.4 = US$1.00).

Results

Clinic sessions were held as scheduled. The once-per-month posts completed 98 percent of scheduled sessions while the twice-a-month and weekly groups completed 97 percent and 96 percent, respectively. Mean duration of the clinic sessions held by the monthly and twice-per-month group was 2.9 hours (standard deviation = .84 and .73, respectively). Mean duration for the weekly group was 2.8 hours (standard deviation = .67). About 73 percent of the family planning talks scheduled for the monthly group were actually completed compared to 66 percent for the twice-monthly and weekly groups. There was no drop-out among physicians, supervisors, or administrative staff.

During the year of the experiment, the 42 posts held 1,136 clinic sessions and received 11,196 visits, including 5,371 family planning visits. A total of 1,705 women accepted a family planning method at the posts. Approximately 77 percent were IUD acceptors, 15 percent accepted pills, and 8 percent accepted barrier methods.

There was a total of 4,768 IUD visits, including 1,387 IUD insertions (a 214 percent per session increase over the previous year, due to the administrative improvements mentioned above), 63 removals, and 3,318 routine IUD revisits. There were also 414 pill visits and 189 barrier method visits. Approximately 89 percent of all family planning visits were IUD-related.

About 87 percent of all IUD insertions were referred by CBD workers and 5 percent by supervisors. Distributors brought virtually all IUD clients to their own posts, regardless of session frequency. Supervisors were each responsible for several posts, and usually sent clients to higher-frequency posts. Only 5 of the 14 once-per-month posts received supervisor IUD referrals, whereas all twice-per-month and weekly posts received referrals.

Table 1 presents, by frequency and post, total visits, non-family planning visits, family planning visits, program acceptors, and IUD insertions. There were 2,054 total visits in once-per-month posts, 3,501 in twice-per-month, and 5,641 in weekly posts. Output increased linearly with session frequency, but in lesser proportion than the increase in number of sessions held. Differences among the three frequency groups are statistically significant for all outputs.[1] Depending on the variable selected, twice-per-month posts had 1.5–2.1 times the output of once-per-month posts, and weekly posts had about 1.3–1.6 times the output as twice-per-month posts.

Table 1 also presents the mean number of total visits, family planning visits, non-family planning visits, program acceptors, and IUD insertions per session by frequency. No significant differences among treatments were found for IUD insertions, program acceptors, or family planning visits per session. However, differences in non-family planning and total visits per session were statistically significant.[2] Differences in total visits resulted from differences in the number of non-family planning visits per session. Although frequency was not a determinant of the number of family planning clients per session, it was a determinant of non-family planning visits and, therefore, of total visits.

Two measures of cost-effectiveness were derived. *Observed cost-effectiveness* was calculated from the actual results of the study, in which both costs and outputs varied by treatment group. Table 2 shows observed costs by component,

Table 1. Community-based distribution back-up program activity by total, post, and session, August 1985 to July 1986

Variable	Once per month	Twice per month	Weekly	All frequencies
		Frequency		
Total number of posts	14	14	14	42
Total number of sessions	165	317	654	1136
Mean hours per session	2.9	2.9	2.9	
Client visits				
Total	2054	3501	5641	11196
Non-family planning	1150	1777	2898	5825
Family planning	904	1724	2743	5371
Program acceptors	353	577	775	1705
IUD insertions	213	449	725	1387
Visits per post				
Total	146.7	250.1	402.9	266.6
Non-family planning	82.1	126.9	207.0	138.7
Family planning	64.6	123.1	195.9	127.9
Program acceptors	25.2	41.2	55.4	40.6
IUD insertions	15.2	32.1	51.8	33.0
Visits per session				
Total	12.4	11.0	8.6	9.9
Non-family planning	7.0	5.6	4.4	5.1
Family planning	5.5	5.4	4.2	4.7
Program acceptors	2.1	1.8	1.2	1.5
IUD insertions	1.3	1.4	1.1	1.2

percent distribution of costs, program income, total net cost, net cost per unit of output, and the index of net cost per unit. Session costs were the highest component costs, followed by administrative costs. Total net costs were highest in weekly posts and lowest in monthly posts. For all visit and acceptor indicators, posts operating twice a month had a lower cost per unit of output than did monthly or weekly posts. Cost per visit was US$3.39; per family planning visit, $6.88; per program acceptor, $20.56; and cost per IUD insertion was $26.42. The once-per-month frequency was 7–38 percent less cost-effective, depending on the variable selected, and the weekly frequency was between 2 and 23 percent less cost-effective. Cost-effectiveness differences between twice-per-month and weekly posts were small for client indicators other than program acceptors.

Lower per-session costs for weekly posts did not translate into lower visit and acceptor costs because the weekly posts had fewer visits per session than twice-per-month posts. Lower session costs mean lower visit costs only when clients fill sessions to capacity. For all groups, session costs were greater than post, patient, or administrative costs.

In the *projected cost-effectiveness* model we asked how many posts operating once a month, twice a month, or weekly, the program would need to produce 11,200 visits (an obviously attainable target), and how much they would cost to operate. Setting a level of output and then calculating the cost needed to

Table 2. Observed cost-effectiveness in December 1986 US dollars

Variable	Frequency		
	Once per month	Twice per month	Weekly
Start-up costs	$1,509 (18%)	$1,509 (12%)	$1,509 (7%)
Session costs	3,227 (39%)	6,364 (51%)	13,039 (63%)
Patient costs	759 (9%)	1,379 (11%)	2,115 (10%)
Administrative costs	2,677 (33%)	3,347 (27%)	4,016 (19%)
Total costs	8,172 (100%)	12,599 (100%)	20,679 (100%)
Program income	(424) (738)	(1,125)	
Net cost	7,748 11,861	19,554	
Net cost per:			
Session	46.96	37.42	29.90
Visit	3.77	3.39	3.47
Family planning visit	8.57	6.88	7.13
Program acceptor	21.95	20.56	25.23
IUD insertion	36.68	26.42	26.97
Index of net cost per:*			
Session	125	100	80
Visit	111	100	102
Family planning visit	125	100	104
Program acceptor	107	100	123
IUD insertion	138	100	102

Note: Total percent may not equal 100 due to rounding. * Twice a month=100.

achieve it eliminates possible errors in cost-effectiveness ranking due to scale effects. Theoretically, any output can be considered for decision-making. INPPARES managers were interested in the total program and selected visits as the most appropriate expression of this interest. The projection of costs is not a simple expansion. Economies and diseconomies of scale were identified and included in the projected cost-effectiveness analysis.[3]

The results of the projection are shown in Table 3. In order to achieve approximately 11,200 visits per year at observed efficiency levels, 78 once-per-month posts, 44 twice-per-month posts, and 28 weekly posts would be required. Net cost of twice-per-month posts was lowest, followed by weekly and once-per-month posts. Figure 1 shows that at all frequencies, cost per unit of output (total visits) decreases as output increases.[4] As in the observed model, projected total net costs were lowest in the twice-per-month posts. The twice-per-month system would be the most cost-effective for all indicators except cost per session. Cost per visit would be $3.17; per family planning visit $6.44; per family planning acceptor $19.24; and $24.72 per IUD insertion. The once-per-month frequency would be between 7 and 38 percent less cost-effective, depending on the indicator (equal to observed results), and weekly would be 6–28 percent less cost-effective (compared to 2–23 percent for observed results). The projection had no impact on the differences between once-per-month and twice-per-month posts observed earlier. However, the cost-effectiveness differences between twice-per-month and weekly posts increased as a result of the simulation.

Table 3. Projected cost-effectiveness (based on 11,200 total annual visits)

Variable	Once per month		Twice per month		Weekly	
			Frequency			
Start-up costs	$7,315	(17%)	$ 4,683	(12%)	$ 3,445	(8%)
Session costs	15,576	(37%)	18,308	(48%)	24,990	(61%)
Patient costs	4,127	(10%)	4,407	(12%)	4,256	(10%)
Administrative costs	14,917	(36%)	10,518	(28%)	8,032	(20%)
Total costs	41,935	(100%)	37,916	(100%)	40,723	(100%)
Program income	(2,311)		(2,362)		(2,271)	
Net cost	39,624		35,554		38,452	
Net cost per:						
Session	44.03		35.03		29.15	
Visit	3.54		3.17		3.38	
Family planning visit	8.04		6.44		6.95	
Program acceptor	20.58		19.24		24.60	
IUD insertion	34.10		24.72		26.29	
Index of net cost per:*						
Session	126		100		83	
Visit	112		100		107	
Family planning visit	125		100		108	
Program acceptor	107		100		128	
IUD insertion	138		100		106	

Note: Total percent may not equal 100 due to rounding. * Twice a month = 100.

The distribution of projected costs is also shown in Table 3. A comparison of the observed and projected cost distributions demonstrates that at widely varying levels of program scale (for example, there were 14 actual monthly posts versus 78 projected monthly posts, and so on), cost distribution remains almost the same. Session frequency determines cost structure.

Cost and output calculations are subject to error and may vary over time and between programs. To test the robustness of the cost-effectiveness rankings, sensitivity analyses were conducted by changing the values of program cost components and family planning outputs, and measuring the impact of these changes on the rankings.

Seventeen components ranging from training costs to the useful life of IUD insertion kits were varied. Twice per month remained the most cost-effective option, even when costs were alternatively halved, doubled, and tripled. The rankings were insensitive to changes in the costs of individual inputs because most components accounted for only a small percentage of total program costs.

The sensitivity of cost-effectiveness rankings to changes in output was tested by reducing the number of IUD insertions in twice-per-month posts while holding the number of insertions in weekly posts constant. Insertions in twice-per-month posts were reduced until the cross-over point was reached and weekly posts became the most cost-effective alternative.

Cost-effectiveness was sensitive to output. Unlike costs, relatively small changes in output produced changes in cost-effectiveness rankings. The cross-

Figure 1. Visit cost at different output levels, by post session frequency

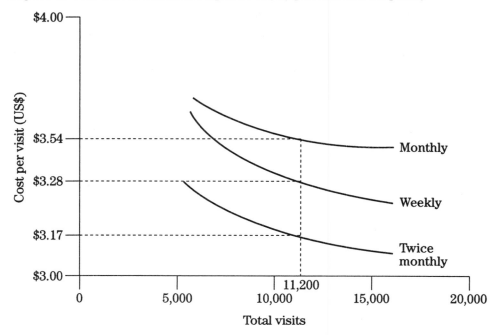

over point for IUD insertion cost-effectiveness was reached when the number of insertions in twice-per-month posts was reduced by 7 percent. The cross-over point for family planning visits was reached when insertions were reduced by 9 percent, and the cross-over point for total visits was 16 percent.

Observed output was used in making cost-effectiveness projections. The correctness of the assumption of real differences in observed output despite lack of statistical reliability was tested by examining post performance over time. Following the experiment, all posts were placed on a twice-a-month schedule, and output remained at projected levels for two years. Between October 1986 and September 1988, the mean number of insertions per session was 1.38 (s.d.=.38). The mean number of family planning visits was 6.74 (s.d.=.95), mean non-family planning visits, 4.43 (s.d. = .65), and mean total visits, 11.17 (s.d.=1.0).

Discussion

This study shows that session frequency has an important impact on the costs, effectiveness, cost structure, and cost-effectiveness of a rotating medical post system. However, efficiency of family planning services was not influenced by frequency. It appears that program norms produced IUD referral patterns that eliminated variation between frequencies. Two distributors worked at every session. Almost all IUD insertions came from distributor referrals, and distributors usually brought clients only when they worked. This resulted in little variation in insertions per session, regardless of post frequency. Since most family planning visits were related to IUDs, frequency did not influence family planning visits per session.

Frequency did influence the efficiency of non-family planning visits, and thereby indirectly influenced total visits per session. No referral fees were paid for non-family planning visits, and most of these clients came to the post without a distributor. Non-family planning clients with access to lower frequency posts had to concentrate their visits in fewer sessions than women using higher frequency posts.

Frequency was a major determinant of total costs because session costs were much greater than post costs. Frequency also influenced cost-effectiveness: increasing frequency from one to two sessions per month produced economies of scale in post and administrative costs, as did increasing frequency from two sessions a month to once a week. But since efficiency declined at the weekly frequency, cost per unit of output increased relative to the two-sessions-per-month posts.

The observed and projected models produced the same cost-effectiveness rankings, but the projection added important information for administrative decision-making. It produced total cost estimates for a program operating at a single frequency, and demonstrated that cost-effectiveness differences between twice-per-month and weekly posts would increase. The finding indicates that cost-effectiveness analysis of family planning programs needs to go beyond observed results. Cost-effectiveness should be projected so that scale effects can be taken into consideration.

INPPARES selected twice-per-month sessions for its medical post program because the trends in efficiency and cost-effectiveness favored this frequency. Other factors were also considered. Monthly sessions were rejected because they produced too many non-family planning visits. The once-a-week frequency was rejected because it would have meant reducing the number of posts, and INPPARES was reluctant to diminish its geographic coverage.

Program utilization suddenly increased at the end of 1988, and many posts had more clients than could be served during a single session. INPPARES switched the most popular posts to weekly sessions, the most cost-effective frequency for posts functioning at capacity.

Also as a result of the study, two other private family planning organizations with CBD programs in Lima, APROSAMI and PROFAMILIA established back-up posts operating twice a month. There are now more than 140 posts operating in urban marginal areas of Lima. The system was also extended to Arequipa, Trujillo, Cusco, and Iquitos, the largest cities in Peru after Lima.

Family planning agencies in Bolivia and Paraguay tested posts operating at a weekly frequency as a less costly and more cost-effective alternative to permanent clinics in both rural and urban areas. The weekly frequency was selected because managers decided that, for small pilot programs, effectiveness was more important in the short term than cost-effectiveness. In Quito, Ecuador, the city government plans to open twice-per-month posts during 1990.

Frequency is one of the few variables truly under the control of program managers and can be an important tool for the rational and equitable provision of services. Frequency of performing family planning activities can be adjusted to a number of factors, including demand for services, availability of resources, and political considerations. A program can begin offering services relatively infrequently, and then increase as demand builds. Alternatively, if high initial demand is expected, services can be offered frequently at the start of a program and decreased if demand is lower than anticipated.

Program administrators may wish to cover more communities than their budgets appear to allow. In this case it may be possible to increase the number of family planning units by decreasing session frequency, with little or no overall loss in program effectiveness and efficiency.

Because it can be so readily controlled by administrators and influences important program variables such as output and costs, the study of frequency should be extended to examine its impact on family planning acceptance and continuation, and on user characteristics. Frequency of services availability may be related to such poorly understood factors as opportunity costs for users, source substitution, and ultimately to overall contraceptive prevalence and method mix.

Reference

Foreit, James R. and Karen G. Foreit. 1984. "Quarterly versus monthly supervision of CBD family planning programs: An experimental study in northeast Brazil." *Studies in Family Planning* 15, 3.

Notes

1. IUD insertions: $F=11.3$, d.f. 2,26, $p<.01$; program acceptors: $F=6.2$, d.f. 2,26, $p<.01$; family planning visits: $F=10.8$, d.f. 2,26, $p<.01$; non-family planning visits: $F=21.6$, d.f. 2,26, $p<.01$; total visits: $F=17.2$, d.f. 2,26, $p<.01$.

2. IUDs per session: $F=.73$, d.f. 2,26, $p>.05$; program acceptors: $F=3.1$, d.f. 2,26, $p>.05$; family planning visits per session: $F=1.2$, d.f. 2,26, $p>.05$; non-family planning visits per session: $F=8.4$, d.f. 2,26, $p<.01$; total visits per session: $F=4.4$, d.f. 2,26, $p<.05$.

3. The model generated economies of scale in transportation costs. These were largely determined by the difference between posts. As the number of posts in the marginal urban areas of Lima increases, the average distance between them decreases, mak-

ing it possible for a van and driver to visit more posts per day. We estimated that the INPPARES coverage area was 410 square kilometers. Assuming a uniform geographical distribution of posts, the distance between them is equal to the square root of the total area divided by the number of posts. Using the coverage area, and estimates of upper and lower bounds on the number of visits one can make per day, we obtained the number of posts visited in one month from the linear least-squares regression $pm = a + bd$, where pm is the number of posts visited in one month by one driver and d is the distance between posts in kilometers. The estimation yielded values of $a = 78.11$ and $b = -7.79$ ($R^2 = .84$). We used a similar logic to calculate how kilometers per post visit changes with distance between posts. We obtained the number of kilometers per post per session from the equation $km = a + bpd$, where km is the number of kilometers per post per session and pd is the number of posts visited in one day. The estimation yielded values of $a = 38.61$ and $b = -6.72$ ($R^2 = .95$). The model produced a distance per post of 18.4 km per session for once per month, 20.4 for twice per month, and 22.4 km for weekly frequencies. The data were then used to calculate transport costs.

During the year of the experiment, the number of sessions missed varied somewhat by frequency, due to random factors. In contrast, the projection assumed that posts of each frequency would only cancel sessions on holidays (ten working days per year). A simple expansion of observed results for once-per-month posts requires 76 posts to produce 11,200 visits. Because the projection increases the number of missed sessions for once-per-month posts, it requires two more posts to produce the same number of visits. Also, the projection model requires only 44 twice-per-month posts to obtain 11,200 visits rather than the 45 posts obtained by simple expansion, because the number of missed visits is lower than actually observed.

4. Figure 1 is not accurate at the extremes of the curves, and differs slightly from Table 3.

Acknowledgments

The authors are indebted to Dr. Karen Foreit for her comments and extensive use of red ink on earlier drafts of this paper, and for the assistance of Sonia Ortiz, Jose Garcia-Nunez, and Peggy Levvitt during the experiment. We also wish to thank Dr. Marcia Townsend, who was with USAID Office of Population, Research Division at the time of the study, and was project monitor for the study. Funding for this project was provided by the USAID Office of Population. The study was conducted as part of the Population Council INOPAL project, Operations Research to Improve Family Planning and Maternal–Child Health Service Delivery Systems in Latin America and the Caribbean (USAID contract DPE-3030-C-00-4074-00) as Population sub-grant C185.01A.

Increasing Use of Reproductive Health Services in a Peruvian Clinic

Federico R. León, Aníbal Velásquez, Lissette Jiménez,
Adolfo Reckemmer, María E. Planas, Rubén Durand,
and Alicia Calderón

Programmatic issue: *The need to identify strategies to increase clinic revenues by increasing the use of existing services.*

Programmatic process/components: *The process manipulated was information given to clients. INPPARES increased the availability of non-family planning reproductive health services. These services were underused, and the organization was searching for a promotional method that would increase the demand for services and increase revenue to help cover costs. The organization wished to determine whether a simple pamphlet distributed to new clients by the clinic receptionist would increase demand and revenues.*

Research design: *An experimental design was used. In a single clinic, a month's clinic sessions were matched on the day of the week and randomly assigned to intervention (use of the pamphlet) and control conditions (no pamphlet). Dependent variables included the number of services purchased at intervention and control clinic sessions, the number of services purchased by individuals participating in experimental and control sessions within 30 days of the session, and money paid for the services used by the study groups.*

Findings: *Distribution of pamphlets reliably increased use of reproductive health services both at the clinic session at which the intervention occurred and within 30 days of clients' receiving the pamphlet. Were the intervention to be implemented on a system-wide basis, introduction of the pamphlet was estimated to be capable of increasing INPPARES revenues by approximately $40,000 per year.*

Program response to findings: *INPPARES decided to distribute pamphlets at all agency clinics.*

Discussion: *The study demonstrated how a low-cost promotional tool, administered within the service-delivery point can increase service use and revenue. The study also reminds us that initial demand for new reproductive health services may be low and that programs will have to promote them. A major* *limitation of the study is that it does not tell us if the prices charged for the underused services allowed the program to break even or generate a profit that could be used to subsidize other services. A next step for INPPARES would be to determine if the services could be sold at break-even or profitable prices. Methodologically, the study shows that meaningful field experiments can be conducted in as little time as one month, and that use of experimental designs are possible, even when the research is being conducted in only one service-delivery point.*

Increasing Use of Reproductive Health Services in a Peruvian Clinic

Federico R. León, Aníbal Velásquez, Lissette Jiménez,
Adolfo Reckemmer, María E. Planas, Rubén Durand,
and Alicia Calderón

Introduction

Over the past few years, many family planning organizations in developing countries have taken steps to implement the Cairo Agenda (United Nations, 1995) and expand their services to include other aspects of reproductive health. In so doing, they have dedicated human resources and infrastructure to provide reproductive health services that in the past were seldom offered. These organizations now face the challenge of increasing use of the newly available services.

Many family planning clients are still unaware of the other reproductive health services available. The Peruvian IPPF affiliate, INPPARES, expanded the services of its largest Lima clinic, Patres, in 1995. Nevertheless, when clients were asked in 1996 to name new services they would like to see the clinic offer, 34 percent mentioned treatment of STDs, cancer screening, antenatal and other reproductive health services that were already offered by the clinic (Velásquez et al., 1996).

Lack of client knowledge about and the consequent use of newly installed capacity has serious financial implications, especially for organizations in the process of becoming independent of external support. At a time when international donors are phasing out their financial assistance, idle infrastructure is a needless drain on limited resources.

Interactive Pamphlet as a Solution

Velásquez et al. (1997) proposed an information, education, and communication (IEC) solution to the use of reproductive health services offered by Patres. The authors developed a pamphlet that clinic clients could use to help decide if they needed any of the reproductive health services available on site. Based on an algorithm developed in Mexico and Guatemala (Vernon and Ottolenghi, 1996), the pamphlet asked the client (1) whether she had been screened for cancer in the past year; (2) if she or her partner had STD symptoms; and (3) if she had

© 1998 by The Population Council, Inc. Reprinted with permission.

other reproductive health problems. The folder informed the client about the appropriate services offered by Patres. Clinic receptionists were trained to give the pamphlet to each new client and explain its contents using a flipchart.

Velásquez et al. (1997) tested this approach over ten days chosen at random from 6 March through 4 April 1997 and used the other ten working days of this period as a control. The purpose of the study was to determine if the interactive IEC strategy would increase use of the clinic and increase clinic revenues. Unfortunately, the results were confounded by a concomitant price reduction of the promoted services, which made it impossible to isolate the impact of the pamphlet from the impact of the reduced prices. Thus, INPPARES decided to repeat the study, this time avoiding contamination, to test the hypothesis that the pamphlet would increase service demand and clinic income.

Methodology

As in the original study, 20 calendar days were randomly assigned to the intervention and control conditions. However, in contrast with the previous approach, prices were left unchanged. The study employed a true experimental design with cohort data (the aggregate of clients coming to the Patres clinic on a given day) as the units of analysis.

All working days (Monday through Friday) of four successive weeks from 13 October through 7 November 1997 were chosen as units of study. A stratified random assignment of calendar days to experimental conditions was conducted to ensure that the days of the week were equally represented in the experimental and control groups (for example, two Mondays when pamphlets were distributed and two Mondays when they were not).

The study was limited to new clients[1] whose first visit occurred during the study period and included the first clinic visit and any subsequent visits during the following 30 days. On the days chosen for the intervention, each new client entering the clinic was directed to the admissions counter, where a trained receptionist handed her the pamphlet and explained its contents using a flipchart. The pamphlet offered early detection of gynecological cancers, diagnosis and treatment of STDs, as well as general medical, pediatric, and psychological counseling. Once the client asked for the service(s) she wanted, the receptionist entered her personal data in the clinic's computerized database, and sent the client to the cashier to pay for the services. The cashier, in turn, entered the amount paid for each service.

The procedure was the same on control days, with the difference that the client was not given a pamphlet or an explanation by the receptionist. The same service prices were charged on intervention and control days: approximately US$7 for reproductive health, family planning, or other health consultations, and more for ecography, IUD insertion, and other, more complex clinical procedures.

Upon completion of the intervention period, four sets of client data were retrieved from the clinic's database: (a) number of services purchased on the day on which the clinic history was opened; (b) total amount paid on that day; (c) number of services purchased by the client over the following 30 days; and (d) total amount paid during the follow-up period.

Results

Group Equivalence

As Figure 1 shows, Monday, Wednesday, and Friday were the days on which most new clients came to Patres. The counterbalanced presence of weekdays in intervention and control groups, however, controlled this variable. Thus, no significant differences were found in number of new clients registered on intervention and control days: daily totals ranged from 18–39 in the intervention group (mean: 26.2, median: 23.5) and from 17–32 in the control group (mean: 25.1, median: 26.5).

Services and Payments on First Visit

Figure 2 shows the mean number of services purchased on the first visit per client cohort and reveals that the intervention group purchased more services than did the

Figure 1. Daily fluctuation in number of new clinic clients, Lima, Peru, 1997

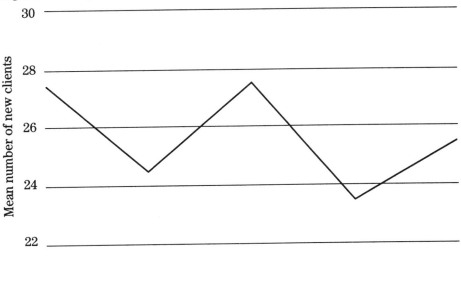

Figure 2. Mean number of services per clinic client, by date, according to intervention and control groups, Lima, Peru, 1997

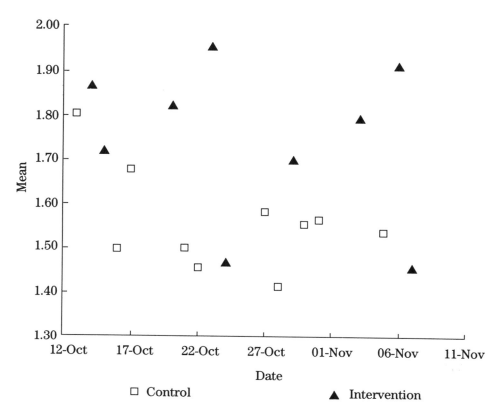

control group. Owing to the nonnormal distribution of the means, a nonparametric statistic, Mann-Whitney's U, was selected to test the difference between the distributions. U with N = 20 was equal to 19.5, significant at the $p < 0.01$ level (one-tailed).

The overall cohort means for the intervention and control groups were, respectively, 1.77 and 1.56, and the medians were 1.80 and 1.54.

Overall means and medians for the amount paid on the first visit were 40.73 and 40.22 *soles* (about $15) in the intervention group and 31.0 and 29.97 *soles* ($11) in the control group. Mann-Whitney's U was equal to 20, significant at the $p < 0.02$ level (one-tailed).

In sum, the intervention proved to be effective, significantly increasing the number of services purchased by 13 percent and the mean amount spent by 28 percent.

Follow-up

Figure 3 shows the means and medians obtained in the analysis of the follow-up data. A 64 percent difference in number of visits and 67 percent in revenue was

Figure 3. 30-day follow-up: Means and medians for number of clinic services purchased and amount paid, per treatment condition (N = 10), Lima, Peru, 1997

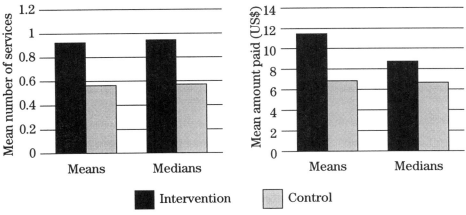

Note: 2.7 soles = $US1.

observed among new clients making subsequent visits in the month following study enrollment. Mann-Whitney Us were 20.0 for services and 19.0 for revenue, significant, respectively, at the $p < 0.02$ and $p < 0.01$ levels (one-tailed), suggesting that the pamphlet continued to motivate the purchase of services after the client left the clinic.

Impact on Clinic Revenues

To control for fluctuations in cohort size, a constant daily number of new clients was set at 25.6, the observed mean of all observation days. Multiplying this mean by the mean price paid per day, during the month of the intervention and the 30-day follow-up period, the Patres clinic earned a total of US$6,810 from the experimental group and $4,785 from the control group. The difference ($2,025) can be attributed to the effects of the pamphlet over the ten intervention days. We can assume that, had the pamphlet been given to both groups, that is, for a total of 20 days, the increase in revenue to the Patres clinic would have doubled ($4,050). If this trend were maintained for one year, INPPARES would increase revenues by about $48,600.[2] The cost of the intervention includes printing the pamphlet and the time taken by the admissions clerk to explain its use. At most, total costs in one year would come to $6,800,[3] meaning a net gain of at least $42,000 that could be obtained by Patres in one year from the use of a simple pamphlet.

Discussion

Like many other family planning NGOs striving to implement the Cairo agenda, INPPARES faced the challenge of increasing the use of recently expanded reproductive health services. Lacking a carefully developed new-product introduction strategy, and suspecting its clinic providers were not screening family planning clients for reproductive health needs, it sought a compensatory IEC solution to a situation in which resources were not being fully used. Introduction of an interactive pamphlet that asked questions about the client's health and informed her about the various services available resulted in increasing the number of services purchased by new clients of the Patres clinic on their first visit by 13 percent, and in increasing the number of subsequent visits in the following month by 64 percent.

The observed change in clients' purchasing behavior suggests that the intervention increased clinic visitors' awareness of the reproductive health services offered by the clinic and their awareness of their own need for reproductive health services. The interactive pamphlet gives information about both the existence of services and the need for such services.

Shrinking donor contributions to family planning programs in Latin America are forcing NGOs to become more self-sufficient. As an organization in the process of becoming more independent of external support, INPPARES not only used the pamphlet as a way to improve the cognitive availability of reproductive health services to family planning clients but also as a vehicle of income generation to increase its financial sustainability.

In implementing the new strategy, INPPARES successfully broke with the tradition of relying on physicians and other professional staff to induce changes in clients' behavior. Receptionists are low-cost workers from whom high levels of compliance with the task can be expected. Finally, the study demonstrated that an NGO may find programmatic solutions that integrate institutional goals usually viewed as requiring opposite courses of action. Generally, efforts to improve access to services are viewed as antagonistic to those used to increase the financial sustainability of programs. In this study, an interactive pamphlet improved clinic revenues and simultaneously increased awareness about reproductive health problems and services.

The results of the study convinced INPPARES managers to use the pamphlet-based system on a routine basis, and the organization made provisions for its reprinting. The system is now being used routinely by Patres and will be inaugurated in all 12 of INPPARES' clinics. Furthermore, INPPARES is planning to use the solution tested here in outreach efforts targeting potential clients. Family planning promoters who perform educational activities in the community will distribute the pamphlet to potential clients outside the clinics.

Finally, INPPARES learned from the study that Tuesdays and Thursdays are the days on which fewer clients come to Patres, and is devising ways to take advantage of this trend, such as programming staff meetings and other administrative activities requiring the participation of professional staff on these days.

Notes

1. INPPARES defines a new client as any person for whom a new clinical history is opened, either a first-time visitor to the clinic or someone returning after a period of five years or longer.

2. Notice that this figure may be an underestimate because it is based on a yearly projection made from only 20 working days per month and it ignores the possibility of giving the pamphlet to women who are clients of the clinic in addition to new clients.

3. This estimate takes into account the reduction of the unit-cost of printing the pamphlet for a one-year clientele. Receptionists dedicated seven minutes with each new client to the task of explaining the use of the pamphlet.

Acknowledgments

This study is a follow-up of a research project devised by Aníbal Velásquez, Adolfo Reckemmer, María Elena Planas, and Rubén Durand with the technical assistance of Ricardo Vernon that was sponsored by the Operations Research Workshop of the Institute of Population Studies (IEPO) of Universidad Peruana Cayetano Heredia (Lima, December 1996), funded by the United States Agency for International Development. The authors appreciate the detailed editorial advice of Jim and Karen Foreit and the comments of Bob Miller on an earlier manuscript.

This is an English version of an article published in Spanish in 1998: "Incrementando la utilización de servicios de salud reproductiva en una clínica de Lima," in *Investigación de Operaciones en Planificación Familiar y Salud Reproductiva: Conceptos, Métodos, y Casos*. Lima: IEPO and Population Council. Federico R. León and M. Chu, eds. The project was financed by the United States Agency for International Development, Office of Population.

References

United Nations. 1995. *Draft Platform for Action*. New York: United Nations.

Velásquez, Aníbal, N. Ostolaza, T. Williams, and James R. Foreit. 1996. "Encuesta de satisfacción de usuarias en la clínica Patres de INPPARES." Lima: INPPARES. Unpublished.

Velásquez, Aníbal, Lissette Jiménez, Adolfo Reckemmer, and María E. Planas. 1997. "Algoritmo de oferta sistemática de servicios de salud reproductiva." Lima: INPPARES. Unpublished.

Vernon, Ricardo and E. Ottolenghi. 1996. *Algoritmo y guía para la oferta sistemática de servicios de salud reproductiva (ALGOSISSAR)*. Mexico: Population Council.

QUALITY OF CARE

Introduction

James R. Foreit

All of the operations research themes in this book are influenced by social values, and the most ideological of all is, arguably, quality. In health care, quality is defined as a program attribute that relates to whether the right thing is done and whether it is done well (Aday et al., 1993). Quality has always been a family planning program issue, and the theme of quality of care has always been present in OR, most obviously in studies testing the safety of non-physician provision of contraceptives, and in assessing the affects of program norms (see, for example, Rosenfield and Limcharoen in the Impact section and Foreit et al. in the Resources section of this book). Quality concerns did not move to center stage until the 1990s, however, when the priority of many family planning programs began to shift from reducing population growth rates to improving the reproductive health and reproductive rights of individual women (Family Care International, 1994). The concept of quality of care helps meet the new priority because it combines elements of patients' rights with attempts to improve reproductive health outcomes.

In the 1990s, programs have made public commitments to quality: Detailed definitions of family planning quality have been produced, quality-improvement techniques have been borrowed from industry and applied to programs, and some research has been conducted on the topic. OR efforts have been dominated, however, by diagnostic studies describing the level of quality in a given program. Little operations research has been conducted to improve the treatment of clients or to demonstrate that higher-quality service delivery produces better outcomes than lower-quality service delivery. Therefore, one of the objectives of this introduction is to suggest topics for intervention research that may influence directly the quality of family planning services.

Presently, programs, donors, and women's health advocates focus on three aspects of family planning program quality that may be summarized as voluntarism (Bulatao, 1998), humane treatment of clients, and appropriate and competently provided services. *Voluntarism* means that responsibility for decisionmaking remains with the person using the program, that women and men are not coerced into using family planning or into choosing a specific method, and that clients are given enough information to make an informed choice of contraceptive method.

Humane treatment means that program staff provide care that is compassionate and considerate. They do not strike, shout at, ignore, or otherwise mistreat the client. It also means that they respect the client's modesty, answer clients' questions, and address common complaints such as excessive waiting time, lack of privacy, and uncomfortable surroundings.

Voluntarism and humane treatment need no further justification because they are human rights. Thus, in OR studies, we can treat them as dependent or outcome variables. Operations research can help programs increase voluntarism and humane treatment of clients by working with managers to define these outcomes operationally and to make changes in program processes that improve them. For example, most programs require signed informed-consent forms before sterilizations are performed or postpartum IUDs inserted. This indicator of voluntarism might be expanded to include comprehension of the information on the form or proof that the patient had received counseling before undergoing the procedure. Informed method choice could be measured by scores on standardized tests of clients' knowledge of contraceptive methods, and clients' participation in method selection could be evaluated through observations of the client–provider interaction or through "mystery client" visits. Program processes and activities that might be manipulated to improve voluntarism include provider training and patient education and counseling. The humane treatment of clients can be measured through a number of existing techniques. An operational analysis technique, patient-flow analysis, can be used to measure waiting time and to identify the bottlenecks contributing to excessively lengthy waits. Mystery clients and observations and interviews with program users can be used to obtain information about mistreatment. Provider education and supervision may be promising avenues for increasing humane treatment of clients in programs.

The third element of quality of care, *appropriate and competently provided services* refers to services that, when correctly provided, can have important impacts on users' reproductive health status and on their ability to control their own fertility. The hypothesis to be tested in OR studies is: The more appropriate the services and the more competent their provision, the greater the health and fertility outcomes and impacts. When referring to family planning services, "appropriate and competent" means, at a minimum, that a program provides a range of contraceptives adequate to serve the needs of different segments of the client population (Potter, 1971; Jain, 1989), that clients are taught their correct use, and that providers are able to administer the methods they distribute correctly and to follow up on contraceptive users (Bruce, 1990).

Appropriate and competent service provision is best treated as a program input or an independent variable, because we justify the cost and effort involved in improving this element by increased program outcomes and impacts, and ultimately an improved benefits-to-cost ratio (Sheps, 1955; Donebedian, 1980;

Chelminsky, 1993; Nash, 1995). Managers face a complex challenge when dealing with appropriate and competent service provision. They must determine how much to invest in specific quality improvements, for example, relative to how much in program expansion. The question is not, should the program be of better quality, but how much better and what kind of improvement (Bulatao, 1998).

The basic OR challenges are to identify which quality improvements affect outcomes and to determine the cost of the outcome improvement. Operations research should begin with determining the outcomes that the program should be designed to improve. Once the desired outcomes have been identified, the program should take into account whether improving quality might help to achieve that outcome. When it has been determined that improving quality has the potential of achieving the desired outcomes, the relationship between quality and outcomes should be tested prospectively with an experimental design.

When quality is treated as an independent variable, two types of indicators must be considered, those that measure the level of quality being provided, and those that measure the degree to which outcomes are affected by quality. Both types are relevant to the study of appropriate and competent services. The level of quality offered by a program has been measured by different kinds of indicators ranging from simple ones that try to capture a single aspect of quality (for example, providers' scores on a standardized test to demonstrate technical competence), to scales that attempt to measure the overall level of quality offered by a service-delivery point or program by combining simple indicators (Mensch et al., 1996).

A number of outcome measures are available to the OR researcher studying quality as an independent variable. These include such commonly used indicators as fertility change, contraceptive prevalence, and family planning continuation rates, as well as less frequently used measures of contraceptive morbidity and fulfillment of individuals' fertility desires. A common validity problem in quality of care research is the confounding of quality and access. Access indicators are often used as quality indicators, with the result that we are measuring levels of access rather than levels of quality (see, for example, Brown et al., 1995; Mensch et al., 1996). Access is a construct that is distinct from quality (see section three in this volume). Moreover, access is a precondition for quality: Without access, quality is irrelevant. When access to services exists, the research challenge is to demonstrate that improving quality results in better outcomes than those obtained through access alone.

Client satisfaction is sometimes proposed as an outcome of improved quality (Donebedian, 1980; Bruce, 1990). Most attempts to measure satisfaction with family planning services directly have been unsuccessful, however, resulting in reports of unvaryingly high levels of satisfaction in virtually all circumstances. As conceptualized in the marketing literature, satisfaction is manifest in brand loyalty, repeat business, and word-of-mouth advertising. Similarly, in the health literature, satisfaction is manifest in better compliance and good word-of-mouth advertising (MacStravic, 1991). By extension, satisfaction measures in family planning programs might include adoption of family planning methods, continuation of family planning, and, ultimately, contraceptive prevalence.

The number of quality of care studies in the OR literature is still relatively small, and individual studies often suffer from one or more of the problems discussed above. The three papers included in this section have been selected as being representative of OR on quality in family planning programs. As is typical of the larger quality literature in OR, two of the three papers use the Bruce (1990) definition of quality in organizing the research. This definition is based on the work of Donebedian (1980) who examined quality in the United States medical care system. Bruce specifies six quality elements including (1) choice of methods; (2) information given to clients; (3) technical competence; (4) interpersonal relations; (5) continuity of use; and (6) appropriate constellation of services.

The first reading in this section is a situation analysis conducted in Senegal (National Family Planning Program of Senegal). Situation analysis is a frequently used tool for measuring how well a program is functioning. Typically it combines direct observation of provider–client interactions with inventories of equipment and supplies and interviews with providers and clients at a given time. It has also been used extensively for studying the quality of services (Miller et al., 1997). In reporting on program quality, situation analyses generally use the six categories included in the Bruce framework.

Situation analysis does not examine the relationship between quality and outcomes. Rather it measures the level of quality present in a family planning program at a specific time. The Senegal report contains information on clients' waiting times and other indicators of humane treatment, as well as measurements of indicators of the quality of services and provider practices assumed to influence health and fertility outcomes.

The second reading is a report from MEXFAM, a Mexican NGO (Vernon et al.) on the application of continuous quality improvement (CQI), one of several methodologies that involve program staff in defining and carrying out quality improvements in family planning programs. Other methodologies include service quality improvement (SQI) and COPE (client-oriented, provider-efficient). They, as well as CQI, are adaptations of quality-assurance systems used in medicine and total quality management systems used in business (Askew et al., 1994). A common element in most of these techniques is that groups of employees are formed that meet periodically to discuss job-related problems and propose solutions.

The MEXFAM study is, to some degree, atypical of operations research reports. It is not a conventional diagnostic or intervention study, but rather a description of the implementation of an extensive program-improvement effort that was simultaneously expected to institutionalize the use of OR by the organization. It is also one of just two papers in this book (the other being Nazzar et al., in the Conduct section) based primarily on qualitative research techniques.

The final paper in this section is a study of the relationship of quality and outcomes conducted by the Guatemala Ministry of Health (Vernon et al.), one of very few intervention studies in the family planning quality of care literature. It is also one of the few published studies in the OR literature that reports negative results—the failure to confirm the research hypothesis. The study attempted to determine the effect of improving the quality of supervision on program outcomes. It uses a prospective, quasi-experimental design and reports the effect of an intervention based on the COPE methodology on the production of couple years of protection. Although the intervention was not successful, reports of negative results are important in OR because they help shape our understanding by identifying specific interventions that may not affect specific outcomes.

References

Aday, Lu Ann et al. 1993. *Evaluating the Medical Care System: Effectiveness, Efficiency, and Equity*. Ann Arbor, MI: Health Administration Press.

Askew, Ian et al. 1994. "Indicators for measuring the quality of family planning services in Nigeria." *Studies in Family Planning* 25, 5: 268–283.

Brown, Lisanne et al. 1995. "Quality of care in family planning services in Morocco." *Studies in Family Planning* 26, 3: 154–168.

Bruce, Judith. 1990. "Fundamental elements of the quality of care: A simple framework." *Studies in Family Planning* 21, 2: 61–91.

Bulatao, Rodolfo A., consultant. 1998. Personal communication. June 19.

Chelminsky, E. 1993. "The political debate about health care: Are we losing sight of quality?" *Science* 262: 525–528.

Donabedian, Avedis. 1980. *Explorations in Quality Assessment and Monitoring, Volume I, The Definition of Quality and Approaches to Its Assessment*. Ann Arbor, MI: Health Administration Press.

MacStravic, R. Scott. 1991. *Beyond Patient Satisfaction*. Ann Arbor, MI: Health Administration Press.

Miller, Robert et al. 1997. *The Situation Analysis Approach to Assessing Family Planning and Reproductive Health Services. A Handbook*. New York: The Population Council.

Mensch, Barbara et al. 1996. "The impact of the quality of family planning services on contraceptive use in Peru." *Studies in Family Planning* 27, 2: 59–75.

Nash, David B. 1995. "Accountability for hospital quality: The role of clinical practice guidelines." In Norbert Goldfield and David B. Nash (eds.). *Providing Quality Care: Future Challenges*. Ann Arbor, MI: Health Administration Press.

Sheps, Mindel C. 1955. "Approaches to the quality of hospital care." *Public Health Reports* 9: 877–886.

Situation Analysis of the Family Planning
Service-delivery System in Senegal

National Family Planning Program of Senegal,
Ministry of Health and Social Action, and
Africa Operations Research and Technical Assistance
Project II, Population Council

Programmatic issue: *The purpose of the study was to identify areas of service-delivery strengths and weakness in the Senegalese program.*

Program processes/components: *The study included an assessment of the condition of the infrastructure, logistics, availability, and quality of services.*

Research design: *All 180 National Family Planning service-delivery ponts (SDP) were included in the study. Data collection included inventories of supplies and equipment, a survey of providers, exit interviews with clients, and observation of client–provider interactions.*

Findings: *As well as providing information on the availability of services and supplies in the SDPs, the report includes a discussion of the elements of the Bruce framework as they applied to the findings of the study. Important program strengths included providing clients with written reminders for their next appointment and telling them where to go for method resupply. Quality weaknesses included lack of observance of program norms and poor provider training and client counseling. Overall, satisfaction was very high; more than 96 percent of clients reported that they were satisfied with the services and information they received.*

Program response to findings: *Dissemination seminars were held in different parts of Senegal for providers and managers. Many of the attendees stated they would institute changes in their service-delivery points to improve quality.*

Discussion: *The degree to which the changes were actually implemented and their results will require a comparison between this study and a future situation analysis. Most situation analyses are conducted on a stand-alone basis. Their value increases, however, if situation analysis is used as part of a cycle of operations research or technical assistance activities to improve quality and other aspects of program functioning. As part of a program of research or technical assistance, situation analyses can be used as pre- and post-test measures for assessing program improvement.*

Situation Analysis of the Family Planning Service-delivery System in Senegal

National Family Planning Program of Senegal,
Ministry of Health and Social Action, and
Africa Operations Research and Technical Assistance
Project II, Population Council

Introduction

Fertility trends in Senegal have paralleled those in sub-Saharan Africa as a whole. The most recent Demographic and Health Survey (1992–93) placed Senegal's current total fertility rate (TFR) at 6.0 children per woman, indicating a consistent decline from the 1978 World Fertility Survey TFR of 7.1 children. Despite progressive efforts on the part of the Senegalese government, the country's high fertility and growth rates have been accompanied by serious health problems, and, like many West African countries, Senegal has only recently become concerned with demographic issues and their impact on economic development.

Policy developments favoring the expansion of family planning began in 1980, when a French law prohibiting the distribution and use of contraceptives was revoked. This initiative cleared the way for major donors, such as the United States Agency for International Development (USAID) and the United Nations Population Fund (UNFPA), to begin their population programs in 1981 and 1982, respectively, covering all ten regions of the country. In 1988, the Government of Senegal officially adopted a population policy, which served as a preamble to the creation of the country's National Family Planning Program (PNPF) in 1991.

The PNPF plays a central role in the coordination and implementation of family planning and maternal and child health activities nationwide. However, it is currently undergoing a period of transition because it is called upon by the Ministry of Health and Social Action (MSAS) to readdress its priorities and resources to improve the quality of FP service delivery. Although previous evaluations have provided some indication of how to improve the quality of services, no study has provided a comprehensive diagnosis of the situation, and no specific interventions based on reliable data have been formulated to date.

Reprinted with the permission of the Population Council from *Situation Analysis of the Family Planning Service Delivery System in Senegal (Condensed Report)*, 1995.

Objectives

The 1994 Senegal situation analysis (SSA) study is the first of two major studies programmed by the PNPF in collaboration with the Population Council's Operations Research/Technical Assistance (OR/TA) Project II. The study's immediate objectives are to: (1) provide descriptive information on the availability, functioning, and quality of family planning services in Senegal, and to identify particular strengths and weaknesses of the national program; (2) formulate strategic recommendations for the Program on Child Survival and Family Planning, a five-year program funded by USAID; and (3) identify and provide indicators of quality to the Ministry of Health and Social Action.

Methodology

Three sampling units are employed in a situation analysis (SA) study: the service-delivery point (SDP), the staff at each SDP, and the clients. Standard data-collection instruments covering all sampling units include:

- an inventory of supplies, equipment, and other facility features;
- an observation of provider–client interactions;
- an interview with family planning clients;
- an interview with family planning staff;
- an interview with maternal and child health clients.

The data-collection instruments were customized for Senegal during the spring and summer of 1994, and were pretested in July of the same year. Data collection took place from 1 August to 30 September 1994. Whereas situation analysis studies were originally intended to generate basic descriptive information, the study objectives have increasingly included more sophisticated analysis as well as research and hypothesis testing. Currently, operations research projects at the Population Council attempt to address a substantive methodological issue in each new study. The Senegal situation analysis study has three main distinguishing characteristics:

1 *Census of service-delivery points:* Unlike most previous SA studies, where large and representative samples were selected for analysis, in Senegal, teams visited each one of the 180 functional SDPs providing family planning services. All family planning service providers and clients who were present on the day of the survey were interviewed, as well as several maternal and child health (MCH) clients. During the visits, 180 inventories (one per SDP) of equipment and supplies needed for family planning service delivery was completed, along with observations of 1,123 service-delivery interactions, and interviews with 837 clients and 361 SDP staff members.

2 *Experimental approaches:* One of the innovative aspects of the present study is the inclusion of special questions concerning abortion and reproductive intentions. Women were asked about their abortion history using direct and indirect approaches, to assess whether different ways of asking questions concerning abortion has an effect on response rates. The second experimental approach involves a panel of women who were selected and interviewed about their reproductive intentions. The panel will be followed and reinterviewed during the second situation analysis study to determine whether they were able to meet their objectives.

3 *Control of observer bias:* In order to investigate whether the presence of an observer biases the providers' performances during consultation, research teams made consecutive return visits of up to two or three days, particularly at clinics with high case loads.

Results

Study results are presented in three sections: The first describes the sociodemographic characteristics of family planning and MCH clients; the second depicts the functional capacity of SDPs; and the third delineates the six basic elements of the quality of care at SDPs based on the Bruce-Jain quality of care framework.

Sociodemographic Characteristics

Client age varies between 15 and 49 years, with a median age of 29 years for FP clients and 26 years for MCH clients. The great majority of women interviewed are married, and more than half are monogamous. Fifty-two percent of FP clients and 37 percent of MCH clients are educated. Virtually all women interviewed are Muslim.

Fertility levels are high in both populations: 53 percent of FP clients and 35 percent of MCH clients have at least four children. Nonetheless, the number of living children by group varies between 0 and 11. Approximately one out of three women were breastfeeding at the time of the survey. The median age of the latest child is 24 months.

The study reveals that a demand exists for spacing children as well as for limiting their number. In fact, 26 percent of FP clients and 19 percent of MCH clients do not desire any more children. Among those who wish to space their next birth (61 percent of FP clients and 77 percent of MCH clients), the desired interval is about three years or more. However, only 4.8 percent of MCH clients were using a contraceptive method at the time of the survey.

The methods most commonly accepted by new FP clients are the pill (51 percent), injectables (24 percent), and the IUD (19 percent). Among revisiting clients, the methods most frequently accepted are the pill (59 percent), followed by the IUD (26 percent), and injectables (11 percent). The recent introduction of Norplant® implants as part of a pilot project at five SDPs explains the use of this method by 5 percent of new clients, and 1 percent of revisiting clients.

Functional Capacity of SDPs

The systematic collection of data at the SDP permitted insight about the functional capacity of each SDP in accordance with the following five elements:

(a) *Facilities and equipment:* Facilities and infrastructure at the SDPs are considered satisfactory. Seventy-nine percent of SDPs have a separate room or area for examinations. The research team judged that in 85 percent of the SDPs, the examination room had visual privacy, 81 percent had auditory privacy, 88 percent were clean, and 84 percent had adequate light. A lower proportion (67 percent) had adequate water in the examination areas.

Figure 1 shows the proportion of clinics lacking the "minimum"[1] equipment necessary for providing FP services. Whereas more than half of the clinics are missing the minimum number of specula, that 22

Figure 1. Percentage of SDPs lacking the minimum equipment necessary to provide FP services, Senegal, 1994

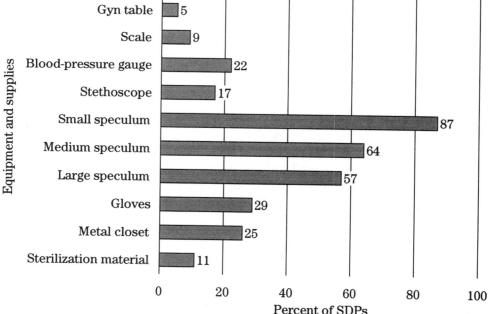

N = 180.

Source: Senegal Situation Analysis inventory, 1994.

percent of SDPs are missing a blood-pressure gauge, 17 percent are missing a stethoscope, and 11 percent are missing a set of sterilization materials is significant.

(b) *Contraceptive supplies and logistics:* Although oral contraceptives and barrier methods (condoms and spermicides) are available at all SDPs, the IUD and injectables are available at 78 percent and 63 percent of the SDPs, respectively. In the six months preceding the study, stockouts of combined oral contraceptives were common, occurring in roughly 8 percent of clinics providing the main brand, Lofemenal. Injectables had the highest frequency of stockouts, experienced by more than 20 percent of SDPs, due, in part, to UNFPA's being the sole provider of injectables at the time of the study.

Fifty-two percent of SDPs visited had a record-keeping system in place for tracking and ordering contraceptive supplies. In 51 percent of SDPs, contraceptives were stored correctly by expiration date, and 79 percent of SDPs had storage areas that protected supplies adequately. The data indicate that although many clinics have available space and store their contraceptives appropriately, management aspects of storage and ordering could be improved.

(c) *Personnel training and experience:* In Senegal, 361 staff members were interviewed for the study. The majority of them were midwives (60 percent), with some community health agents (14 percent) and nurse's aides (13 percent). Approximately three out of four service providers reported that their training had been insufficient for them to provide adequate FP services. In addition, Figure 2 reveals the need for diversified training, given that more than half of the providers (62 percent) claimed to have received training in clinical FP, but very few in IEC technique (24 percent), FP counseling (26 percent), or HIV/AIDS counseling (13 percent).

Of the staff who provided a family planning method during the three months preceding the survey, 88 percent had provided Lofemenal pills, 82 percent had provided Ovrette (progestin-only) pills, 75 percent had provided condoms, and 68 percent had provided spermicides. More than 50 percent had provided IUDs and injectables, whereas fewer than 10 percent had provided voluntary surgical contraception (VSC).

(d) *IEC materials and activities:* Figure 3 indicates that IEC is one of the weakest points of the Senegal FP program. Although a large majority (82 percent) of SDPs had MCH and FP posters available, the proportion of clinics with other IEC materials was very low. The data also

Figure 2. Percentage of personnel trained by type of training, Senegal, 1994

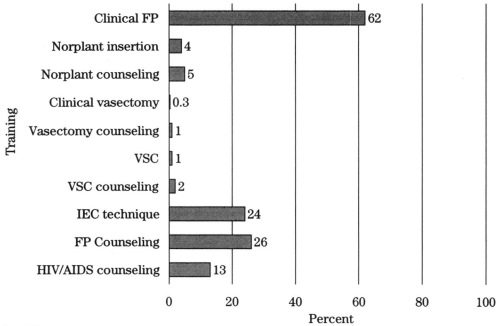

N = 361.
Source: Senegal Situation Analysis, FP staff interviews, 1994.

reveal that IEC activities in the SDPs are practically nonexistent; only 6 percent of the SDPs visited held a FP talk on the day of the visit. Furthermore, 60 percent of SDPs had no visible sign announcing the availability of FP services.

(e) *Management and supervision:* The management and supervision of FP activities at all SDPs present important weaknesses. Only 6 percent of SDPs had job descriptions and defined responsibilities for the staff, 8 percent had a program of activities, and 2 percent had an established objective as to the number of clients to serve at any given time.

According to norms of the PNPF, each SDP should receive one supervisory visit every three months. Unfortunately, only 38 percent of the SDPs had been visited by a supervisor during the three months prior to the survey (Figure 4). Thirty-three percent had not been seen by a supervisor in seven months or more, and 18 percent had not had supervision at all.

The great majority of SDPs (94 percent) have a monthly statistical report of FP activities. In the 30 days prior to the survey, however, only 65 percent had sent the report to a supervisor. The lack of feedback on the

Figure 3. IEC materials and activities available at the SDPs, Senegal, 1994

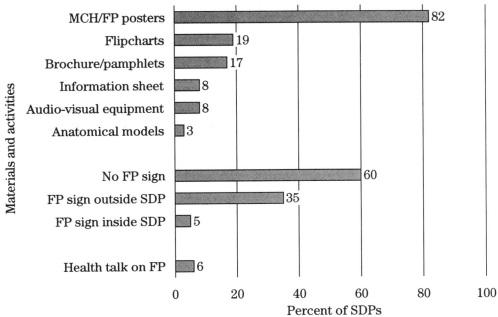

N = 180.
Source: Senegal Situation Analysis inventory, 1994.

quality and supervisors' use of these reports may be a factor that discourages service providers from complying with the reporting procedure.

Quality of Care

This section deals with the quality of care provided by SDPs, as defined by the six elements of the Bruce-Jain quality of care framework. The data are measured through observations of client–provider interaction and subsequent interviews with FP clients and service providers.

Choice of Methods

If the client desires to space her next pregnancy, more than three providers out of four recommend the pill or the IUD. Prejudice regarding the use of injectables exists among FP service providers in Senegal; they claim it is offered as a method for limiting the number of births. In general, first-visit clients come in with a desired method in mind (53 percent). In more than half of these cases, the method they are considering is the pill. Other than condoms and spermicides, which are low in demand, clients' personal choice of the pill or injectables is the most often respected (81 percent). Clients' choice of the IUD is respected only in 67 percent of the cases.

Figure 4. Time since the last SDP visit by a FP supervisor, Senegal, 1994

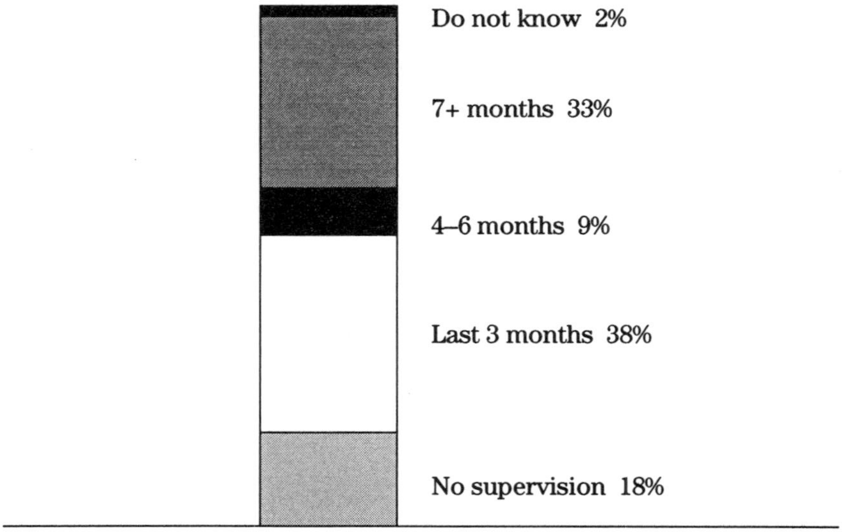

Do not know 2%

7+ months 33%

4–6 months 9%

Last 3 months 38%

No supervision 18%

N = 180.
Source: Senegal Situation Analysis inventory, 1994.

Although medical tests conducted prior to the provision of a contraceptive method are no longer required, close to one-fourth of the providers still request them. A urine test, blood test, and Pap smear are the most commonly requested tests for prescribing the pill. A significant number of providers attach certain prejudices to the distribution of specific methods. More than half of the providers claim that a woman should have at least one child before she receives a method. Because, in Senegal, injectables seem to be associated with infertility, providers indicated that a woman should have at least three children in order to receive this particular method. More than 80 percent of the providers interviewed stated that a minimum age of 17 years and a maximum age of 37 years is necessary for a woman to receive the pill. The minimum age, however, is higher for the IUD (19 years) and injectables (25 years). Finally, although only 10 percent of providers would require that a woman be married in order to prescribe a contraceptive method for her, a more substantial proportion (34 percent) claimed to request the husband's approval, particularly for the pill and the IUD. Few providers encourage a particular method (13 percent). The methods most commonly encouraged by providers are the pill, followed by the IUD and injectables.

Information Given to Clients
A client's knowledge of her contraceptive options depends not only on the mere mention of a method, but also on the degree of information provided to her. The pro-

vider should focus on determining the client's needs and presenting the range of methods available, along with their contraindications, advantages, and disadvantages.

Figure 5 shows that service providers ask 56 percent of new clients about their reproductive intentions and 48 percent about their preferred contraceptive method. Only 44 percent of revisiting clients were asked about problems they have had with their current method. Among those who did report having problems, only 17 percent were offered the possibility of changing the method.

The data reveal that not all methods are mentioned systematically to new clients. The pill was mentioned to 75 percent, the IUD to 54 percent, injectables to 42 percent, and the condom to 25 percent of clients (not shown).

New clients receive more information about the method selected than do revisiting clients who have changed to a new method. Information that is most commonly provided concerns how to use the method and how to follow-up (Figure 6). More than 50 percent of new clients did not receive any information on the side effects or disadvantages of the method selected, nor on precautions or the possibility of changing methods if any problems arise.

Figure 5. Questions spontaneously asked by the service provider during consultation, Senegal, 1994

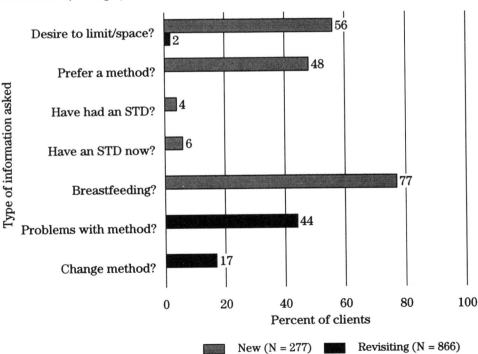

Source: Senegal Situation Analysis, observations, 1994.

A comparison of the results above with data emerging from individual interviews with clients reveals that clients have, in general, retained limited information regarding the method selected. Clients' knowledge about the methods they use is particularly low with respect to minor and major side effects.

Technical Competence

During data collection, team members recorded the medical procedures followed during client examinations, including the observance of protocols and aseptic measures used in performing a pelvic exam and while providing a clinical method (that is, IUDs and implants).

The great majority of providers ask their clients about the date of their last menstruation, and proceed to weigh them and take their blood pressure. Pelvic and breast examinations are more frequently performed on new clients (72 percent and 69 percent, respectively). Acknowledging and addressing a client's problem with a particular method remains an important element of method continuity (see Figure 7). Data from this study reveal that in such cases, only 17 percent

Figure 6. Information given to FP clients about the new method accepted, Senegal, 1994

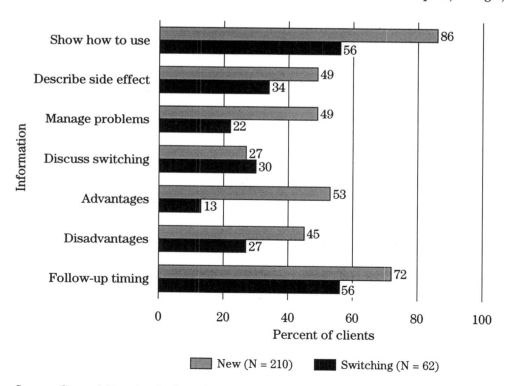

Source: Senegal Situation Analysis, FP client interviews, 1994.

of providers asked the client to change to another method, 2 percent referred clients for treatment, and another 15 percent neglected the problem altogether.

Among observed pelvic exams with revisiting clients, a sterile speculum was used 80 percent of the time, and sterile gloves 65 percent of the time. Only 10 percent of providers washed their hands before performing the exam. Approximately 80 percent of clients are not informed that they will undergo a pelvic examination, and only 30 percent of new clients and 42 percent of revisiting clients are informed of the results (not shown).

Providers (mostly midwives and nurses) are well informed on how to use each of the three main contraceptive methods: the pill, the IUD, and injectables, as well as on their minor side effects. However, the level of knowledge on these methods' major side effects represents a significant weakness in their training.

Interpersonal Relations

The section on interpersonal relations refers to the interaction between the provider and the client. Difficulties in measuring this element have been acknowledged by previous researchers. In the Senegal situation analysis study, data-col-

Figure 7. Provider response to clients with problems, Senegal, 1994

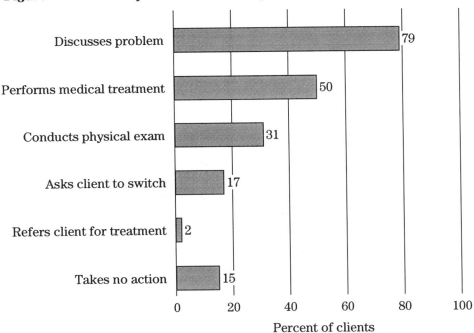

N = 251.
Source: Senegal Situation Analysis, FP client observations, 1994.

lection teams attempted to measure interpersonal relations through a number of indicators: client satisfaction, duration of the consultation, and the proportion of clients who received the desired information.

An index of client satisfaction was developed based on the client's perception of her interaction with the service provider and the overall organization of the SDP. More women indicate satisfaction with the organization of services (59 percent) than with their interaction with the service provider (53 percent). Waiting time was the most common reason for clients' dissatisfaction with the organization of services. Indeed Figure 8 indicates that 58 percent of clients wait between 30 minutes and two hours or more to receive FP services. In general, consultation time was found to be short, particularly when compared with clients' waiting time. The median duration of a first visit is 12 minutes, and of a control visit is five minutes. Overall, client satisfaction is high; 96 percent indicated that they received the information and services they desired.

Mechanisms to Encourage Continuity

The Senegal situation analysis study indicates that clients usually receive important information to encourage continuity. In fact, all new clients were told when to return for resupply, and virtually all clients (96 percent) were given a written reminder. Furthermore, almost all clients (99 percent) were told where to go for resupply. These findings indicate that this is a particular strength in the Senegal National Family Planning Program.

Figure 8. FP clients' waiting time before consultation, Senegal, 1994

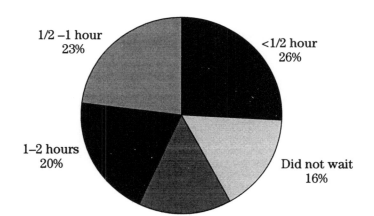

N = 1,038.

Source: Senegal Situation Analysis, observation, 1994.

Provider practices with respect to informing the client about method re-supply or control visits may also play an important role in encouraging continu-ity. In Senegal, the norm dictates that new clients receive one cycle of pills. The data indicate that 71 percent of providers respect this norm. Thirty-four percent of revisiting clients continue to be provided with a single cycle of pills, obliging them to revisit the clinic every month for resupply.

Appropriate Constellation of Services

At virtually all public service-delivery points, FP services are offered within the context of a wide range of services. In fact, on average, four different types of services were reported to be offered each day. That an SDP claims to offer a service, however, does not mean that the service is truly integrated into FP pro-vision. For instance, among MCH clients, family planning was discussed in only 36 percent of interactions. One-fourth of the SDPs visited belong to SANFAM, whose mandate in the private and parastatal sectors is to provide FP services only.

Figure 9 presents information on the frequency with which other health issues are discussed during FP client consultations. Overwhelmingly, providers

Figure 9. Other health issues addressed by the service provider, Senegal, 1994

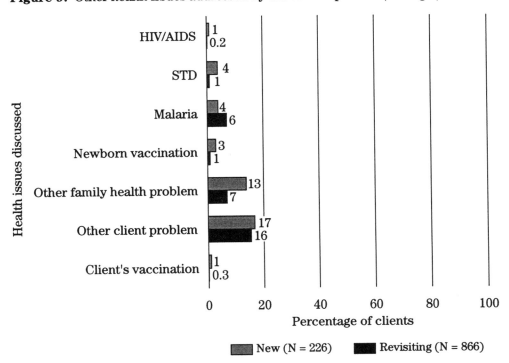

Source: Senegal Situation Analysis observations, 1994.

and clients are not discussing other important health issues. Concerns about HIV/AIDS were discussed in only 1 percent of observed new client visits. Furthermore, although 92 percent of SDPs claim to offer consultations regarding STDs, new clients were asked about current STD symptoms in only 6 percent of observed interactions (STD history was discussed in only 3 percent of new client interactions).

Recommendations

The recommendations proposed by the Senegal situation analysis study were first formulated by participants at a one-day national dissemination seminar and later refined by staff members of the PNPF and the Africa OR/TA Project II. The following is a synthesis of the seminar recommendations:

Functional Capacity of SDPs

- Improve the infrastructure in the rural sector, particularly the availability of water.
- Provide FP training to all medical doctors and ensure their involvement in FP activities at all levels.
- Assure training of all personnel in clinical FP, counseling, IEC techniques, and management.
- Standardize and implement refresher training courses.
- Ensure that all SDPs have the minimum equipment necessary to provide FP services.
- Implement the use of the FEFO (first expiration, first out) system to stock contraceptives.
- Develop a forecasting system for contraceptive procurement and adopt a standard logistics system.
- Encourage SDPs to provide all of the authorized contraceptive methods.
- Encourage all SDPs to plan FP activities on an annual basis and in systematic fashion.
- Develop a guide for supervision and implement regular supervisory visits of all SDPs every three months.
- Train service providers in the use and maintenance of records and statistical information.
- Define responsibilities of the different levels (national, regional, and district) in terms of their overview of FP activities.
- Equip all SDPs with more IEC materials, and encourage the use of these materials during training.
- Integrate IEC activities in the provision of FP services at all SDPs.

Quality of Care

- Encourage service providers to reduce medical and nonmedical barriers in the provision of contraceptive methods and observe standard norms more closely.
- Encourage service providers to respect scheduled hours of services;
- Standardize prices of contraceptive products.
- Emphasize the need for an integrated training curriculum and for the reorganization of services.
- Provide training on client counseling and integrate counseling as part of daily FP activities.

Impact and Use

The results of the Senegal situation analysis study were presented at a two-day dissemination seminar in January 1995, which involved national representatives from the MSAS and the PNPF, major funding agencies, nongovernmental organizations working in family planning in Senegal, and FP staff representing the regions. A second presentation of the results took place at a five-day workshop in January/February 1995 on the implementation of the USAID/ Senegal Child Survival and Family Planning Project. At this workshop, study results served as a basis for recommending project strategies, identifying key areas for operations research, and developing quality of care indicators. Following the workshop, a secondary analysis of the SA data was conducted to define quality of care indicators that would serve to evaluate the project in the next five years.

In an effort to maximize the impact of the study and the use of the findings, a series of regional dissemination seminars was held during the second half of 1995, covering all ten regions of the country. During these activities, regional medical doctors, midwives, and supervisors were presented with SA results pertinent to their districts and to their region as a whole. Participants were organized in working groups by districts and encouraged to formulate their own recommendations. This activity was followed by group presentations and vigorous discussions, because some of the recommendations had a direct impact on providers' daily practices. This dissemination process culminated in the use of study recommendations to develop regional workplans for 1996 and the development of ten individual final reports representing each of the regions.

Note

1   The "minimum" equipment necessary to provide FP services, as defined by the PNPF during data analysis, includes: one gynecological table, one scale, one blood-pressure

gauge, one stethoscope, one metal closet, one set of sterilization materials, at least ten gloves, and at least six of each of the different types of speculum.

References

Association Ivoirienne pour le Bien-Etre Familial (AIBEF). 1992. *Analyse Situationnelle du Programme d'Extension des Services de Planification Familiale en Côte d'Ivoire.* New York: The Population Council.

Bruce, Judith. 1990. "Fundamental elements of the quality of care: A simple framework." *Studies in Family Planning* 21,2: 61–91.

Cerulli, Annamaria, Diouratié Sanogo, Gil Cusack, Bill Emmet, and Paulette Chaponnière. 1995. *Activités pour la Survie de l'Enfant et la Planification Familiale au Sénégal: Revue de la Littérature et Recommandations pour la Recherche et les Programmes Futurs.* Dakar: The Population Council and Management Sciences for Health Projet Survie de l'Enfant/Planification Familiale au Sénégal (USAID).

Fisher, Andrew, Robert Miller, Ian Askew, Barbara Mensch, Anrudh Jain, and Dale Huntington. 1994. "The situation analysis approach to assessing the supply side of family planning programs." Paper presented at the annual meeting of the American Public Health Association, Washington, DC, 30 October–3 November.

Fonds des Nations Unies pour la Population (FNUAP). 1991. *Mission de Revue du Programme et de Développement de Stratégies en Matière de Population au Sénégal.* Rapport final. Volumes I et II. Dakar: FNUAP.

Ministère de la Santé Publique et de l'Action Sociale. 1994. *Programme National de Planification Familiale au Sénégal.* Dakar: Direction de la Santé Publique.

Ministère de la Santé et de l'Action Sociale. 1994. *Politique et Normes des Services de Planification Familiale au Sénégal.* Thiès: Ministère de la Santé et de l'Action Sociale.

Ministère de la Santé du Bénin. 1994. *Analyse Situationnelle du Programme de Planification Familiale au Bénin.* Rapport préliminaire. New York: The Population Council.

Acknowledgment

This project was financed by the United States Agency for International Development, Office of Population.

PREFATORY REMARKS

Institutionalizing a System of Continuous Quality Improvement

Ricardo Vernon, Pedro Manuel Acosta,
Jesús Vertiz, Ilse Salas, Alma Bermúdez, and
Alfonso López Juárez

Programmatic issue: *Can continuous quality-improvement (CQI) techniques be successfully applied to family planning programs?*

Program processes/components: *CQI is applied to all program processes and components by organizing quality-improvement teams in all administrative departments and clinics.*

Research design: *Qualitative techniques, including focus groups, document reviews, and interviews with managers, were used to monitor the introduction of CQI in the MEXFAM agency.*

Findings: *By design, the implementation of CQI involved careful organization and lengthy training for all staff involved. Both managers and workers reported that CQI had made the organization more client centered and had increased workers' problem-solving ability and job satisfaction. Participation in the teams was excellent, and a large number of problems were identified and solved. Most solutions involved improving clinic amenities such as reducing waiting time and making waiting rooms more comfortable. Some interventions also improved program revenues and made some processes like accounting and reporting more efficient. Despite careful preparation, many quality-improvement teams failed to measure the changes in outputs and outcomes resulting from quality improvements and could only report changes in inputs.*

Program response to findings: *The study helped MEXFAM identify areas needing strengthening in its CQI system. The agency's CQI experience was sufficiently positive to convince Management Sciences for Health, a US-based technical assistance organization, to adapt the MEXFAM training materials for wider use.*

Discussion: *The study presents evidence that CQI techniques increase the humane treatment of clients and result in improvements in program amenities, but the study failed to produce clear evidence that CQI improved* *program outputs or outcomes. More research in this area is needed, as are studies that use CQI to improve voluntarism.*

Implementing CQI techniques requires a long-term commitment on the part of workers and managers and relatively good labor–management relations. These conditions may be hard to satisfy in many developing-country situations, and CQI may ultimately be more applicable to private, nonprofit and for-profit providers rather than to large governmental institutions like health ministries.

Institutionalizing a System of Continuous Quality Improvement

Ricardo Vernon, Pedro Manuel Acosta,
Jesús Vertiz, Ilse Salas, Alma Bermúdez, and
Alfonso López Juárez

Introduction

The purpose of this project was to combine the improvement of quality of services at MEXFAM, a private, nonprofit Mexican family planning organization, with the institutionalization of operations research in the same agency. The project attempted to accomplish both objectives by adapting business and industrial quality-improvement techniques to the family planning context.

MEXFAM, the Mexican International Planned Parenthood Federation (IPPF) affiliate, provides services through 27 centers, including seven clinics and 20 units that operate a variety of nonclinical programs. Resources and personnel deployed vary greatly by center. Some have a single paid person to coordinate volunteers, whereas others have large paid staffs. In 1993, MEXFAM's clinics provided services to 297,000 new family planning clients and, through its nonclinical programs, services to an additional 238,000 new clients.

Improving the quality of services is an important agency objective, and management was particularly interested in quality-improvement systems originally designed for business and industrial settings. MEXFAM decided to adapt the continuous quality-improvement technique (CQI), which involves forming discussion groups of employees who meet regularly to consider job-related problems and propose solutions. An advantage of CQI is that it can be applied to administrative systems such as logistics and accounting as well as to production units. The need to become more efficient, to reduce operating costs, and to increase income was also an important factor in MEXFAM's selection of CQI.

Over the years, MEXFAM had conducted a number of operations research projects with external assistance. The organization was interested in making its use of OR as a managerial problem-solving tool more routine, but was unable to afford the expense of a dedicated research unit. CQI also seemed to offer a way

---

© 1998 by The Population Council, Inc. Reprinted with permission.

to institutionalize the ability to conduct OR. Continuous quality improvement may be considered an operations-analysis technique. It is concerned with the improvement of program operations; it uses a systematic, qualitative methodology; and it relies on the process of problem identification, solution generation and testing, and results dissemination.

The Population Council's Latin American Operations Research Project provided financial and technical assistance to the project to learn if CQI could be implemented successfully in a family planning program. MEXFAM conducted the test of CQI in the greater Mexico City area.

The CQI Methodology

The CQI system identifies problems and relies on employees to generate solutions and evaluate success. At meetings, workers identify job-related problems, which may involve an examination of organizational statistics, costs, and so forth, or a simple exchange of views of salient problems. Once problems are identified, the group considers alternative solutions and selects the one that seems best. The solution is then implemented and evaluated, and results of the quality-improvement activity disseminated within the organization. Both process and outcome improvement can be measured, and either qualitative or quantitative measurements can be employed. CQI usually takes a long time to implement and requires the sustained participation of the workforce, from the lowest to the highest levels, to be successful.

The CQI technique includes cross-function and quality-improvement teams. Cross-function teams are composed of individuals working in different functional areas or at different administrative levels. They identify problems that involve more than one department. In contrast, quality-improvement teams are composed of people who work in the same location and solve problems in a specific clinic or department. Successful implementation of CQI requires that all members of the organization be trained in the technique, that suggestions be implemented, and that staff be rewarded for solving problems. Finally, CQI has a consumer, rather than a producer orientation. In family planning, organizations must provide services that consumers want, and workers must strive to please the client.

Training

CQI was tested in the MEXFAM Mexico City headquarters and in seven centers, five of which were in the Mexico City metropolitan area. Training of agency staff took place between 1991 and 1994. In study locations, all managers attended three courses on CQI that provided them with an introduction to the technique and methods for identifying problems. Quality-improvement team leaders attended four courses that lasted between 20 and 40 hours each.

The MEXFAM evaluation department was given the task of coordinating CQI activities. The department head attended a 200-hour diploma course in continuous quality improvement. All employees participating in cross-functional and quality-improvement teams were each given 20 hours of training in ten sessions over a period of three months. In the final months of the project, as MEXFAM started to emphasize quality of medical care, 116 community physicians in six new centers were each given 30 hours of training.

Quality Teams

To direct quality-improvement activities, a quality-management team and a quality-support team were created. Cross-functional teams were created, and each of the participating centers established quality-improvement teams.

The Quality Management-information System

To assess progress and manage the CQI process, a simple management-information system (MIS) was designed and implemented.

Commitment and Rewards

To demonstrate commitment to quality improvement, the agency decided to publish quality-improvement items in the MEXFAM newsletter and to hold an annual "quality day" for employees to give them the opportunity to present the results of their work and receive quality-improvement awards.

Results

Implementation of CQI

Between 1991 and 1994, 25 teams were established, including nine at MEXFAM headquarters and 16 in centers. Fifteen groups were involved in service delivery and the remainder in support services such as accounting and evaluation. Four of the groups were cross-functional teams. Teams were established at different times and functioned for two to 40 months during the study period. Approximately 91 percent of employees in study sites participated in quality-improvement teams. Teams held a mean of 1.1 meetings per month. The mean number of suggestions for improvement per team was 13.5, and the mean number of suggestions per participating employee was 1.4. The techniques most commonly used to select problems for improvement included brainstorming, analyzing processes with flowcharts, and obtaining opinions from clients. Several service-delivery quality-improvement groups placed suggestion boxes for clients in clinic waiting rooms or conducted small, frequent surveys to assess the satisfaction of clients and collect complaints.

During the course of the project, two issues of MEXFAM's monthly bulletin were devoted to quality of care and quality-improvement topics. The monthly and weekly house organs regularly published articles devoted to quality improvement, and Quality Days were held in 1992 and 1994.

At focus-group meetings held to evaluate CQI implementation in 1993, most quality-improvement-team participants felt that communication between workers had been improved and reported that participation in teams improved job satisfaction.

Quality-improvement Activities

A mean of ten improvement suggestions were implemented per team. In clinics, the great majority of problems selected required improvements of amenities such as upgrading waiting rooms by providing more chairs, water carafes, plants, reading materials, and videos. Less frequently, quality-improvement teams carried out more complicated interventions such as reducing waiting time, remodeling the clinic, and changing logistic procedures to improve availability of medical supplies.

Administrative quality-improvement groups focused mostly on problems of noncompliance with reporting norms and on reducing the amount of time devoted to routine activities. The accounting and evaluation quality-improvement teams, for example, improved the timeliness and quality of reports delivered from logistic areas by changing the paper flow and reporting periods and providing centers with report templates.

Cross-functional teams dealt with more complex problems. A budget-control group, for example, was able to improve the accuracy of expenditure projections; and the financial control cross-function team was able to implement, for the first time, all recommendations made by external auditors.

Observations indicated that teams under-reported quality-improvement activities and had problems measuring the effect of solutions tested. Recording and reporting quality-improvement activities was the responsibility of quality coordinators, and supervisors were often too busy to follow through on the task or assigned quality-improvement reporting a low priority. Therefore, the impact of most improvements is unknown.

Quality-improvement teams also competed for scarce resources with other program activities; not all quality-improvement activities could be approved for financing, which often lowered morale among team members, and made some reluctant to participate in improvement activities. Many managers were frustrated with the improvement process, because often teams did not report that tangible benefits (increase in program users, revenues, and so forth) were accruing as a result of their activities.

Quality-improvement Case Study

In for-profit organizations, concern with quality is driven by the belief that improvements in quality improve profits. Although it is a nonprofit organization, MEXFAM faces the problem of recovering an ever-larger share of operating costs. The following case study reports the results of a quality-improvement activity designed to increase revenues by improving quality. The project was carried out in the Nezahualcoyotl clinic located in metropolitan Mexico City. Clinic staff suggested and designed all improvements. The project won a second-place award at the 1994 Quality Day.

In January 1993, the Nezahualcoyotl clinic raised service fees by 25 percent to recover a larger portion of its operating costs. To counter the possibility of client loss as a result of the price increase, the clinic implemented the following quality improvements:

- putting paper sheets on examining tables and changing them after every user;
- providing free vaccinations for children;
- providing free dextrose analysis and blood-pressure readings;
- providing free oral rehydration salts;
- putting contraceptives in paper bags to increase clients' privacy;
- remodeling the clinic;
- installing television sets in waiting rooms; and
- requiring that staff wear uniforms so that clients can identify them.

The changes were accompanied by clinic-promotion activities, including community leafleting and the installation of an electric sign outside the clinic.

Revenues increased from 15,000 pesos (US$5,000) per month before the price, promotion, and quality changes to 26,000 ($8,500) after the changes. Increases in revenue are only partially attributable to price increases. Promotion and quality improvement resulted in an increase in clinic visits. For example, the number of new family planning clients increased by 13 percent, and gynecological visits increased by 19 percent.

Discussion

Implementation of CQI was a long process. The technique was successful in producing a focus on clients in MEXFAM that is manifest in the improvements of amenities and the addition of new services. CQI also improved internal reporting, accounting, and other systems, and improved the finances and attendance of at least some centers. Overall, management feels that CQI strengthened the initiative and problem-solving capacity of staff and strengthened the sustainability of the agency.

A disappointment for MEXFAM was the inability of teams to monitor the results of many quality-improvement efforts. Despite efforts to enable the evaluation unit to prepare and assist quality-improvement teams in assessment of outcomes, training and assistance in measurement was one of the most serious implementation weaknesses. Thus, with the exception of projects attempting to improve agency revenues, most of the information available from teams was limited to changes in inputs.

Despite weaknesses in the CQI system, MEXFAM management and staff were sufficiently satisfied to expand it to all of the organization's centers. Management Sciences for Health (MSH), a United States-based technical assistance organization, adapted MEXFAM materials used in the test and has assisted many Latin American organizations to implement CQI.

Quality-improvement systems use very broad definitions of quality. Upgrading of many processes, such as improving paper flow and accounting procedures, are also considered by CQI to be quality improvements. A lesson learned about CQI is that successful quality-improvement efforts such as the one conducted by the Nezahualcoyotl clinic actually involve factors other than quality. Nezahualcoyotl staff, for example, also increased promotion. Finally, both clients and providers tended to identify quality with amenities like short waiting times and comfortable waiting rooms. Whether quality teams will, over time, go beyond improvement of amenities remains a topic for further research.

References

Deming, W. Edwards. 1986. *Out of the Crisis*. Cambridge, MA: Massachusetts Institute of Technology, Center for Advanced Engineering Study.

Imai, Masaaki. 1990. *Kaizen. La Clave de la Ventaja Competitiva Japonesa*. Compañía Editorial Continental, S.A. de C.V. México. (*KAIZEN: The Key to Japan's Competitive Success*. New York: Random House [in English]).

Ishikawa, Kaoru. 1985. *What is Total Quality Control? The Japanese Way*. Prentice Hall.

MEXFAM. 1989. Final technical report. *The Use of Operations Research as an Administrative Tool*. Mexico City: MEXFAM and The Population Council, Mexico.

Philip Crosby Associates. 1987. *Quality Improvement Process Management College*. Philip Crosby Associates.

Acknowledgment

This project was financed by the United States Agency for International Development, Office of Population.

A Test of Alternative Supervision Strategies for Family Planning Services in Guatemala

Ricardo Vernon, Anne Staunton, Mario García,
Juan José Arroyo, and Raul Rosenberg

Programmatic issue: *Does supervision that stresses quality improvement lead to improved outcomes?*

Program processes/components: *Supervision is a chronic problem in family planning programs. Because they are costly, supervisory visits to SDPs in government programs are made very infrequently, and when made, they tend to be idiosyncratic in purpose and content. The study attempted (1) to reduce supervisory visit costs and (2) to improve program output through a systematic attempt to improve quality.*

Research design: *Quasiexperimental with two alternative supervision strategies. "Indirect supervision " and "self assessment" were compared with the program's traditional supervision process. "Indirect supervision" included replacing one of the two routine supervisory visits to health posts with a district-level group meeting. The content of supervision included training of providers in areas chosen by the supervisor or the providers, including quality, reproductive risk, and contraceptive prescription. "Self assessment" substituted a workshop in the modified COPE initiative for one of the two annual supervisory visits. Dependent variables included cost per supervisory visit and number of CYP produced by the SDP.*

Findings: *About 80 percent of problems identified by SDP staff were corrected within one year of being identified. No reliable differences were found in CYP. Indirect supervision was less costly than either the traditional or self-assessment methodologies.*

Program response to findings: *Study results could not be implemented. Shortly after the project was implemented, reductions in donor funding forced the Ministry of Health to drastically reduce its supervision program.*

Discussion: *The study is a good example of the kind of prospective intervention studies that are needed in the study of quality. The paper examined both costs and outcomes. The COPE-based supervision strategy did not appear to effect program outcomes, and it was more costly than an alternative supervi-*

sion strategy. Given the popularity of techniques such as COPE, an urgent need exists to conduct more studies to determine if they are effective and cost effective in improving health and fertility outcomes.

A Test of Alternative Supervision Strategies for Family Planning Services in Guatemala

Ricardo Vernon, Anne Staunton, Mario García,
Juan José Arroyo, and Raul Rosenberg

Supervision of family planning programs is important for two main reasons: to find out what is happening at the clinics and to renew the enthusiasm of staff. Supervisors should help staff perform better by offering support, training, and assistance with resources and logistics, and by providing monitoring and evaluation (Wolff et al., 1991). In large, decentralized service-delivery systems, such as the Ministries of Health (MOH), supervision is the principal way in which central administrative units are able to focus the activities implemented by their regional operational counterparts. Because family planning competes with many other health programs that are assigned a greater priority, the motivational function of supervision is crucial.

Supervisors working in Ministries of Health often find it difficult to provide motivation, guidance, and training services because the units needing such supervision are numerous and the distances between health units are great. In the case of the Family Planning Unit (FPU) of the Ministry of Health of Guatemala, standards require that each of the nine national supervisors visit an average of 100 health centers and posts twice a year. In addition to these visits, supervisors prepare reports, program and evaluate activities, and serve as instructors in MOH training courses for service-delivery personnel. Thus, supervisors normally visit two or three health units a day, staying in each just long enough to complete such routine tasks as gathering service statistics and resupplying contraceptives and other program materials. During their visits, most supervisors usually have a brief interview with the manager of the health clinic or post and do not interact with, train, or motivate the family planning service-delivery personnel. They have little opportunity, therefore, to detect and solve problems, or to achieve quality and productivity improvements.

For these reasons, the FPU decided to conduct an operations research project to test alternative supervision strategies. Ideally, these schemes should allow supervisors to complete routine activities while providing greater opportu-

Reprinted with the permission of the Population Council from *Studies in Family Planning* 1992. 25,4:232–238.

nity for motivating and training staff, as well as for improving low family planning productivity and what family planning program managers perceive as the inadequate quality of services. Budgetary constraints require that the alternative supervisory schemes should not be more expensive than the current strategy. The results of the operations research project conducted by the FPU are presented here.

Alternative Strategies Tested

The FPU tested two alternative supervisory strategies designated "indirect supervision" and "self-assessment."

Indirect Supervision

The indirect supervisory strategy consisted of replacing one of the two annual supervisory visits with a brief (four-to-six-hour) group meeting attended by the supervisor and all family planning service-delivery personnel in the district.[1] During these meetings, the supervisors completed routine activities, including the collection of service statistics and the resupply of contraceptives and forms. In addition, they devoted some time to training in subjects that they or the service-delivery staff felt were necessary, including quality of care, contraceptive methods, and reproductive risk. This first meeting was followed by the supervisor's visit to the individual health centers and posts within the following three to six months. In the beginning of the second year of the study, another district meeting was held, and an immediate follow-up visit was carried out to assess service-delivery conditions and collect data.

The FPU management perceived the supervisor's interacting with and training of the service-delivery personnel as the main advantages of this strategy. In addition, by not having to visit every health post and center, supervisors could use their time more productively, improving the cost-effectiveness of their activities by saving travel expenses. However, the MOH also worried that this strategy would result in a loss of "presence" of family planning at the service-delivery level, ultimately reducing the productivity of personnel.

Self-assessment

The self-assessment strategy was based on an adaptation of the COPE strategy tested by the Association for Voluntary Surgical Contraception (AVSC) in Africa in hospitals providing sterilization services. The COPE strategy calls for organizing a session with service staff in which, with the aid of checklists, personnel identify service-delivery problems for improvement.[2] Once problems are identified, hospital staff draft a self-improvement plan that lists the actions to be taken, the persons responsible, and the time frame allotted for carrying them out. In subsequent visits, the supervisors assess the degree of improvement and assist the service-delivery personnel to overcome problems that were not solved (see Dwyer et al., 1990 and Lynam et al., 1993).

To implement the self-assessment strategy, the FPU substituted one of the two annual visits to each unit with a two-day workshop at the district level on quality of care and the use of self-assessment checklists. The supervisors of the different districts, who had previously attended a five-day course on both subjects, served as the workshop instructors. The initial workshops were held from March through May of 1992. All district service-delivery staff were invited to these meetings. The workshops included a session on quality of care, a discussion of self-assessment checklists, and instruction on filling them out. Each attendee filled out a checklist identifying the main problems in his or her service-delivery outlet that could be solved by the staff working there. The group discussion followed, during which the staff of each center or post selected the five or 10 most important problems in their out let that could be solved with the resources at hand. Finally, the teams from each outlet developed a self-improvement plan in which actions to be taken as a group were mapped out, persons responsible for carrying out each action identified, and a schedule for each action established. The workshop ended with such routine activities as the collection of service statistics and the resupplying of contraceptives.

In the subsequent visit to each outlet, the supervisor determined what progress had been made in solving the problems selected at the workshop, provided assistance in overcoming obstacles, and carried out routine administrative tasks. A second workshop was conducted at the beginning of the second year (from April through June of 1993), followed by an on-site inspection of the outlets to assess conditions and collect data.

The self-assessment checklists used in the workshops were based on the norms of the MOH of Guatemala (Ministerio de Salud Pública y Asistencia Social, 1989 and 1990), the quality of care framework developed by Bruce (1990), and, especially, the list of quality of care indicators developed by a subcommittee of the United States Agency for International Development (Helzner et al., 1990). The self-assessment checklists enumerate 77 problems or conditions divided into seven sections, one for each quality of care element and an additional one for supervision and evaluation. The providers are asked whether they consider each of the items a problem in their outlet, and, if they do, whether they can solve it with resources at hand. After a group discussion, the most important problems are selected, and a self-improvement plan is drafted. A copy of the self-assessment checklists can be found in *The Family Planning Manager* (1993).

The FPU perceived as advantages of this supervision strategy the focus on quality of care, which was considered a problem in health centers and posts, and the use of a structured instrument, which had been observed to be more effective than unstructured supervision in projects in Peru and Guatemala (León et al., 1990; Santiso et al., 1989). In addition, the strategy involves staff in the identification and solution of their own problems, which is considered critical for effective supervision (Benavente and Madden, 1993). It allows service-delivery personnel to focus on family-planning activities over an extended period of time and structures the actions of all staff. The strategy helps supervisors deal with substantive issues in interactions with services-delivery personnel. Through the checklist, personnel learn about quality of care and the importance of satisfying the needs of their clients.

Methodology

The project employed a quasi-experimental, nonequivalent control-group design. Six areas were selected as project sites based on such criteria as the interest and support of the area chiefs. In each area, five districts were randomly selected. Finally, two of these five districts were assigned at random in each area to Experimental Group 1 (indirect supervision), two were assigned to Experimental Group 2 (self-assessment), and the remaining district was included as part of the control group.

Thus, a total of 12 districts participated in each experimental group and six districts participated in the control group. Table 1 presents the districts and the number of health outlets included within each area in each experimental group.

In the control-group districts, supervisors carried out their activities in the traditional manner during their semiannual visits to the service-delivery outlets. In each experimental district, the strategies were implemented in the health center and in all its dependent posts. (Districts usually have one health center and from one to 10 health posts.)

Dependent Variables

The dependent variables measured included (1) impact on the productivity of service-delivery outlets in terms of contraceptives distributed and of couple-years of protection (CYP);[3] (2) the effectiveness of the supervision strategies in terms of the percent of outlets supervised; (3) the cost-effectiveness of the different supervision strategies (money spent per supervised unit); and (4) the satisfaction of workers and of family planning users attended to under different supervision schemes. In addition, for the self-assessment group, the number of problems selected and solved by participating outlets were measured.

Data-collection Instruments

The number of contraceptives delivered and CYPs offered by each outlet were obtained from the Kardex used by each supervisor for his or her units. In the Kardex, the supervisor registers the number and type of contraceptives available

Table 1. Areas, districts, and number of health-care outlets, by experimental group, Guatemala, 1991–93

| | Experimental group | | | | | | Control group | | |
Area	Indirect supervision districts	Health centers (N)	Health posts (N)	Self-assessment districts	Health centers (N)	Health posts (N)	Control group districts	Health centers (N)	Health posts (N)
Baja Verapaz	San Jerónimo	(1)	(1)	Salamá	(1)	(8)	Purulá	(1)	(2)
	San Miguel Chicaj	(1)	(1)	Rabinal	(1)	(5)			
El Progreso	Morazán	(1)	(1)	San Agustin	(1)	(4)	San Antonio		(3)
	Jicaro	(1)	(3)	Sanarte	(1)	(6)	La Paz	(1)	
Jutiapa	Santa Catarina Mita	(1)	(2)	Jutiapa	(1)	(7)	Moyuta	(1)	(6)
	Jalpatagua	(1)	(4)	Atescatempa	(1)	(3)			
Escuintia	Palín	(1)	(0)	La Gomera	(1)	(6)	Tiquisate	(1)	(5)
	La Democracia	(1)	(1)	Nueva Concepción	(1)	(7)			
San Marcos	Tecum Umán	(1)	(6)	Malacatán	(1)	(2)	Sibinal	(1)	(2)
	San Pedro Sacatepequez	(1)	(7)	Tejutla	(1)	(5)			
Quiché	Joyabaj	(1)	(2)	Sacapulas	(1)	(5)	San Andrés Sacabajá(1)		(1)
	Uspantán	(1)	(4)	Santa Cruz Quiché	(1)	(1)			
Total (N)	Districts (12)	(12)	(32)	Districts (12)	(12)	(59)	Districts (6)	(6)	(19)

Source: MSPAS, Quiché, 1992.

Table 2. Mean number of contraceptive methods and couple-years of protection (CYP) distributed per health-care outlet, by experimental group, according to time period, and the difference in distribution between the second time period and the first, Guatemala, 1991-93

	Period: 15 April–14 April		
Group/method	1991–92	1992–93	Difference
Self-assessment (N=50)			
Pills	303.95	300.43	–3.52
Condoms	720.37	757.85	37.48
Tablets	186.98	87.36	–99.62
IUDs	3.11	4.58	1.47
Total CYP	40.24	43.03	2.79
Indirect supervision (N=33)			
Pills	294.23	321.80	27.56
Condoms	857.07	933.68	76.61
Tablets	161.84	191.48	29.64
IUDs	7.82	8.79	.97
Total CYP	52.36	57.98	5.62
Control (N=10)			
Pills	392.99	308.55	–84.44
Condoms	770.46	749.61	–20.85
Tablets	111.60	84.08	–27.52
IUDs	1.68	0.65	–1.03
Total CYP	43.27	33.71	–9.56

at the time of his or her visit, the number of contraceptives given to clients for resupply purposes, and the number delivered by the outlet to clients between the previous and current visits. To adjust for the different dates in which the visits (or workshops) were made, a monthly average was obtained for the different intervisit periods, and the total number of CYPs offered during the periods 15 April 1991 to 14 April 1992 and 15 April 1992 to 14 April 1993 were calculated.

The number of service-delivery outlets supervised was obtained from the records kept by the supervisors in each visit.

Costs for each strategy were estimated from FPU accounting records. Costs included supervisors' and drivers' salaries and per-diem expenses, fuel and vehicle maintenance, travel and per-diem expenses for workshop participants, and workshop materials. The FPU kept a record of expenses incurred for visits to each area, rather than of those incurred for each district. A set of rules was established thereby to divide the expenditures among the different groups. Personnel costs, travel, per-diem expenses, and maintenance costs were divided according to the estimated time supervisors spent in each district, and for the number of service-delivery outlets visited. For workshop materials and travel and per-diem expenses for workshop participants, expenditures could be assigned directly to the corresponding districts.

The satisfaction of workers and users of service-delivery outlets was measured by surveys with 71 service-delivery providers working in a random sample of 17 health centers and 21 health posts, and of 327 MOH current contraceptive users who lived within a 15-block radius of these outlets.

Finally, improvement in quality of care was measured by the number of problems selected for improvement that were solved. (During their visits to outlets, the supervisors recorded in a copy of the self-improvement plans whether each problem had been improved or not.)

Results

The impact of the supervisory strategies on the productivity of family planning services was measured in terms of contraceptives and couple-years of protection provided by service-delivery outlets during the period 15 April 1991 to 14 April 1992 (the year before the experiment) and 15 April 1992 to 14 April 1993 (the year of the experiment). Only service-delivery outlets for which complete information was available for both periods were included in the analysis. Table 2 shows that only the group testing indirect supervision had an increase in the distribution of all methods (pills, tablets, condoms, and IUDs). In the self-assessment group, increases were observed in the use of IUDs and condoms, but the use of pills and vaginal tablets decreased. In the control group, a decrease in the distribution of all methods was observed. In couple-years of protection, the increase between periods was 7 percent for the self-assessment group and 11 percent for the indirect supervision group. The control group showed a decline of 22 percent. However, none of the observed differences between groups was statistically significant.

Further analysis showed that the productivity improvements in health centers testing self-assessment was larger than in those testing indirect supervision. In contrast, indirect supervision was more effective in health posts than was the self-assessment strategy. No improvements were observed either in health centers or health posts in the control group.

Effectiveness and Cost-effectiveness

Table 3 shows that the self-assessment group had the highest proportion (99 percent) of health-care outlets supervised through workshops and meetings in the first semester of the first year of activities. About 86 percent of outlets in the indirect supervision group received supervision. The control group had the lowest proportion (60 percent) of units supervised (not visited or visited when the service-delivery staff was not available). In the second year of activities, participation in the indirect supervision meetings improved to 96 percent while participation in the self-assessment group decreased to 77 percent. Information on the follow-up of health-care outlets in the control group was not available for this period.

Table 3. Percent of supervised health-care units and cost per supervised unit, by strategy, Guatemala, 1991–93

Experimental group	Total units 1992 (N)	Supervised units (N)	Percent of units supervised	Total costs (US$)	Cost per supervised unit (US$)
Indirect supervision	(44)	(38)	86	3,688	97
Self-assessment	(71)	(70)	99	7,963	114
Control	(25)	(15)	60	1,777	118

During the first year of activities, the indirect supervision group had a cost-effectiveness of US$97 per health-care outlet, compared to $114 in the self-assessment group and $119 per unit in the control group. Thus, both of the alternative supervision strategies were more cost-efficient than traditional supervision.

Satisfaction of Workers and Clients

To study workers' satisfaction with their jobs and family planning clients' satisfaction with the services they received, a small survey was conducted in a sample of 38 health-care units and in the communities where they were located. A total of 71 providers and 331 women were interviewed.

Active MOH family planning clients, regardless of experimental group, reported that they were satisfied or very satisfied with the services and that service providers were friendly, easy to understand, and trustworthy. Workers also had a favorable attitude toward family planning and were satisfied with their work as community-service agents, even though they felt that the family planning program was not sufficiently supported by the MOH authorities. Among the few differences observed between the experimental and control groups was the proportion of women reporting that they were using the method they wanted to use and clients' perception of waiting time for services. In both cases, women served by units in the experimental group seemed to be better satisfied than women in the control group. Women in the experimental groups also were slightly more likely to say that they were satisfied with the method they were using and with the services received, and to report that the service-delivery personnel were friendly and easy to understand. However, none of these differences was statistically significant.

Problems Selected for Improvement and Proportion Solved

The MOH personnel attending the quality of care workshops in the self-assessment group planned to carry out a total of 345 improvements to overcome quality of care problems. The largest proportion of problems selected for solution (40 percent) involved information, education, and communication (IEC). Problems related to provider-client relationships (14 percent), technical competence (11 percent), constellation of services (10 percent), continuity and follow-up (9 per-

Table 4. Problems frequently selected and solved by health-care outlet staff within six months of initial workshop, Guatemala, 1992

Problem (N=345)	Total times selected (N)	Percent resolved	Solutions
No display/showcase for methods	(27)	55	Developed materials, demonstration samples
No follow-up of drop-outs	(24)	38	Made home visits; held talks in district health centers; instituted coordination with NGOs
No or few family planning health talks	(16)	56	Held health talks each week; instituted coordination with NGOs
No posters promoting family planning	(15)	40	Developed materials; posters
No training in method prescription	(14)	29	Provided information/ counseling; supervision; evaluation; district-level training
No posters about availability and schedule of services	(12)	75	Developed materials; promoted family planning services
Shortage of forms/ administrative supplies	(11)	64	Asked for support from district/area/family planning unit
Lack of awareness of clients' needs and opinions	(9)	75	Practiced informal surveys at clinics; talked with clients about their needs and opinions
Lack of integrated care with primary health care/ maternal and child health care	(4)	100	Held staff meetings; provided supervision
Storage and expiration of methods	(3)	100	Sought support from supervising MD; included information in training, supervision

cent), and choice of methods and program supervision and evaluation (each 8 percent) were selected less frequently.

During follow-up visits to service delivery outlets, the supervisors gathered information about the extent to which the previously identified problems had been solved. Table 4 shows a sample of frequently selected problems that were solved by the time of the first follow-up, three to six months after the initial workshop. Most of the solutions implemented required only simple interventions, such as making a contraceptive-method display, improving the follow-up of users, or giving informational talks in waiting rooms. In general, the data showed that the more complex the required solution, the lower the probability that the problem would be solved. Problems frequently selected but infrequently solved included a dearth of talks presented to men in the community and a lack of family planning referrals from community volunteers. However, a few solutions were found for complex problems, including the construction of a much-needed bathroom at one health-care post.

By the time of the first follow-up, 38 percent of the 345 selected problems had been solved. After one year, when the next supervisory visits were made, nearly 80 percent of all planned improvement actions had been taken. At six months, the problem-solving effectiveness of the different districts ranged between 5 percent and 60 percent; after one year, they ranged from 33 percent to 100 percent in effectiveness.

Discussion

The question the project was designed to answer was whether more efficient supervision systems could be developed for the Family Planning Unit of the MOH of Guatemala. The results showed that either supervision strategy could be fruitfully employed by the FPU. Service-delivery outlets under both strategies showed greater increases in productivity that the outlets in the control group. In addition, these new strategies were more cost-effective than the traditional supervision strategy. Even more important, both new strategies allow supervisors more direct and substantive contact with service-delivery staff.

Even though the self-assessment strategy was marginally less cost-effective and had a slightly lower impact on the productivity of health-care outlets than did indirect supervision, the advantage of facilitating greater staff involvement by emphasizing and structuring day-to-day tasks in a long-term plan should not be overlooked. This advantage would seem to be especially important for Ministries of Health, which manage many health programs of higher priority than those related to family planning. An additional bonus of the self-assessment strategy was the public relations value achieved by its quality of care focus, and the interest that this topic raised among service providers and government officials. By stressing the importance of satisfying client needs, the FPU was able to show that its main interest was the welfare of women, an important message where some service providers continue to view family planning with reluctance, and where most programs emphasize quantity over quality.

If the FPU were to institutionalize the self-assessment strategy, the checklists used should change from time to time in order to give service providers a sense of novelty. In following supervision rounds, the FPU could use checklists that are focused on the improvement of such specific areas as referral systems, promotion of services or of particular methods, training of providers, the involvement of men in the program, methods for reaching rural populations, and targeting of efforts to reach women with unmet needs. In these cases, the methodology used in this experiment could be used.

Notes

1. The administration of the MOH of Guatemala is organized into 24 health areas or *jefaturas*. The area chief, a physician, works with a team usually consisting of a nurse, a social worker, a rural health technician, an expert in environmental health, a bookkeeper, and one or two administrative personnel. Each member of this team acts as supervisor for his or her respective personnel at the health-district level. An area contains between two and 15 districts that consist of a health center and its surrounding health posts. Centers are staffed by one or more physicians and other health personnel. Family planning methods offered in centers include the IUD, pills, condoms, vaginal tablets and suppositories. Health posts rely upon nurses and nurse assistants and provide pills and condoms, vaginal tablets, and suppositories. Clients requesting the IUD are referred to health centers or area hospitals. Only a few MOH hospitals currently provide sterilization services.

2. Because of the characteristics of the project, the term "self-assessment" is used here to mean the evaluation of service-delivery processes and conditions by means of the project's checklists. Self-assessment is a process that includes but is not restricted to the use of self-assessment checklists.

3. The conversion factors used were one CYP = 100 condoms or 100 vaginal tablets or 13 pill cycles. One IUD insertion = 2.5 CYP.

References

Benavente, Jaime and C. Madden. 1993. "Improving supervision: A team approach." *The Family Planning Manager* 2,5.

Bruce, Judith. 1990. "Fundamental elements of the quality of care: A simple framework." *Studies in Family Planning* 21, 2: 61-91.

Dwyer, J., Jeanne Haws, Grace Wambawa, Mofoluke Babawale, and Frances Way. 1990. "COPE: A self-assessment technique for improving family planning/voluntary sterilization services." Paper presented at the 118th annual meeting of the American Public Health Association, 1-4 October, New York.

The Family Planning Manager. 1993. *Pocket Guide for Service Improvement, a Supplement to The Family Planning Manager.* October/November/December.

Helzner, Judith et al. 1990. *Report of the Subcommittee on Quality Indicators in Family Planning Service Delivery.* Submitted to the USAID's Task Force on Standardization of Family Planning Program Performance Indicators. New York: International Planned Parenthood Federation/ Western Hemisphere Region.

León, Federico, James Foreit, Rosa Monge, Eduardo Mostajo, Sonia Ortíz, and Miguel Ramos. 1990. "An experiment to improve the quality of care in a Peruvian community based distribution program." Final technical report. Lima, Peru.: Instituto Peruano de Paternidad Responsable (INPPARES) and The Population Council.

Lynam, Pamela, Leslie McNeil Rabinovitz, and Mofoluke Shobowale. 1993. "Using self-assessment to improve the quality of family planning clinic services." *Studies in Family Planning* 24, 4: 252-260.

Ministerio de Salud Pública y Asistencia Social (MSPAS). 1989. *Programa Nacional de Salud Materno Infantil. Manual de Normas y Guías de Atención Materno Infantil. Puestos y Centros de Salud.* Guatemala, Guatemala: MSPAS.

——. 1990. *Evaluación del Proceso de Actividades de la Unidad de Planificación Familiar del Ministerio de Salud Pública y Asistencia Social.* Guatemala, Guatemala: MSPAS Unidad de Planificación Familiar.

——. 1992. *Inventario de Unidades.* Guatemala, Guatemala: MSPAS.

Santiso, Roberto, M. Mendieta, and Sandra Rosenhouse. 1989. "Improving the performance of distributors in APROFAM's CBD programs in indigenous areas." Final technical report. Guatemala, Guatemala: Asociación Pro-Bienestar de la Familia de Guatemala (APROFAM) and The Population Council.

Wolff, James A., Linda J. Suttenfield, and Susanna C. Binzen. 1991. *The Family Planning Manager's Handbook: Basic Skills and Tools for Managing Family Planning Programs.* Hartford, CT: Kumarian Press.

Acknowledgments

This project was funded by The Population Council's INOPAL II (Family Planning and Maternal Child Health Operations Research for Latin America and the Caribbean) project under contract with the United States Agency for International Development. The authors gratefully acknowledge the suggestions and assistance of Carlos Brambila, Jim Foreit, and Nancy Murray.

CONDUCT

Introduction

Tomas Frejka

The papers presented in the previous sections have described OR projects that attempt to improve family planning programs. The papers in this section are concerned with the same objective; however, they also deal with problems related to the conduct and the application of operations research. The main issues are:

- *assemblage of critical data*: assembling of relevant background social, economic, environmental, political, cultural and other knowledge that is critical for the optimal design and functioning of programs and projects;
- *unplanned events*: realistic planning of OR projects, taking into account that during all phases, particular factors may turn out to be different from those originally assumed;
- *research design*: selecting an appropriate research design to test the impact of a new service-delivery approach;
- *utilization of program experience*: accumulating of organizational and managerial experience of family planning program providers at all levels during the OR project and using this experience to improve the functioning of family planning programs;
- *scaling up*: expanding small or pilot projects for broader application; from a few communities or facilities to regional, national, or cross-national levels; and
- *generalization*: generalizing knowledge gained from a number of OR projects on identical themes, so that the gained experience and knowledge can be used to inform policy decisions, for planning, and in the operation of programs.

Assemblage of critical data: In the absence of background knowledge, a good chance exists that a project will have some basic flaws and therefore fail. The absence of this knowledge can entail unintended and undesirable consequences. Aspects of the project may be offensive to the clients, difficult for the providers to implement, or damaging for local, regional, or national government leaders. To maximize the chances of success of a project, the authors should have relevant information at hand. Typically, this information may include books analyzing or describing the respective country or region in political, sociological, or anthropological terms, the results of diagnostic studies, and information from local staff as well as from local political leaders.

Often, background information is gathered informally from easily available sources and is implicitly and automatically applied when a project is designed and planned. In other cases, existing knowledge is collected and systematically organized as background material prior to the design and planning of the project under consideration. Occasionally, a special effort is considered necessary for collecting a body of knowledge before the project can be designed, planned, and implemented. Such was the case with the Taichung project (see, in the Impact section, Berelson and Freedman, and Freedman). The baseline survey prior to the project served not only the purpose of gathering data for comparison and eventual evaluation of impact, but, equally important, it served "also as a guide for program action" (Berelson and Freedman). The paper on the Navrongo experiment presented in this section (Nazzar et al.) illustrates the breadth and depth of knowledge that was assembled so that a culturally appropriate health and family planning program for a traditional community could be designed and implemented.

Unplanned events: Foreseeing specific developments that will interfere with the implementation of a planned OR project is difficult. The most common general occurrences causing problems in the implementation and subsequent evaluation are: (1) that the interests of the researchers may come into conflict with those of the managers while the project is in progress; for example, program managers may make decisions based on preliminary results before the project has run its course; (2) that a second unplanned intervention is introduced confounding the results of the study; and (3) that the intervention may reach the control group prior to the completion of the study, making evaluation of the results of the intervention impossible.

Problems in the implementation of a project can stem from personnel issues. Research staff hired and trained for the project may leave and their replacements may not be fully qualified to conduct the project appropriately. Sometimes service-delivery personnel ignore research protocols; for example, they may fail to assign clients to experimental and control conditions randomly and thus may contaminate the results. Personnel hired and trained for the project may be of lesser quality than was expected or exert more initiative and independence than is desirable, thereby affecting the results. Interference may also originate in the social, political, economic, or natural environment surrounding the project. A drought, an earthquake, or an economic or political crisis may affect the physical conditions of the project or the performance of program workers.

The Fisher and Carlaw paper in this section vividly illustrates a number of these problems, all of which occurred in a single project. To some extent, preventing events from interfering with the outcome of a project is made possible by building flexibility into the project, by anticipating disturbances that may occur, or by using research techniques, such as random assignment, that are robust enough to survive problems in the program environment.

Research design: Design selection is closely related to the need for realistic planning. In a field setting where unplanned events may occur, selecting a research design that can survive many unanticipated events can provide satisfactory, meaningful, and policy-relevant results. Fisher et al. argue in their paper reprinted here that applying a quasi-experimental rather than a more powerful experimental design will frequently accomplish the desired objective. They propose the principle of three multiples, that is, using multiple sources of data, multiple measurements over time, and multiple replications of the study intervention. The fulfillment of such requirements may present difficulties, however. For instance, there may be insufficient financial resources, time, or availability of suitably trained personnel to carry out multiple measurements.

Utilization of program experience: Program managers accumulate valuable experience during the course of their work in many different aspects of family planning service delivery. This experience is a valuable source to be used in the design and implementation of OR projects. Close cooperation of managers and researchers contributes to the quality of OR projects, and the results of the research are more likely to be employed and scaled up. A good example of manager–provider participation in the OR process is discussed in the MEXFAM paper by Vernon et al. in the Quality of Care section of this book. Through participation in the continuous quality-improvement process, staff are enabled to design and implement OR projects with a minimum of outside assistance.

Although managers and providers bring essential experience to OR projects, it is also true that working on an operations research project can be a valuable experience for managers and providers, even in areas unrelated to the project's intervention. Although the originally planned project discussed in Fisher and Carlaw experienced so many unanticipated negative events that they posed severe threats to the validity of the evaluation of the project, a series of unanticipated positive experiences were gained. As a result, important changes were made in the management of the Nepal family planning program, such as the decision to decentralize training, to expand the role of field-workers, and to involve local leaders in family planning committees.

Scaling up: Whatever an OR project's substance, considering whether it can be used elsewhere and whether it has broader application is relevant, that is, whether what works in one community can also work in other communities. Frequently, the preparations, quality of staff, extent of supervision, and attention to detail applied in an OR project may be difficult to replicate on a regional or national scale. Thus, the gained experience may have to be applied with a lesser amount of resources per unit of service or per client. A number of papers in this volume deal with various aspects of these issues (see, in this volume, Berelson and Freedman, Faúndes-Latham et al., Rosenfield and Limcharoen, and Freedman). Financial and organizational problems also emerge when pilot projects are expanded. The report on a project in India (to offer small monthly cash incentives for a limited period to see if doing so would lead to an increase in the knowledge and use of temporary methods of contraception among rural women in an environment where only sterilization was being promoted intensively) discusses the issue of sustainability when a project is scaled up. Stevens and Stevens provide a detailed exposition of this project that was originally implemented on a small scale. The project subsequently went through a series of experimental variations and eventually was expanded from private to public facilities and to larger urban and rural areas.

Generalization: When several projects have been undertaken on the same or similar issues in comparable settings, a joint evaluation of such projects may yield stronger conclusions with wider applicability than findings from a single study alone. Vernon analyzed six operations research projects dealing with the promotion of vasectomy in three Latin American countries where the target population was young and comparatively well-educated men and came up with a number of important findings that can be used to design and implement potentially successful services: that mass-media promotional strategies have tended to be effective, especially in large cities where high-quality clinic services are available; that certain campaign themes have been shown to be effective, namely that vasectomy, particularly performed without a scalpel, has many advantages over female sterilization; and that men elect vasectomy out of love for their wives and concern for their health.

Developing a Culturally Appropriate Family Planning Program for the Navrongo Experiment

Alex Nazzar, Philip B. Adongo, Fred N. Binka,
James F. Phillips, and Cornelius Debpuur

Although levels of mortality and fertility in rural Sahelian populations rank among the highest of any setting in the world, little is known about feasible strategies for addressing these critical problems. Basic health and family planning technologies have been developed and are available at low cost, but profound social, economic, and institutional obstacles prevent the delivery of even the most basic technologies to target groups. While commentators often recommend community involvement for such settings, practical examples of how to achieve this are rarely documented in the policy or scientific literature.[1] Instead, policy documents engage in vague exhortations to "improve supervision," "strengthen management," or "encourage community participation" that have no meaning to service managers who face such severe budgetary, bureaucratic, and social constraints on progress that little more is possible than what has been done in the past. Recognizing the need for practical guidance from field research on this issue, Ghana's Ministry of Health (MOH) designated one rural district of one of its two northernmost regions as a special experimental area. Located in Kassena-Nankana District of the Upper East Region, the Navrongo Health Research Centre (NHRC) is equipped to assess the health and family planning service needs of rural communities, develop new approaches to village-based care, and assess the impact of experimental schemes.[2]

The Navrongo setting represents a challenging context for the introduction of health and family planning services. Literacy levels are low, women's autonomy is constrained, poverty is pervasive, and mortality levels remain high, even by West African standards. Customs associated with the traditional sedimentary lineage system and strong extended family ties tend to emphasize the importance of childbearing early in marriage. Religious beliefs, economic institutions, social organization, and marriage customs all lend support to high-fertility

Reprinted with the permission of the Population Council from *Studies in Family Planning* 1995. 26,6: 307–324.

norms. Further obstacles to service-delivery operations are geographic features of the locality that limit the coverage of the health-care system. Settlements are generally isolated from roads, communication, electrification, and markets. Clinics have been constructed in Navrongo town and outlying subdistrict health centers, but caseloads of fixed service points are low, because travel costs are prohibitive for most households. Reliance on traditional medicine remains the norm; clinical facilities are overstaffed and underused.[3]

The Phase I Pilot Study

The MOH launched a series of investigations in 1993 designed to clarify reasons for the poor coverage of health and family planning services in rural Ghana, and to identify feasible options for improving community-based health-care delivery. Community-based distribution (CBD) in Ghana has involved traditional birth attendants (TBAs) as local contraceptive sales agents and distributors. Various assessments have indicated that this approach was not working. To determine why CBD had failed and what could be done to address this problem, a series of diagnostic studies and field investigations were launched. They also sought to discover whether the new program of action, the Community Health and Family Planning Project (CHFP), would be acceptable to the communities served.[4] This research program, constituting Phase I of the Navrongo experiment, involved consulting communities to determine if the highly developed traditional structure of rural African communities can represent an organizational resource for establishing effective community health services. This pilot program was launched in March 1994 in three villages of Kassena-Nankana District. A pilot service-delivery system was implemented and modified over time, and a social research system was conducted to gauge community reactions to pilot services, clarify the nature of social resources for improving operations, and guide strategic change in the service-delivery model.[5]

This Phase I activity was designed to develop the service-delivery system of a large-scale experiment to be launched in Phase II. Phase I of the Navrongo experiment represents an application of open-systems theory to the practical problem of developing appropriate human service organizations for rural African populations. Open-systems perspectives emphasize the importance of adapting formal organizations to the broader institutional environment.[6] In this view, effective family planning programs are adapted to the social environment, because fostering reproductive change involves interaction with individuals and groups about matters that are strongly influenced by social norms and institutions.[7] The Navrongo project aims to generate practical experience in adapting operations to the social environment. While African social institutions inhibit the process of fostering reproductive change, social organization also represents a powerful resource for getting service work done. Placing services in traditional communities involves much more than distributing contraceptives. Phase I has, therefore, involved analyzing the structure of Navrongo's society and the climate of its reproductive and health beliefs and practices, diagnosing the constraints these place on achieving program objectives, and proposing appropriate ways to respond to these constraints.

Research is based on 12 focus-group discussion (FGD) panels, each comprised of 8–12 respondents, convened prior to Phase I operations. Six different types of participants were included: Women younger than 30 years, older women between the ages of 30 and 45, wives of compound heads, young men, opinion leaders, and heads of compounds in rural Kassena-Nankana District. Sessions were designed to elicit discussion of reproductive beliefs and preferences, the value of children, and household decisionmaking.[8] In-depth interviews were held among chiefs, lineage heads, landlords, and soothsayers in the baseline period.[9] In-depth interviews were repeated at 90-day intervals after the onset of service operations. In addition, detailed field observations were compiled to include open-ended, in-depth interviews of service providers, their supervisors, chiefs, and elders to gauge reactions to service-delivery operations. The regimen of focus-group interviews was repeated in the course of Phase I. This appraisal is based on the initial interviews, baseline in-depth interviews, and follow-up interviews of community leaders.

Results of in-depth interviews and FGDs were reviewed by a strategic planning committee comprised of the District Health Management Team (DHMT), the project social scientist, and special pilot service-delivery workers.[10] Since Navrongo Demographic Surveillance System (NDSS) interviewers and supervisors are particularly knowledgeable about the Kassena-Nankana people, these research workers were convened as a special focus-group team to comment on proposed plans and strategies.

Project social scientists extracted lists of sociocultural constraints from the FGDs and from the in-depth interview data. These constraints were grouped into four general themes, and the strategic planning committee was invited to identify related programmatic obstacles and possible strategies for responding to them. This article discusses the results of the first six months of the strategic planning process, addressing with particular attention the challenging problem of organizing the family planning component of a community health program. Constraints to family planning practice reviewed in this analysis are embedded in interlocking health, gender, and development determinants of reproductive behavior.[11] The search for feasible operational strategies, therefore, extends beyond developing contraceptive accessibility to more general consideration of how traditional communities are appropriately served by outreach programs.[12]

Obstacles to Program Success

Fertility has been high and unchanging for at least a generation.[13] Women consign considerable importance to having children early in marriage, with the belief that many children are required if both sons and daughters are to survive.[14] Focus-group discussants are typically aware of the particular infectious diseases that are the leading causes of death. As one compound head noted:

> In recent times you people are always talking about *adog-maake*.[15] As we are in this area, we don't know anything about adog-maake. Why do I say this? During the days of our fathers, there was a sickness called *katsuwar* [measles] that could come into a compound and kill all children. Now if you say you want to limit your children, measles is dreadful and can even kill ten children at a go. So how can we limit the number of children? In Naga here, this problem still exists, so if you have five children, it is good for you to continue having children, because our eyes have seen in Naga here how our children have been killed by this sickness. I have one wife, and if she is able to deliver ten children, I will continue. I will not agree to adog-maake. I'm already suffering, but I will not agree to adog-maake.

High mortality, prevalent infectious disease, and related security concerns represent the most commonly discussed nexus of factors that women and men cite as constraining their interest in family planning. As one weeping woman noted, in relating her experience:

> It is true that if you give birth to two or three children, it is okay, but because our children are dying, that is why we give birth to many children.

The leading causes of death are well known to villagers: Acute respiratory infections, malaria, measles, diarrhea, and cerebrospinal meningitis, in that order. These risks are compounded by seasonal hunger, nutritional adversity, and widespread poverty, and are all viewed as contributing to the risks associated with infectious disease.

Existing public health services have done little to mitigate these concerns. While health conditions may well have had an impact on some causes of morbidity, perceptions of risk have yet to change.[16] Communities continue to rely upon traditional healers, traditional birth attendants, and soothsayers for health services, rather than upon allopathic medical practitioners. A few families use modern medicine for their health problems, but costs are prohibitive for most families, and distances to health facilities are, for most, insurmountable. Modern health care is something provided at distant places by people who are culturally removed from the village health system at prices that village members cannot afford. As a result, use of the formal health-care system is rare.

The problems of prevalent ill health and high mortality are compounded by ecological conditions of the study district. Declines in rainfall in recent decades and the poor quality of soil in the area have resulted in diminishing yields for the subsistence farmer. With compound farms averaging between one and a half to two acres, the success of a family farm is critical to the nutritional needs of the compound. Hunger and nutrition-related disease such as vitamin A deficiency, kwashiorkor, marasmus, and pellagra are common, especially among children.[17] Several insightful analyses have documented ways in which African religious customs have evolved in response to high mortality.[18] Focus-group studies indicate that religious customs and beliefs emphasize the spiritual importance of progeny, lineage, and descent. A person with many children will have souls on this earth to commune with in the afterlife; whereas the soul of a childless man or woman will dwell in a wasteland of spiritual isolation. As focus-group respondents noted (a male opinion leader and male compound head, respectively):

> We want to have children so that our generation will not be lost. One would like to have children, grandchildren, and great grandchildren so that your name will not be forgotten after your death, as we have not forgotten our ancestors, forefathers, and fathers.

Lineage is a matter of particular spiritual importance:

> If you have children, you expect some, if not all, to continue the line of your father's line, especially the reasonable ones, because we have inherited idols, and shrines from our fathers, which is useful to society. So if they continue with our father's lines, all these will not get lost.

Although high fertility represents a rational response to adversity and mortality, many women nonetheless claim to want access to family planning. Such decisions are not governed by individual women, however; these matters are the prerogative of husbands and kin. Even matters so minor as taking a child to a clinic require the concurrence of husbands, mothers-in-law, and compound heads, a phenomenon that we have termed "gatekeeping." Few women acquire any formal education, and most are illiterate, preventing employment of Kassena-Nankana women in the modern economy, and diminishing the role of migration as a source of exposure to extrafamilial ideas and institutions. Isolation of women from external ideas is profound, in part because few roads, amenities, or radios exist; in part because of linguistic isolation; but most importantly, because so few women have acquired formal education.

The problems of young women are particularly acute. Arranged marriage among teenagers is virtually universal and is accompanied by a dowry payment. Although premarital fertility is believed to be low, fertility soon after marriage is highly desired. Thus, high adolescent marital fertility rates occur in a population where maternal mortality is known to be extremely high for first-born children. These problems are compounded by the stigmatization of women, their limited access to prenatal and delivery services, and the high incidence of reproductive tract infections.

A further constraint on the practice of contraception is imposed by a pervasive lack of male support for fertility regulation. This, in turn, is related to the widespread practice of polygyny, infrequent spousal communication about reproductive issues, and low levels of spousal trust that have been documented in reference to traditional settings elsewhere in Africa.[19] Men view their wives and children as property. Children bring prestige to men and their wives, not only as a tradition, but also through the system of land allocation. A large, extended family has a claim on correspondingly large tracts of farmland; a large compound with many children will have land to till and laborers for working the fields.

Decisionmaking in Kassena-Nankana society subordinates individual preferences to the collective will of family, kin, and community. For example, few women view travel for health or family planning services as something that they are free to pursue, unless husbands, compound heads, and mothers-in-law are consulted and their approval is obtained. Decisions about health care are particularly subject to the opinions of others.

Women's roles not only constrain their autonomy, but limit their means of communication about reproductive matters. They rarely discuss their reproductive preferences with their husbands, and many view their husbands as the key decisionmakers about such matters. Many individuals expressing support for fertility regulation also express the view that they cannot discuss their preferences openly with others, because rumors about such matters can be embarrassing. Women, in particular, are reluctant to initiate such discussions.

Traditional religious practices interact with male dominance in ways that further complicate the introduction of family planning among the Kassena-Nankana. Fertility is considered a spiritual matter of such central importance to families and lineages that soothsayers must be consulted about all questions concerning future childbearing. A woman with concerns about her fertility is obligated by tradition to raise this issue with her husband, who, in turn, must discuss with the compound head the matter of a consultation with a soothsayer. The soothsayer engages in incantations that are believed to lead to spiritual exchanges with the ancestral lineage. The male-dominated process of religious consultation thus restricts the reproductive autonomy of women Spirits symbolize the male lineage; male soothsayers, male lineage heads, and compound heads practice religion on behalf of women.[20]

Societal restrictions are further compounded by the ecological setting. Apart from the small town of Navrongo, the district is entirely rural with a settlement pattern that is so diffuse that no other villages or towns of consequence exist. This situation hampers the development of communications, electrification, and other amenities. The economy is dominated by subsistence farming. Although most compounds now have access to traditional markets for trading, goods traded in these markets consists mainly of grain, animals, and domestic products; economic activity remains premodern.

Supply-side Constraints

Primary health-care and family planning programs in Ghana are not new. Ghana was the second country in Africa to promulgate a national population policy and ranks among the earliest countries to adopt regional initiatives for improving primary health care. Yet, health-care services are rarely used, and preventive programs seldom reach the people in greatest need. At the heart of the problem is the tradition of organizing health services according to the technological requirements of dealing with clinical problems—an institutional philosophy that characterizes health-system bureaucracies everywhere.

At the top of the hierarchy are the teaching hospitals and regional hospitals where the most complex surgery is conducted, and specialists are resident. Next in importance are the district facilities where hospital care is provided to those who can reach facilities and afford to pay for ambulatory care (known as Level C). Third in rank are the clinics dispersed in rural areas, and staffed entirely by paramedics (Level B). Finally, at the periphery, are village health posts that are staffed by volunteers or organized by outreach workers (Level A).[21] The result of this structure is an institutional culture that is fundamentally shaped by the requirements of treating illness rather than of preventing it. Resources are committed in top-down fashion to static facilities. Staff, in turn, are assigned to facilities, provided housing to remain where they have been assigned, and denied resources that would enable them to provide community-based care.

The Clash of Institutional Cultures

This official top-down style is poorly suited to fostering the involvement of traditional community organizations in family planning.[22] Primary institutions of family, kin, chieftaincy, and paramountcy are of overwhelming importance; secondary institutions organized by the government for human services are of no practical significance to rural families. Thus the organization of community initiatives through the Ministry of Health represents a clash of institutional cultures—the categorical aims of a top-down bureaucracy collide with the nonbureaucratic style of traditional village governance.

The Ministry of Health's attempts to develop volunteerism are a case in point. Tapping community support for primary health care by enlisting volunteers in the program proved to be a promising lead that has failed completely. The Ministry recognized that it could not afford to post primary health-care providers in every village of Ghana, but could afford to backstop the work of village volunteers. Accordingly, several thousand village health workers (VHWs) have been recruited, trained, and equipped to provide basic health services. Clearly, the training for VHWs has been too brief, with too little emphasis on the harm that they can bring to a community by peddling antibiotics. Without a career ladder leading out of their volunteer role, VHWs have little incentive to function as volunteers and no supervision to ensure that they do no harm. The challenge is to identify a productive role for volunteers that recognizes their need for incentives to sustain their involvement, but bases the incentive system on services that actually benefit the community.

Contributing to this problem is the official policy of treating VHWs as if they were an unpaid cadre of the MOH. Communities were consulted when VHWs were selected, but were not involved in their supervision in any way. Focus-group discussions indicate that considerable hostility to this program exists and that the VHW program should be disbanded. Volunteerism remains an important value among the Kassena-Nankana. A need exists to review the role of volunteerism to clarify ways in which it can be broadened to include traditional committees, chiefs, and elders in supervisory roles, with technical support from MOH community health nurses (CHNS).[23] At present, village volunteers do not work at all, or if they do, they operate as completely independent unsupervised agents for marketing drugs.[24]

Respondents believe that an appropriately redesigned volunteer scheme could fulfill a need if the volunteers could be trained and equipped with safe and effective pharmaceuticals, so that family planning is not the obvious purpose of sales exchanges:

> When you are going to buy family planning drugs, and your colleagues see you, they will laugh at you. They will say, "Oh, I know this man is going to buy the drug for his wife."

The Lack of Effective Outreach

Other operational problems have hampered the introduction of community health services. CHNs have been community workers in name only. In general, the two-year training program for CHNs has not served them well, because it is too theoretical with too little practical training and no follow-up in service delivery. Work routines are not community related. Outreach services are not reliably scheduled. Communities, in turn, never know what to expect from the system, and have learned to keep their hopes to a minimum. Villagers have little reason to trust the system or to expect it to address their concerns and needs. In the absence of a coherent outreach system, the population is almost completely unexposed to service delivery. The distribution of contraceptives at convenient locations would improve the accessibility of services, but social constraints would persist. If distribution alone is pursued, no mechanism exists through which the systemic restrictions to behavioral change are addressed by the program.

As noted above, male dominance of the society, economy, and family is so profound that the women reached with services have no social, religious, or familial support for fertility regulation. Simply distributing supplies at convenient clinical outlets fails to address the social structure that limits reproductive autonomy more generally. By failing to address the institutionalization of high fertility, community-based distribution of contraceptives represents a less promising approach to introducing reproductive change among the Kassena-Nankana than has been the case in less structured societies elsewhere. Services are oriented to facilities and technologies rather than to the needs of people and communities. Work routines, logistics systems, resource allocation, operational rules, and guidelines correspond to passive health-care facilities rather than to the requirements of achieving coverage, quality-oriented services, and sound community relations. The problems of high fertility and mortality persist. The challenge to be confronted in this experiment is to achieve a fundamental reorientation of MOH staff and activities, presently focused on facilities, to a more genuine focus on the health and family planning problems of the community.

Resources for Meeting the Challenge

Although the CHFP faces daunting obstacles to the launching of its program and to achieving success, various resources are available that can be marshaled for the program. Of particular importance to the future of family planning in Kassena-Nankana District are the existing demand for services, the social structures that can be employed for contraceptive supply, and the staff and equipment that are already available.

Emerging Demand

Survey research suggests that some demand for family planning exists in the study area. More than one-fourth of the currently married women in the study area state that they want no more children, a proportion that increases with age and parity in the fashion that is so often observed in surveys conducted elsewhere. Survey responses thus suggest that desire for family planning exists, especially among older, high-parity women or young women who have had several closely spaced pregnancies. When currently married women are interviewed about their preferences and intentions to practice contraception, nearly half indicate an interest in fertility regulation. Nearly 30 percent say they intend to

adopt a method soon (Debpuur et al., 1994). Surprisingly low proportions of respondents state that they are unsure about future use.

Focus-group discussions suggest ways in which economic changes in the
recent past may have fostered emerging demand. Both men and women expressed concerns about the consequences of high fertility, and ways in which traditional fertility values are anachronistic. Often this line of discussion is couched
in terms of what discussants feel is ideal, and was the norm in the past, but is no
longer feasible, given today's circumstances.

Discussions of the economic or labor value of children illustrate this point.
Increasingly, families see the value of children as deriving less from what they
contribute as farm laborers than from their wages earned in distant cities and
towns. Sending children away to earn money for the family is recognized as a
strategy that works best if one or two children are well educated and have good
jobs. Moreover, the investment in children works better if few children are given
opportunities than if many children are reared in the hopes that one or two will
succeed in life.[25] But educating children is expensive, and the problems of financing the schooling of children are mentioned frequently in focus-group discussions on this issue. No only are uniforms, books, and desks often too costly for
households, but the investment is sometimes questioned on quality grounds.
Discussants note that schools are typically poorly maintained, teachers are
poorly trained and uncommitted, and schooling detracts from other tasks that
children can readily perform. But such discussions arise in the context of parents' expressing aspirations for children that are, in a genuine sense, nontraditional. Some people say that they want to have a few well-educated children who
can go somewhere else, earn a good living, and send money home. Faith in the
value of education is new in this society. Nonetheless, such views are emerging
as a factor in perceptions of the value of fertility regulation.

Discussions of such notions are typically expressed in terms of how the
past generation differed from the present. Many uneducated children sent off to
cities for economic gain are seen as unreliable supporters of parents, and are
characterized by respondents as "thieves" who are not as trustworthy as educated children capable of finding wage income:

> Formerly, giving birth to a large number of children was the norm,
> but these days if you give birth to a large number of children you are
> going to suffer. What is good for this generation is to have three chil-
> dren and make sure they all go to school. If you have many children,
> they are going to get lost. They are likely to be thieves and jobless.

Thus, the notion that children are assets is subject to considerable qualifi-
cation among respondents. Under ideal circumstances, a child is a source of
security, but in practice, only a few can be trusted to carry out familial obliga-

tions. Some argue that to ensure security, many children are needed so that a few "good sons" will go somewhere, succeed in some way, and support their elderly parents. Others counter this view:

> People are now trying to marry only one wife and limit the number of children they deliver in order to be able to look after them well, because, if there are many children in your family, at this time of the year (dry season), there is no job here. All our children leave and go to Kumasi, and when they get there, there are no jobs. They have to steal.

Issues arise, moreover, that indicate possible changes in the way the Kassena-Nankana view the traditional economy, as well as shifting views on the economic role of children. In focus-group sessions, respondents often talk about high fertility as something that was appropriate in the past, but is ill-suited to the rigors of contemporary survival. For example, elderly men often speak of how land was once plentiful, but is now scarce:

> Before family planning came, we had very good rains and our farms produced maximum yields. We were getting good food yields from our farms; we were also having some sheep, goats, and cows. We attempted to marry every beautiful woman that came our way and have lots of children. Recently, family planning has come and some people are seeing that it is good to have one wife and few children, because there is no land to farm and feed the children.

Others relate this scarcity of land to population growth, and turn to the issue of seasonal shortages, famine, and adversity in the manner of village Malthusians. Interpreting such statements is difficult, because, clearly, they do not express the dominant view, and the notion that fertility should be regulated and children spaced for the economic well-being of parents is new to this society. Common ground exists in discussing such issues, however, and may indicate altered economic perspectives that can set the stage for reproductive change.

A basis for optimism is implied by results from the apparent desire for family planning expressed in the baseline survey. The true meaning of such responses is subject to challenge on the grounds that women may not have understood the question or that contraception is unlikely to be practiced to control fertility in the Western sense. Nonetheless, survey responses may indicate an emerging demand for family planning that is also evident in focus-group discussions. Many couples are clearly receptive to the concept of contraception.

Cultural Resources for Supplying Contraceptives

The Kassena-Nankana have a highly structured social organization in which lineages and chieftaincies define hierarchical relationships, and networks define important lateral linkages across lineage groups. Both represent important resources for organizing family planning services. Traditional women's networks are formed for trade purposes, music groups for traditional performances, and other types of associations are formed for various purposes. The CHFP has not yet identified these networks, but they are believed to be important bases for communication and interchange.

More important than networks, however, are the social organizational roles of the hierarchical lineage and chieftaincy system. Each of the villages of Kassena-Nankana District has a royal lineage and a chief who serves his people. According to tradition, the chief mediates disputes and attempts to solve all of the community's social problems. He also represents the community to outside authorities. The chief is consigned the place of honor at any occasion, and is engaged in a dialogue with his people on a continuous basis. A simple meeting place lies outside the chief's compound where he holds audiences and serves as judge (and jury) for matters raised by those seeking his help. The chief rules through his council of elders or lineage heads. He symbolizes village unity and attempts to quell conflict and prevent factionalism. In addition, he serves as the ritual head of the community's religious activities. Chiefs are selected by a council of elders of the royal lineage on the basis of character and devotion to service. Once a chief has been installed, he becomes the reigning chief for life.

In all, Navrongo has 12 paramount chiefs. In visiting these chiefs to discuss family planning, the authors were immediately impressed by the degree of authority that they exercise, and the unusual sophistication they evince about social programs, health, and development. Our initial concerns about opposition to family planning have proved to be unfounded. All paramount chiefs in Kassena-Nankana District have been involved actively in development programs, politics, or large-scale farming.[26] All strongly support family planning. One has volunteered extensively with the Planned Parenthood Association of Ghana.

As a group, the chiefs function in the manner of collaborating members of the CHFP study team—advising the project on strategy, organizing community action, and participating in program deliberations. They, in turn, convene meetings with project staff, divisional chiefs, and lineage heads on matters requiring the attention of the community. These meetings and discussions have four vital functions for the project: First, chiefs and elders can call meetings, known as *durbars*, for communicating information on subjects requiring collective action to the entire community. Second, arriving at agreements with chiefs legitimizes activities that might otherwise be controversial, thereby preventing needless conflict Third, activities organized by the chief translate directly into educational and communication activities that would be complicated and expensive to organize without their support. Finally, participation of the chiefs permits delegation of duties to the community, responsible action in support of the program, and collective participation in the process. Early activities have focused on obtaining housing for CHNs donated by the community, but a much broader program of collaboration is envisioned for the future.

Durbars organized by the chiefs have proved to be particularly useful to the CHFP, because the speeches, songs, and dialogue at such meetings build credibility for field-workers and emphasize themes that worker advise conveners to focus on. As the pilot project has progressed, durbars have increasingly become a mechanism for health communication, strategic planning, and gauging community reaction to activities.

Untapped Programmatic Resources

While MOH resources for primary health care are severely limited, resources are a lesser problem than the inefficient deployment of staff and equipment: four fully functional community subdistrict clinics are available, 32 CHNs who have been trained for two years in paramedical services, three four-wheel-drive vehicles, an outreach clinical staff, pharmaceuticals, and more. These usual resources of the Ministry, if mobilized properly, can reach a far greater proportion of the population than has been the case in the past. Detailed plans were required to clarify the work routines of CHNs, communities, and supervisors. This clarification required planning logistics, purchasing equipment, and developing management information systems (MIS), culminating in the relocation of CHNs. Early in the pilot outreach process, preliminary work plans were seen to be inflexible: Seasonal rains are associated with seasonal planting and harvesting activities. Work plans were, therefore, adapted to seasonal conditions.

Findings from the Strategic Planning Process

When operational planning must confront so many interlocking problems simultaneously, forming an interdisciplinary team to inventory all problems—whether large or small—and to develop strategies to deal with the problems is helpful. Although this is an ongoing process that has yet to incorporate focus-group data on community reactions to the micropilot project, qualitative studies on fertility norms, behavior, and beliefs have been weighed to identify appropriate actions to take in order to deal with constraints on reproductive change.

Plans for Outreach

The tables that follow report, in the left-hand column, themes and issues that emerge from community focus-group studies that collectively comprise constraints to achieving program objectives. At this stage, fieldwork has concentrated on obtaining a general appraisal of community structure, fertility beliefs and norms, and attitudes toward contraception. The present assessment does not report opinions about the service-delivery operation, and is, therefore, preliminary; it does not include community advice about service operations that the micropilot project will eventually convey. Nonetheless, strategic planning has been a continuous process, involving ongoing operational review of all research activity.

Following the first phase of this study, results were shared with supervisory staff of the Ministry for discussion and review (column 1 of the tables). Initial attention was focused on obtaining an inventory of operational problems relating to these issues (column 2 of the tables). In the course of this review, a proposed strategic response was developed, appearing in column 3 of the tables These strategies have been implemented in the three pilot villages. A final step, to be completed, involves convening focus-group participants to react to the service regimen shown in column 3, advise the Ministry on strategic change, and scale up the Navrongo experiment.

As shown in Table 1, the population is dispersed, isolated, and poor, having little exposure to the health-care delivery system. Reaching the population requires an investment to clarify where people are and to purchase the equipment that could be used to reach them. None of this operational planning is in place in the typical northern Ghanaian district. However, in the Navrongo system, all compounds are mapped and numbered, permitting plans to be drawn up on outreach work routines. Dialogue with community leaders established that CHN relocation would require community liaison and chieftaincy support for the scheme. CHNs required housing that did not exist. Communities were requested to construct a traditional compound for each nurse with volunteer labor and community-donated supplies. This requirement established community ownership of the outreach program.

Seasonality of rainfall and crop planting and harvest is associated with seasonal patterns of adversity, employment, mobility, and availability of cash. The operational design requires adaptation to these circumstances and to rules of work that depart from standard Ministry of Health office hours and work routines.

Plans for Marshalling Cultural Resources

Table 2 represents an inventory of the less obvious features of the socioeconomic context for the experiment. Stating that the population is traditional, for example, is insufficient. What this term means and how operations should be adjusted to the social context must be made clear. This clarification has involved developing detailed guidelines on how to work with chiefs and elders, how to relate to community work routines and supervisory cycles, and how to involve traditional leaders in maintaining program accountability to the community and sensitivity to community concerns. The aim of this activity is to employ traditional institutions as a

Table 1. Ecological constraints on family planning systems development, related operational constraints, and CHFP strategic responses, Kassena-Nankana District, Ghana, 1994

Ecological constraint	Related operational constraint	Strategic response
Project located in an arid region with dispersed settlement pattern	Public transportation system poorly developed	Design work routines to be home based, or market based, or durbar based, so that travel for services is not required
	Clinics are remote and underused	Develop plans for CHNs for community-based health-care and FP services
	No village-based housing for community health nurses (CHNs)	Consult with communities about CHN posting
	No systematic addresses for residents	Construct community-based housing for CHNs with volunteer labor
	No work routine for outreach	Map compounds, develop addresses, plan outreach scheme
	Shortage of vehicles, spare parts, and fuel for outreach	Purchase motorbikes and train workers to use them. Relocate CHNs to villages
Seasonal farming pattern leading to seasonal adversity, mortality, and fertility	No seasonal health service or operational strategies	Plan more intensive family planning durbars for the peak conception season, malaria prevention for the malaria epidemic season, cerebrospinal meningitis education for the CSM season
	Clients difficult to locate during planting and harvest seasons	Use children as locators. Commence evening work shifts
	Seasonal shortages of cash for paying service fees	Experiment with offering free family planning service coupons in the preharvest season
	Migration of young adults during dry season	Maintain MIS records of migration status

Table 2. Social constraints to the introduction of family planning, related operational constraints, and CHFP strategic responses, Kassena-Nankana District, Ghana, 1994

Social constraint	Related operational constraint	Strategic response
Traditional rural society with profoundly pronatalist social institutions, customs, and norms	Weak role of government and bureaucracy and correspondingly strong role of traditional leadership in community governance	Organize program in concert with traditional leaders Convene councils of chiefs and elders to coordinate program activities, monitor implementation, and maintain worker accountability for operations Organize durbars for health and family planning
Male-dominated lineage system	No health or family planning IE&C program directed to traditional leaders or men	Develop a zurugelu program for chiefs, elders, and husbands Involve community leaders in CHN supervision Involve communities in CHN housing construction
Limited autonomy of women; gatekeeping	Women not allowed to travel for services. MOH not organized to take services to women in their homes	Organize MIS, work routines, and resources so that CHNs can take services to women at their doorsteps Provide outreach to gatekeepers and provide CHN training on building trust Develop means of monitoring women's concerns and needs and of communicating women's concerns to men
Prevalent practice of polygyny Poor spousal communication	Prevalent spousal mistrust leading to concerns about possible role of family planning in fostering infidelity or promiscuity. This, in turn, leads to operational policies restricting individual women and unmarried young people's access to contraceptives	Use trusted outsiders (for example, CHNs) for outreach Develop procedures for training all staff to respect confidentiality and privacy Develop communication themes for durbars that place family planning topics in the open Develop strategies to involve chiefs and elders in making family planning a subject of open discussion Develop means of outreach to men who oppose their wives' interest in health or family planning services

Social constraint	Related operational constraint	Strategic response
Pronatalist religious precepts and traditions	Staff and officials overly concerned about risk-taking in family planning service work	Open promotion of family planning through chiefs, elders, and durbars
		Consult with soothsayers to elicit advice on the design of service operations; cooperate with soothsayers with the aim of building trust and collaboration
Fragile demand	Limited range of service options, CBD limited to the pill	Train clinic, field, and supervisory workers to improve service quality
		Emphasize multiple choice and modify logistics, clinical, and field procedures to ensure a wide range of service options
		Develop services for methods that focus-group reponsdents say are in demand (injectable and long-acting methods not requiring spousal involvement); DMPA outreach; develop NORPLANT® and IUD clinical services
	No service links between health care and family planning	In community education, emphasize role of family planning for spacing births
		Provide service support for continuity of use: treatment of side-effects, outreach to gatekeepers, frequent follow-up
		Focus on building CHN credibility and trust through village IE&C campaigns (as opposed to promoting family planning)
		Retrain all staff in health care and family planning; provide quality-of-care guidelines for both components
		Extend health-care services to homes and communities and add family planning to active health-care outreach

resource for the MOH program (for discussion of this theme, see Warwick, 1988, and Wulf, 1985). Column 3 of the table notes this resource, along with organizational tools that chiefs use to implement their authority: The council of chiefs and elders, durbars, and the *zurugelu* system of traditional action committees. Durbars can be convened to review activities with the communities served, thereby providing an efficient means of dialogue about community needs and reactions to the program as well as a diagnosis of problems.

Durbars are scheduled for market days to provide the maximum degree of coverage and are organized in consultation with chiefs and elders so that a coherent theme motivates the occasion. They are completely open to all who may wish to attend. Divisional chiefs and lineage heads are obligated by tradition to participate. Durbars begin with traditional drumming, dancing, and singing, followed by a procession of elders, divisional chiefs, and the paramount chief. A crowd gathers, and a formal program is announced, although the specifics are often swept away by the spirit of the occasion. Formal speech making ensues, followed by a lively open discussion session. To date, most of the discussion has been dominated by men, although the participation of women employed by the MOH has served to open the occasions to dialogue with women. Strategies are pursued for developing women's participation, such as inviting women's singing groups to perform and encouraging women to speak out on issues that arise.

Three themes are evident from these sessions: First, the Kassena-Nankana people are open to outside ideas, appreciative of MOH initiatives, and surprisingly receptive to the role of CHNs as family planning outreach workers. Speeches typically praise the role of these workers, usually in the context of relating personal experiences about health-care exchanges with them. Our impression is that the CHNs provide an important function to the communities they serve. Men in the study area appear to know little about modern contraceptives, and confusion about family planning abounds. Basic family planning education programs for men are greatly needed. Few men really understand how contraceptive methods work, that they can be used for birth spacing, and that they benefit women. The nature of the participants' questions about family planning and their curiosity suggest that much can and should be done to convey basic health and family planning education through durbars. Finally, if the project is to succeed, motivational programs must be devised for men that are as rigorous as the service programs for women. Young men are not only confused by this program but also are worried that women who use contraceptives will be controlling their reproductive lives., Men feel threatened by this notion and concerned that women will be free to find other partners, or assert their autonomy in other ways. The CHFP has begun the process of reacting to these exchanges, but much remains to be done in the future, and the success of the project will hinge on the outcome of plans in this area.

When outreach workers identify problems in the community, their supervisors consult with chiefs and elders. Also, supervisors note problems in registers for review in monthly District Health Management Team staff meetings. Plans are made and activities are proposed that require DHMT follow-up visits to village chiefs and elders. This scheme aims to develop a dialogue between traditional leaders and program management focused on MOH resources for addressing community problems.

In the course of the review, the finding that women often say they want to practice contraception, but must defer to the decisions of others, is of particular concern. Outreach activities and information must be focused on gatekeepers, not just on women of reproductive age. At the same time, outreach must be designed carefully to ensure contraceptive users' confidentiality and privacy at all times. Focus-group sessions indicate that for contraceptive distribution, CHNs are more often trusted to keep secrets than are villagers.

Strategies are being developed to respond to women's concerns that their husbands and kin are not supportive of family planning Some of this work will be undertaken as an IE&C activity at the community level; some will require outreach. A simple "problem routine" has been devised to permit CHNs to designate individual men for outreach sessions.

Soothsayers wield considerable influence, and are likely to be a source of opposition to the promotion of family planning. To deal with this potential source of misunderstanding of the program, the project has undertaken the simple expedient of consulting soothsayers about the project and its work systems, paying them a small fee, noting their advice, and developing as close an understanding of their concerns as possible in the process.[27] This process of consultation with soothsayers will continue, with the aim of providing the project with an early indication of problems, and a sound line of communication with traditional religious leaders.

Simple adjustments to program strategies may address many of the concerns of the Kassena-Nankana that prevent contraceptive use. Because demand for contraception is primarily a demand for spacing future childbearing rather than limiting fertility, communication and dialogue about the program must be structured in terms that are consistent with these preferences and needs. That the terms for contraception used by the existing family planning program translate as "stopping childbearing"—anathema to the women who are interviewed about such concepts—is troubling. Spacing is well understood among the Kassena-Nankana:[28]

> If your wife has a child, for a short period you feel for sex again and you reach your wife, you are likely to kill the previous child. On the other hand, if your wife has a small baby and you like to have sex, the alternative will be to go after other women. Is this good? So if the family planning is there and you bring it, give it to the man in the

presence of this wife and say, "This is adog-maake medicine we have brought to you. Use it to prevent pregnancy, but when your child is grown, stop and deliver again," then we will like it. This will help our children to grow well.

The picture that emerges from survey research on demand for contraception is complex and laden with contradictions. Women consider large families to be ideal, but, nonetheless, many women want to practice family planning. Personal preferences are consistent with the notion that many women will adopt family planning if services are offered to them; the same women view such decisions as belonging rightfully to others who decide on such matters, and view those others as wanting and needing many children soon. Indeed, as other studies in the region have shown, women want to practice family planning less to limit their fertility than to space childbearing or to substitute for traditional forms of contraception.

The implication of this situation is that an overly simplified women-to-women contraceptive-distribution scheme may work for a while, but will probably fail in the long run. Although many of the ambulatory health-care needs in the study areas can likely be addressed by developing a clinical program based in the compound where CHNs reside, a doorstep component of the program is crucial to offering family planning services. Concerns about the confidentiality of family planning together with social restrictions on women's mobility suggest that a health-outreach approach will be far more acceptable than a categorical contraceptive distribution scheme. What is needed is a comprehensive strategy that fosters ideational and motivational change among the male decisionmakers, and convenient services for individual women that make implementing their preferences as simple as possible. They must be able to trust that service providers will help them with information, counseling, and care if anything goes wrong. A very strong and comprehensive program is required, therefore, given the weak climate of demand.

Plans for Responding to Economic Constraints

Table 3 lists economic restraints to the introduction of family planning, and identifies strategic responses to this situation. To date, many critical issues have not been resolved. Among them is the problem of payment for services, and the social costs that payments pose when the commodity to be purchased is a contraceptive. That prices are low is immaterial to rural women. Payment of any kind requires that women negotiate with their husbands and kin about how money is spent, the purpose of family planning, and the rationale for spending money on contraceptives when so many other family financial problems remain unaddressed. Severe food shortages prevail in the preharvest season, and the cost of a family planning injection would provide enough grain for a meal for eight. Under these circumstances, contraceptives are expensive at any price. Careful research is required to determine the implications of these social, psychological, and familial costs associated with payment. Programs are expensive to run; cost-recovery schemes may incur more costs that far exceed the monetary gains they provide for the program. Coupon schemes for offering free supplies merit experimentation and trial.

Although the population is poor and traditional, economic organization is extensive. The table notes how hardships have impeded the success of health and family planning operations and lists ways in which traditional social and economic institutions can contribute to program success, either as means of community program messages or as mechanisms for organizing the delivery of services. Most men belong to labor cooperatives, formed for collective harvesting and other cooperative activities, and they elect leaders known as *Bia Pe* for this network. Many women form trade networks for marketing activities, as well as lending groups, known as *sousou*, for pooling savings and sharing the burden of adversity. Both types of networks have been used for local grassroots political organization. These traditional networks are potentially valuable resources for organizing health and family planning services and may also provide mechanisms for individual women in need to finance contraceptive supplies.

The CHFP has taken an inventory of these networks, identified their leaders, and constituted a program of volunteer activity for reaching men with family planning information and services. In the local idiom, volunteers are termed *yezura zenna* (YZ), a term connoting a trusted health leader. The YZ serve as the primary health providers of the initiative and are charged with promoting the wisdom of fertility regulation in a male-dominated traditional society.

Plans for Responding to Health Constraints

Table 4 lists some of the health- and mortality-related constraints to the introduction of family planning services. In general, the project will focus on health concerns and promote preventive health measures in concert with its promotion of family planning. The prevalence of reproductive tract infections is unknown in the study population, but services are designed on the assumption that such problems are serious and that outreach must be oriented to identifying and solving them rather than to promoting family planning per se. In time, the CHFP aims to develop as broad a service regimen as possible, but to facilitate the eventual introduction of this package, training emphasizes the importance of listening to women, understanding their problems, and seeking solutions, so that reproductive health technology can be introduced readily as capabilities improve. A people-centered system is more amenable to providing reproductive health services than is a system focused narrowly on modalities or demographic aims.[29]

The Strategic Response

Clearly, the service system that is required will take more planning than simply listing problems and assigning the tasks listed in the tables. A new system of

Table 3. Economic constraints to the introduction of family planning, related operational constraints, and CHFP strategic responses, Kassena-Nankana District, Ghana, 1994

Economic constraint	Related operational constraint	Strategic response
Pervasive poverty	General development problems	Offer convenient, low-cost services
		Develop cost-sharing and coupon schemes to mitigate costs
		Experiment with cost recovery to determine the implications of user fees and recommendations to the MOH
Low levels of development, leading to		Use traditional resources for fostering
Low literacy levels, particularly among women		Volunteerism
Limited exposure to extrafamilial social institutions and ideas	Inadequate infrastructure	Community donations and maintenance of CHN housing
Limited access to transportation, markets, and communication	Inadequate communication, health, and educational systems	Active outreach
No electrification outside of Navrongo town		Open discussion of family planning
	Limited exposure to mass media	Develop music, cultural events, and other activities that communicate family planning and health themes through traditional channels
Agrarian subsistence economy, limited exposure to outside ideas	Limited cash for transportation, service delivery, or social-marketing purchases	Review pricing policies; research the implications of fee structure
		Determine if traditional lending networks can support health and family planning expenses
	No link between Ministry of Health programs and economic development programs for farmers or women	Work with trade networks to build program outreach within traditional economic activities
		Contact women and development programs engaged in lending, political action, and women's organizational efforts
		Identify women's trade networks as possible means of communication, service delivery, or organizational work
	Time constraints on adult farming population during planting and harvest seasons	Attempt to identify collaborative links with other outreach programs for farmers or community development programs

Economic constraint	Related operational constraint	Strategic response
Wealth flows from children to parents Security value of children Labor value of children	No social insurance scheme	Build credibility for health-care program; direct resources to improving child survival Communicate information about the benefits of small families
Limited access to the modern economy	No resource in the women's program for loans for income-generating activities	Undertake field research to identify women's traditional economic and trading networks Seek ways of linking services to traditional communication networks

Table 4. Women's health constraints to the introduction of family planning, related operational constraints, and CHFP strategic responses, Kassena-Nankana District, Ghana, 1994

Health constraint	Related operational constraint	Strategic response
High rates of morbidity, infectious disease, mortality	Constrained drug budgets; Shortage of service resources	Focus on resolving principal health problems of mothers and children
Reliance on traditional healers and soothsayers for health advice	Curative bias in health-seeking behavior; unnecessary delays in seeking treatment for children's infectious diseases	Consult with traditional healers regarding program strategies
Concerns about survival of children that impede acceptance of family planning	Widespread misunderstanding of health and FP modalities; Rumors and false beliefs about pharmaceutical side effects	Promote public education in durbars about immunizations, sanitation, disease prevention, and family planning
Seasonal nutritional adversity	Constrained food-relief budgets; logistics problems	Develop outreach strategy for nutrition education; Use focus-group data to identify appropriate themes concerning population problems
Prevalent reproductive health problems	Poor reproductive health-care diagnostic and referral systems	Improve referral systems and facilities; develop antenatal care screening procedures; improve community outreach services to pregnant women
Female genital mutilation	Lack of programs for reproductive health education	Research reproductive health beliefs, customs, and strategies (no strategy yet developed)
High incidence of obstructed labor	No reproductive health outreach; Few trained midwives or traditional birth attendants	Train CHNs in reproductive health screening; Train CHNs to train TBAs
Prevalent infectious disease	Undeveloped laboratory facilities; limited screening capabilities	Develop syndromic screening procedures; train outreach workers in syndromic referral
High rate of maternal mortality	No functional screening program, poorly trained and equipped delivery attendants, and limited budgets for referral transportation, clinical care, and facilities	Test and develop screening algorithm; Explore community transportation resources for emergency referrals; Conduct Situation Analysis of fixed facilities; Review delivery practices and retrain all midwives and CHNs

operations will be required. The absence of a system of work is the central reason for the failure of family planning and primary health care in the area. In the course of the micropilot project, approaches to supervision and deployment, management information, and community-based operations have been developed to provide systems support for outreach. A woman who wishes to regulate her fertility has no institution in her village to turn to. Therefore, an outreach worker acting alone will almost certainly fail: She will be a source of embarrassment to her clients, at best, and if she is too active in promoting family planning, she will be the subject of derision, rejection, and scorn. Therefore, primary workers require an extraordinary sense of support from the program.

Technical Support

The absence of a basic technical support system for community workers has been the principal barrier to the provision of community health services to the study population. When workers in the study area were asked about factors that hamper their work, the most common issue they raised was the conviction that their efforts would prove fruitless. Supplies are inadequate, fuel is lacking, referral services are not functioning, and services sought by the community are not included in the work regimen. A completed review of this situation identifies the minimum configuration of technical support functions that enable workers to do their jobs. This system has yet to be put into place. It includes technical training for all staff so that the highest quality of service possible may be provided; logistics planning to provide transportation, fuel, and supplies; and the development of management information systems to give workers the information they need to sustain normal work routines. A new technical support system will be instituted to address these problems.

Supervisory Support

Supervisors are engaged in monitoring the system of household coverage, clarifying workers' roles, and solving problems that arise. In training, the supervisors' responsibility to assist the worker (rather than the workers' responsibility to report to the supervisor) is emphasized. Workers, in turn, are trained to identify health problems and assist families with their needs Supervisory training is designed to establish a bottom-up orientation to leadership, stressing problem identification and solution and resource mobilization. Workers confronted with this difficult task need to know that supervisors exist to help them do their jobs. Establishing appropriate work routines involves collaboration with community leaders to maintain accountability for work. By informing community leaders of the detailed work plan for their locality and equipping them with simple reporting procedures for lodging complaints, supervisors involve traditional leaders in the supervisory-support process and demystify work routines.

Peer Support

When CHNs were interviewed about their reaction to community work, they repeatedly expressed concerns about isolation, fear of rejection by the community, and vulnerability to various pressures. Such pressures include being asked to provide drugs for free, to perform services not included in the work regimen, to provide services to undeserving clients, and the like. Technical problems also arise that CHNs are requested to address but are not competent to resolve. Workers should be made aware of mutual problems, solutions, and performance, according to the strategy that has been designed.

Zonal meetings are convened for the purpose of fostering interchange between workers about problems, possible solutions, and peer leadership ideas. The pilot CHNs are being used extensively as trainers, with emphasis on counterpart training, as opposed to classroom instruction. As the project is scaled up, those with experience will be involved in training the new CHNs to be deployed, with emphasis on joint fieldwork. Zonal meetings are monthly staff meetings of the CHNs responsible for a treatment area (eventually eight workers), their supervisors, and occasionally technical staff from the District Health Management Team. In these meetings materials are prepared for community leaders, informing them of the work routine and the problems encountered, and problem reports are provided for the DHMT. These reports are brief notes of any difficulties arising at the periphery that could not be resolved at that level. Problem referral is designed to summon resources to assist the CHNs as needed. Most problems stem from the need for diplomatic attention to the concerns of husbands or of heads of compounds. Problems with CHN living arrangements involve mustering community resources with diplomatic support from senior DHMT staff.

Community Support

Achieving community support requires identifying social institutions that can be used to support program activity. For example, community support for CHNs can be generated by promoting CHN activities during public gatherings. To this end, a coupon has been developed that offers free health and contraceptive supplies in return for paying one visit to a CHN. Nearly 300 of such service coupons were distributed at a durbar, entitling recipients to treatment for minor ailments, free family planning supplies for three months, and other services. The idea is not to promote any particular service, but to enhance the credibility and role of the CHN.

Political Support

Administrators and community leaders may be reluctant to take concerted action if they believe that political or administrative risks are inherent in the promotion of the program. Political leaders, in turn, may be reluctant to extend support if they anticipate controversy. The project has, therefore, included an attempt to build political credibility for operations and to involve local political officials in public gatherings and promotional activities. The aim of this approach is to establish for all parties concerned that activities are being undertaken with the support of all the traditional leaders, technical representatives of the Ministry of Health, and political representatives in local government. Building political support requires dialogue, diplomacy, and strategic planning. It is, nonetheless, an essential element of successful community-based family planning in a traditional African setting. In all gatherings fielded in this project, local political leaders have been briefed on project activities; several are now regular participants in family planning durbars.

Conclusions and Implications

In addition to the strategy that has been designed and developed to reach rural women with services at their doorstep and to communicate with their husbands and traditional village leaders and soothsayers, further work is anticipated in a variety of areas.

First, young married men may oppose this initiative, if concerted efforts are not undertaken soon to discuss their concerns and interests openly in durbars and to direct information campaigns to them. Traditional leaders have been more supportive of this initiative than had been anticipated. The strong partnership that the program managers have built with chiefs and elders will provide the basis for effective communication with young men.

Second, strategies must be developed for reaching men through informal social networks. Although communication through durbars is a useful means of legitimizing program activities among men, outreach to male networks may be a more effective way of reaching them on a continual basis. The value of understanding how male economic networks are formed and led, what functions they perform, and whether such groups can be an effective means of reaching young men is clear.

Third, additional strategies are needed for increasing women's contact with the program. The concept of compound visitation rounds is popular and is having an impact, but the population is dispersed, and the pace of outreach is slowed by the settlement pattern. Roughly 2 percent of the currently married women encountered on the first round adopted a method, all but one of whom chose the injectable contraceptive, DMPA. Similar levels of acceptance were registered in the second round. That only four such rounds can be completed in a year suggests that compound outreach alone will not meet the community's need for services adequately. The CHFP is, therefore, developing an outreach clinic program, scheduling it to coincide with market days, and exploring ways of promoting family planning at public gatherings. In addition, it is researching the nature of women's trade and their communication networks, and taking stock of development program initiatives designed to stimulate the formation of women's economic groups. By augmenting compound visits with promotional and service work through networks, the efficiency of outreach may be improved.

Fourth, the volunteerism component of the project has not been addressed in this phase of the strategic planning process. Further clarification of the social role of the lineage system and male and female peer networks may produce ideas that will lead to an effective volunteer program.

Although prototype systems now in operation are functioning well, not all management systems will be developed totally at the beginning of the full experiment. The project will require four years of fieldwork, not only to test demographic results, but also to provide a continuing field laboratory for developing management systems for health and family planning workers. What has been learned already could have an immediate impact on policy, however. Equipping CHNs with a work system and a motorbike greatly intensifies a public health presence in the community. A single community health nurse provides far more service at lower cost than a fully staffed Level B clinic. District Health Management Teams from neighboring districts of Ghana have visited the project. One district is already replicating the CHN outreach approach. Sound, replicable management strategies can be demonstrated by the CHFP, and translated into action far faster than centrally promulgated policy directives. Such dissemination will be a continuous process, involving field observation and collaboration addressing practical questions about what works best in a difficult setting.

Finally, the micropilot work while criticized by some as a prolonged distraction, has been a valuable tool in the project development process. It has created the capacity to manage and plan the initiative before large-scale supervisory and training tasks overwhelm the agenda. It has focused attention on community liaison, strategic innovation, and planning, minimizing the distractions that are implicit in any districtwide initiative that must be administered by a small technical team. The pilot testing has ensured that all potential problems receive scrutiny and all possible leads and strategies are weighed in order to adapt the program to the ecological, social, economic, and institutional realities of the Navrongo setting.

Notes

1. For a discussion of this issue, see Askew (1989).

2. The design of the Navrongo experiment is described in Binka et al. (1995). The Kassena-Nankan district covers about 1.674 km^2 of the Upper East region of Ghana. The name Kassena-Nankana refers to the two ethnic groups of the district. The Kassena-Nankana belong to the Grussi-Gurma group, one of the major ethnic groups in Ghana. The two groups—the Kassena and the Frafra—were originally distinct and have been fused together over the years into a homogeneous ethnic group with a com-

mon culture. They form part of the Gur linguistic group and speak principally two languages known as *Kassim* and *Nankam*, each with varying dialects Although the languages differ substantially, social characteristics of the two groups are similar.

3. The traditional supports of social institutions for high fertility are reviewed in Adongo et al. (1994) and Fayorsey et al. (1994).

4. Four general recommendations emerged from this series of studies: (1) Central importance is consigned to health care and concerns about the risks that children will die. Family planning should be provided in the context of extending community health services to mothers and children; (2) Focus-group respondents often stress the importance of selecting workers who can be trusted to maintain confidentiality. Studies of this issue consistently show that preselected types of village members, such as traditional birth attendants, are not appropriate. Outsiders are often preferable to village members who cannot be trusted to maintain confidentiality; (3) The existing program for information, education, and communication has led to misunderstanding and confusion. A need exists for careful trial and review of culturally appropriate communication themes; (4) In Ghana, a high value is placed on having contraceptive options. If any method is preferred, it is the injectable contraceptive, and this method has been excluded from CBD initiatives (see Ministry of Health, 1991a, 1991b, 1991c, and 1992).

5. In 1995, a fourth pilot village was added to Phase I to test volunteer-worker schemes. This article describes the initial three-village pilot project.

6. Formal organizations are viewed as open systems in equilibrium with their environment (Katz and Khan, 1978; Perrow, 1978). By implication, understanding how to organize social services requires an understanding of the social system (Hasenfeld, 1978).

7. From this perspective, effective organizations are adaptive—continuously responding to changing needs (see Sarri and Hasenfield, 1978). This perspective has been particularly influential in business and commercial research applications (see, for example, Peters and Waterman, 1982), although some applications of open-systems research are noted in the development literature, as well (see, for example, Paul, 1982; Freedman, 1987a; and Simmons and Simmons, 1987). For this reason, some analysts argue that research is crucial to designing and developing successful family planning programs. While open-systems perspectives are theoretically appealing, little has been done to apply these principles to practical situations and to report on steps and procedures that can be used to develop programs (Freedman, 1987b; Phillips and Greene, 1993).

8. Baseline FGD methods and results are presented in Adongo et al., 1995.

9. The term "landlord" in these societies refers to persons who act as custodians or trustees of land. Landlords neither own land nor rent it to others.

10. The DHMT participants were MOH officers concerned with the supervision of field operations. Clinical supervisory staff were not involved in the strategic planning process. The team consists of the project's principal investigator, who is a public health physician, a nurse supervisor, a public health nurse, and a retired regional public health nurse supervisor. Pilot-study community health nurses participated in the final session of the planning process. Various labels have been applied to this management strategy, the most general of which is "strategic planning" (see Paul, 1987 and 1988)—an approach to developing organizational systems that solve complex problems (see also Korten, 1980 and 1984).

11. In noting these constraints elsewhere in the region, several influential observers have concluded that family planning programs cannot succeed in this context (for example, see Frank, 1987 and 1988; van de Walle and Foster, 1990).

12. Community reactions to the Phase I pilot and the final operational design are reviewed in Antwi-Nsiah et al. (1995) and Nazzar et al. (1995).

13. Knowledge of contraceptive methods is high (82 percent) among the Kassena-Nankana, but ever use of contraceptives is only 8 percent, and current use prevalence is very low at 4 percent (Debpuur et al., 1994). Reasons for nonuse are not precisely understood but are believed to be complex, systemic, and ingrained in traditional cultural institutions (Favorsey et al., 1994; Adongo et al., 1994). The total fertility rate in the study area is 6.0 children per woman of reproductive age. Although this level is low in comparison with levels observed elsewhere in Africa, fertility reduction arises entirely from traditional practices of postpartum spousal separation and lactational amenorrhea, rather than from contraception.

14. The infant mortality rate, at 185 deaths per 1,000 live births, ranks among the highest recorded in the contemporary setting. The health and socioeconomic, religious, and traditional governance systems of the people of Kassena-Nankana District are more typical of neighboring Sahelian countries than of the peoples of Ghana's southern and central regions. Mortality in the Sahelian region is the highest of any subregion in the world (see Hill, 1991). Rates of contraceptive use in the Sahel are the lowest of any region (Ross et al., 1993). Various influential observers have commented on the link between high mortality and the culture of high fertility (Caldwell and Caldwell, 1987; Caldwell et al., 1992).

15. The term *adog-maake* is generally used to mean family planning. Translated literally, it means stopping childbirth.

16. Evidence from the Navrongo Demographic Surveillance System (NDSS) suggests that child mortality may have declined slightly in recent years. This issue is under investigation.

17. Vitamin A supplementation has been shown to reduce child mortality in the study population. Nutritional adversity is implicated in all leading causes of mortality among children (Ross et al., 1995).

18. See, for example, Caldwell (1979). Relatively little has been written about ways in which programs can be designed to mitigate religious opposition. There are a few notable exceptions, however. See, for example, Askew et al. (1992).

19. Research in several settings has demonstrated that polygyny reduces natural fertility. Thus, in the absence of other changes, the nucleation of families and monogamous marriage leads to higher fertility. Polygyny, nonetheless, leads to norms, values, and practices that inhibit the introduction of family planning, sustaining natural fertility at levels far below the biological maximum, but well above levels that policy planners consider optimal. See discussions of this issue in Caldwell and Caldwell (1981, 1987, and 1990). The conjugal bond is thought to be weak in cultural settings where polygyny is widely practiced. This, in turn, leads to household economic arrangements in which the costs of children are borne by mothers, but decisions about reproduction are made by husbands. This characteristic of polygynous unions has been documented in several studies of the African family. See, for example, Kalipeni and Zulu (1993). For a discussion of gender roles in Ghana, see Lloyd and Gage-Brandon (1993).

20. Detailed investigation of the role of religion in reproductive behavior has determined that soothsaying is pursued in reference to childbearing, but not in reference to questions concerning contraception. The behavioral implications of this finding are the subject of continuing investigation (Antwi-Nsiah et al., 1995).

21. For all practical purposes, Level A remains a concept that is rarely implemented.

22. Formal bureaucratic organizations have always lacked historic grounding in Sahelian settings. The late arrival of the British and their attempts to introduce government in territories that are now northern Ghana never led to an established civil bureaucracy in the region. Nor have the institutions of the postcolonial era had a great impact on the lives of northern Ghanaians. Contemporary social, health, agricultural, and educational bureaucracies have only a marginal impact on village life. Reports of efforts to organize the civil service in the locality read much like early accounts of British incursions into southern regions (Rattray, 1932).

23. CHNs are outreach workers of the MOH—paramedics trained in MOH nurse-training centers for two years and assigned to rural subdistrict-level clinics. All CHNs are women.

24. A reasonable question to ask is whether village health workers can serve as the front-line agents of the social marketing program. Such a change would shift their function from antibiotic peddling to the more responsible role of serving the community as sales agents for oral rehydration salts, condoms, and oral contraceptives. One CHN has been approached by a trader who sought supplies for sale in a village. Other CHNs are experimenting with distributing condoms through village sales agents who maintain sales depots in their homes.

25. A useful discussion of this issue appears in the report of the National Research Council (1993). Microeconomists refer to the trade-off between quantity and quality of children, noting that parental aspirations for their children are linked to their own reproductive goals.

26. Surprisingly, little attention has been directed in the past toward involving chiefs and elders in MO programs or activities. Of the 12 paramount chiefs who were contacted, none had ever been visited by a District Health Management Team Officer or CHN prior to this pilot project.

27. This strategy is informed by mystery-client research on the quality of health-care and family planning services (Schuler et al., 1985). In the mystery-client methodology, trained research workers pose as clients at service points, observe the quality of services provided, and report observations to investigators. Given the nature of soothsaying, a more open approach is employed about the nature of the encounter: Service workers are concerned about family planning in the community, and they consult soothsayers about the future of the initiative and its acceptability in this setting. Six soothsayers have been asked to consult ancestral spirits about these matters; all six indicated that the project will succeed if various rites are performed as instructed.

28. See the analysis of this issue by Bledsoe et al. (1994). Based on data from rural Gambia, it suggests that the classical concept of "natural fertility" is inappropriate for West African traditional societies where women consciously regulate birth intervals. Contraception is widely accepted and sought after in rural Gambia, but the use of Western contraceptives has little fertility impact, since the purpose of adoption is to maintain desired spacing intervals that are obtained by other traditional means if contraception is not available.

29. Some cultural practices represent particularly challenging reproductive health issues. For example, female genital mutilation is widely practiced. Its prevalence is unknown and the more general reproductive health implications of this custom require clarification. Feasible interventions to address this issue merit investigation.

Acknowledgments

The Navrongo Community Health and Family Planning Project is funded by grants to the Navrongo Health Research Centre from the Rockefeller Foundation, the Finnish International Development Agency (FinnIDA), and the Africa Operations Research and Technical Assistance Project (OR/TA). The OR/TA Project is a regional program of the Population Council funded by the United States Agency for International Development.

References

Adongo, Philip B., James F. Phillips, Beverly Kajihara, Clara Fayorsey, Cornelius Debpuur, and Fred N. Binka. 1995. "Cultural factors constraining the introduction of family planning among the Kassena-Nankana of northern Ghana." Navrongo, Ghana: Navrongo Health Research Centre, Community Health and Family Planning Project. Unpublished.

Antwi-Nsiah, Cherub, James F. Phillips, Placide Tapsoba, Philip Adongo, Kofi Asobayire. 1995. "Community reactions to the Navrongo experiment." Navrongo, Ghana: Navrongo Health Research Centre, Community Health and Family Planning Project. Unpublished.

Askew, Ian. 1989. "Organizing community participation in family planning projects in South Asia." *Studies in Family Planning* 20,4: 185–202.

Askew, Ian, S. F. Njie, and A. Tall. 1992. "Overcoming religious barriers to family planning in rural Gambia." Paper presented at the annual meeting of the National Council for International Health, Arlington, VA, June.

Binka, Fred N., Alex Nazzar, and James F. Phillips. 1995. "The Navrongo Community Health and Family Planning Project." *Studies in Family Planning* 26,3: 121–139.

Bledsoe, Caroline H., Allan G. Hill, Umberto D'Alessandro, and Patricia Langerock. 1994. "Constructing natural fertility: The use of Western contraceptive technologies in rural Gambia." *Population and Development Review* 20,1: 81–113.

Caldwell, John C. 1979. "Variation in the incidence of sexual abstinence and the duration of postnatal sexual abstinence among the Yoruba." In *Natural Fertility*. Eds. H. Leridon and J. Menken. Liège: Ordina Editions.

Caldwell, John C. and Pat Caldwell. 1981. "The function of child-spacing in traditional societies and the direction of change." In *Child-Spacing in Tropical Africa: Traditions and Change*. Eds. H. Page and R. Lesthaeghe. London: Academic Press. Pp. 73–92.

——. 1987. "The cultural context of high fertility in sub-Saharan Africa." *Population and Development Review* 13,3: 409–437.

——. 1990. "High fertility in sub-Saharan Africa." *Scientific American* May. Pp. 118–125.

Caldwell, John C., I. O. Orubuloye, and Pat Caldwell. 1992. "Fertility decline in Africa: A new type of transition?" *Population and Development Review* 18,2: 211–242.

Debpuur, Cornelius, Alex Nazzar, James F. Phillips, and Fred N. Binka. 1994. "Baseline Survey on Contraceptive Knowledge and Use," Reproductive Preferences and Study Population Characteristics: A Report of Key Findings." *Community Health and Family Planning Project Documentation Note* Number 7. Navrongo, Ghana: Navrongo Health Research Centre.

Fayorsey, Clara, Philip B. Adongo, and Beverly Kajihara. 1994. "Findings and recommendations—The Social Organization in Kassena-Nankara District: Assessing the Context for Reproductive Change in a Traditional African Society." *Community Health and Family Planning Project Documentation Note* Number 10. Navrongo, Ghana: Navrongo Health Research Centre.

Frank, Odile. 1987. "The demand for ferility control in sub-Saharan Africa." *Studies in Family Planning* 18,4: 181–201.

———. 1988. "The childbearing family in sub-Saharan Africa: Structure, fertility, and the future." Paper presented for the joint seminar series on the Determinants and Consequences of Female-Headed Households. New York: The Population Council and International Centre for Research on Women.

Freedman, Ronald. 1987a. "The social and political environment, fertility, and family planning effectiveness." In *Organizing for Effective Family Planning Programs.* Eds. Robert J. Lapham and George B. Simmons. Washington, DC: National Academy Press, Pp. 37–58.

———1987b. "The contribution of social science to population policy and family planning program effectiveness." *Studies in Family Planning* 18,2: 57–82.

Hasenfield, Y. 1978. "Client-organization relations: A systems perspective." In *The Management of Human Services.* Eds. R.C. Sarri and Y. Hasenfeld. New York: Columbia University Press.

Hill, Althea. 1991. "Infant and child mortality levels, trends, and data deficiencies." In *Disease and Mortality in Sub-Saharan Africa.* Eds. Richard G. Feachem and Dean T. Jamison. Washington, DC: The World Bank and Oxford University Press. Pp. 37–74.

Kalipeni, Ezekiel and Eliya M. Zulu. 1993. "Gender differences in knowledge and attitudes toward modern and traditional methods of child spacing in Malawi." *Population Research and Policy Review* 12,2: 103–122.

Katz, D. and R. L. Kahn. 1978. *The Scoial Psychology of Organization.* Second edition. New York: Wiley and Sons.

Korten, David C. 1980. "Community organization and rural development: A learning process approach." *Public Administration Review* 40,5: 480–511.

———. 1984. "Strategic organization for people-centered development." *Public Administration Review* 44: 341–352.

Lloyd, Cynthia B. and Anastasia J. Gage-Brandon. 1993. "Women's role in maintaining households: Family welfare and sexual inequality in Ghana." *Population Studies* 47: 115–131.

Ministry of Health (MOH), Health Research Unit. 1991a. "First make sure our children won't die: An appraisal of community potential to support family planning services in Bolgatanga District." Acrra, Ghana: MOH. Unpublished.

———. 1991b. "Won't it cause infertility?: An appraisal of community potential to support family planning services in Berekum District." Accra, Ghana: MOH. Unpublished.

———. 1991c. "The ability to keep secrets: An appraisal of community potential to support family planning services in Dangbe West District." Accra, Ghana: MOH. Unpublished.

———. 1992. *Contraception and Misconceptions: Community Views of Family Planning.* Accra, Ghana: MOH. Unpublished.

Nazzar, Alex, James F. Phillips, Kofi Asobayire, Olivia Aglah, and Fred N. Binka. 1995. "Developing the Navrongo Project with Community-based Strategic Planning." *Community Health and Family Planning Project Documentation Note* Number 20. Navrongo, Ghana: Navrongo Health Research Centre.

Paul, Samuel. 1982. *Managing Development Programs: The Lessons of Success.* Boulder, CO: Westview Press.

———. 1987. "Community Participation in Development Projects: The World Bank Experience." *World Bank Discussion Paper* 6. Washington, DC: The World Bank.

————. 1988. "Governments and grass-roots organizations: From coexistence to collaboration." In *Strengthening the Poor*. Ed. John P. Lewis. Washington, DC: Overseas Development Council.

Perrow, C. 1978. "Demystifying organizations." In *The Management of Human Services*. Eds. R. C. Sarri and Y. Hasenfeld. New York: Columbia University Press. Pp. 105–120.

Peters, T. J. and R. H. Waterman, Jr. 1982. *In Search of Excellence: Lessons from America's Best-Run Companies*. New York: Harper and Row.

Phillips, James F. and W. Greene. 1993 "Community-based distribution of family planning in Africa: Lessons from operations research." New York: The Population Council Africa Operations Research and Technical Assistance Project. Unpublished.

Rattray, R. S. 1932. *The Tribes of Ashanti Hinterland*. Oxford: Clarendon Press.

Ross, John A., W. Parker Mauldin, and Vincent C. Miller. 1993. *Family Planning Planning and Population: A Compendium of International Statistics*. New York: The Population Council.

Ross, David A., Betty R. Kirkwood, Fred N. Binka, Paul Arthur, Nicola Dollimore, Saul S. Morris, Rosaleen P. Shier, John O. Gyapong, and Peter G. Smith. 1995. "Child morbidity and mortality following vitamin A supplementation in Ghana: Time since dosing, number of doses, and time of year." *American Journal of Public Health* 85,9: 1,246–1,251.

Sarri, R. C. and Y. Hasenfield. 1978. *The Management of Human Services*. New York: Columbia University Press.

Schuler, Sidney Ruth, E. Noel McIntosh, Melvyn C. Goldstein, and Badri Raj Pande. 1985. "Barriers to effective family planning in Nepal." *Studies in Family Planning* 16,5: 260–270.

Simmons, Ruth and George B. Simmons. 1987. "The task environment of family planning." In *Organizing for Effective Family Planning Programs*. Eds. R. J. Lapham and George B. Simmons. Washington, DC: National Academy Press. Pp. 59–78.

van de Walle, Etienne, and A. D. Foster. 1990. "Fertility Decline in Africa: Assessment and Prospects." *World Bank Technical Paper* Number 125. Africa Technical Department Series. Washington, DC: The World Bank.

Warwick, D. P. 1988. "Culture and the management of family planning programs." *Studies in Family Planning* 19,1: 1–18.

Wulf, D. 1985. "The future of family planning in sub-Saharan Africa." *International Family Planning Perspectives* 11,1: 1–8.

Family Planning Field Research Projects: Balancing Internal Against External Validity

Andrew A. Fisher and Raymond W. Carlaw

Family planning programs throughout the world have relied heavily upon field research projects as one means of testing new approaches to the delivery of services. Cuca and Pierce review 96 such projects,[1] and a report by Osborn and Reinke discusses 28 community-based contraceptive distribution efforts funded by the Agency for International Development (AID).[2] Both of these reviews stress the difficulty of trying to implement and evaluate field projects as originally planned. Unanticipated events often force changes in the study design, and research objectives sometimes come into conflict with service delivery objectives.

Field projects are designed to provide data relevant to policy formulation and program change. They are intended to indicate on a small scale the potential impact that a program might be expected to have at a higher or national level. They also serve to highlight the administrative problems and the social and cultural barriers that most family planning and maternal/child health project face in developing countries.

From the standpoint of program managers, field research projects sometimes are seen as opportunities to manipulate the organization and administration of such input as funds, staff, supplies, and equipment. Evaluators, on the other hand, tend to view these projects as experiments designed to measure program outcomes with some degree of confidence. In some instances, the program manager's manipulation of inputs in order to meet service delivery objectives runs counter to the evaluator's desire to maintain tight experimental control in order to meet research objectives. In these situations, service delivery objectives usually take precedence over purely research ones.

If an experimental input, such as a new logistics system, fails to deliver commodities to distribution points, it will probably be changed by a program manager regardless of the effect on the experimental design. If project staff go on strike, increased salary or changed work conditions are more likely to get them back to work than appeals to maintain the original study design and continue working as before. And, if a monsoon flood in the experimental areas

Reprinted with the permission of the Population Council from *Studies in Family Planning* 1983. 14,1: 3–8.

forces project staff to be taken off their regular work to help relief efforts, there is very little the evaluator can do except try to account for these events in the data.

This report discusses the experience of a two year, community-based family planning and maternal/child health project in Nepal. Although the project was planned as a field research experiment to compare one service delivery approach with another, several unanticipated factors forced compromises in the original study design. Unquestionably, these compromises weaken the validity of the inferences that can be drawn from the data. Yet at the same time, the project provided a visible demonstration under actual field conditions of a new approach (for Nepal) to the delivery of health and family planning services. It also provided a rich source of experience for national family planning personnel that subsequently affected program decisions on staff training, service delivery, and involvement of local officials in program activities.

A full description of the many facets of the Nepal project has already been undertaken.[3] It is not our purpose here to repeat this description, but rather to draw upon the Nepal experience as illustrative of the dynamic nature of field projects, the multiple objectives that they serve (some stated but others not), the unforeseen events encountered, and the difficulty of balancing concerns for internal validity over those for external validity. Internal validity is the extent to which an observed relationship between two or more variables within a particular experimental setting is causal. External validity is the extent to which the observed causal relationship found within that particular experimental setting can be generalized to other areas and other populations.

The Gorkha and Dhanusha Project

Started in February 1976 and continued for two years through February 1978, the Gorkha and Dhanusha district project was designed (1) to test a new fieldbased, experiential model of training for Nepal; (2) to compare the work performance of panchayat-based[4] workers against a similar category of clinic-based workers, and (3) to evaluate the effect, if any, that these workers had on the family planning knowledge and contraceptive practice of currently married women.

Gorkha district in the western hill region of Nepal and Dhanusha in the central terai (plains) were selected as project areas because each had previously been included in a four-district, longitudinal family planning knowledge–attitude–practice (KAP) survey. These surveys were begun in 1975, before the start of the experimental project, and continued each year through 1978, after the project ended.[5] Among other purposes, the surveys were intended to provide preproject and postproject measures for evaluation. The two other districts included in the surveys, Kaski in the hills and Parsa in the terai, served as matched controls for Gorkha and Dhanusha. District matching was done on the basis of similar geographic size, density of population, number of hospitals, number of health clinics, ethnic composition, and proportion of males and females with no education.

Before the introduction of the experimental project in Gorkha and Dhanusha districts, basic health and family planning services were delivered in rural areas of Nepal by clinic-based-workers. In theory, the clinic workers visited village homes four days a week. The remaining two days a week they spent in a rural health clinic. In practice, most spent four days a week in the clinic and only two doing home visits. It was seldom possible for them to cover areas beyond a few miles from the clinic. As a result, large areas of the panchayat were left unattended.

In contrast to the clinic model of service delivery, the Gorkha and Dhanusha project introduced a community-based health and family planning service delivery system. Each panchayat worker used his/her own home as a base and devoted a full six days a week to visiting eligible couples, meeting with village leaders, and organizing group meetings. The panchayat workers carried contraceptive supplies, iron and multivitamin tablets, oral rehydration solution packets, and simple medicines, such as aspirin and iodine. They also received a new five-week training course. This course was different in almost all respects from the program given to the clinic-based workers. The clinic workers were given a two-week, didactic, classroom-based course in Kathmandu, while the pachayat workers were given a five-week, experimental, field-based program in either Gorkha or Dhanusha. The course emphasized the development of an effective community health and family planning service delivery team, with the district family planning officer as the leader.

Unanticipated Events

Selection of Project Sites

Gorkha district had a total of 56 panchayats and Dhanusha 69. From each district, 12 panchayats were selected as experimental sites for introducing the panchayat-based health and family panning project. In addition, all six clinic-serviced panchayats in each district were selected as comparison areas.

The selection of experimental panchayats was made by a committee consisting of the chief district officer, the district family planning officer, and one other government official. The support of these and other local officials was considered essential to the implementation of the project. Indeed, the active involvement of local people in family planning and health activities was one of the unstated objectives of the project.

While it was explained to the selection committee that for research purposes there was a need to select experimental panchayats from among the panchayatas in each district that already had been included in the KAP survey sampling framework, the committee felt that this could not be done in all cases. The Gorkha and Dhanusha project was seen by many local officials as a convenient means of extending services to areas that previously had received only minimal or no services. As a result, some of the experimental panchayats chosen by the committee were very remote areas. This made project monitoring and service delivery quite difficult. It also introduced a major change in the original research design. The remote experimental panchayats were definitely not equivalent on the basis of many measures with the more accessible clinic-serviced panchayats that were to be used as comparison areas. Equally important from the standpoint of the original project design was the committee's selection of experimental panchayats that did not coincide with the panchayats in the KAP survey sampling framework. Without the KAP surveys, preproject baseline measures of family planning knowledge, attitudes, and practices were not available, and subsequent postproject measures were difficult to obtain. The selection in both Gorkha and Dhanusha of some experimental panchayats that were either very remote (and thus very atypical) or not include in the KAP sampling framework constituted the first major departure from the original project design and a significant compromise of research objectives in favor of service delivery objectives.

Project Field Staff

When the experimental project was first planned, the intention was to recruit and train 18 panchayats workers and four supervisors for each district. In Dhanusha, only 16 panchayat workers were recruited and trained, and one resigned after a year, leaving 15. Also, of the four supervisors, two were discharged for poor performance after 13 months and their work assigned to the two remaining supervisors. In Gorkha district, all 18 panchayat workers and four supervisors were recruited and trained, but the district family planning officer, a key figure in implementing and monitoring the project, was absent from his post for six months during the first year. He was subsequently replaced by another family planning officer, who was absent from his post for eight months during the second year of the project.

While personnel problems such as these are common in the history of almost any service delivery program, they are poorly tolerated deviations from the controlled world of research studies. The lack of a full field and supervisory staff in Dhanusha and the intermittent availability of top administrative leadership in Gorkha constituted the second major unanticipated event and another disturbance of the original design. From an administrative standpoint, these staff problems were certainly annoying, but at the sane time controllable. From a research standpoint they were changes in study design with probable effect on fieldworker morale and performance and project outcomes such as contraceptive use that simply could not be measured.

Sterilization Camps

During the project period, two large laparoscopy sterilization camps were held in Dhanusha district. Each camp attracted widespread publicity, and each resulted in approximately 1,000 sterilization procedures. While they were considered very successful service delivery activities by the program managers who planned them, they were viewed by the evaluators as a third unanticipated event that in this case represented a history effect[6] to the internal validity of the project evaluation. Such large events in one district make interdistrict comparisons difficult. Each camp required the total commitment of all district workers for about two months.

Routine project activities stopped, including follow-up-services for pill and condom users. Both the experimental panchayat workers and the clinic workers devoted their time and energy to recruiting sterilization clients. It is likely that their efforts, coupled with radio and newspaper publicity, had the effect of increasing people's awareness, knowledge, and acceptance of family planning in Dhanusha district. At the same time, the divergence of staff from their regular work possibly resulted in some loss of confidence among people who had come to depend on them for supplies, and this probably led in some cases to method discontinuation.

Experimental and Comparison Panchayats

During the second year of the project, field reports from both Gorkha and Dhanusha indicated that some of the panchayat workers were operating, at least part of the time, in panchayats neighboring the one assigned to them. Possible these neighboring panchayats were more receptive to the panchayat worker; possibly they were more easily accessible from the panchayat worker's home base; or possibly the panchayat worker believed that the pool of ready acceptors was exhausted in the assigned area. This fourth unanticipated event had several project implications. First, it meant that the panchayat worker did not and could not devote as much time and attention to couples in the assigned experimental panchayats. Second, since some of the neighboring panchayats were also serviced by clinic workers, there was a clear contamination of these comparison areas serviced by clinics. Finally, it seemed very probable that coverage of clinic-serviced panchayats by both panchayat workers and clinic workers may have resulted in dual reporting of clients and thus in inflated service statistics.

Salary Payment

Each month, field supervisors collected the salary envelopes of the panchayats workers form the district family planning office. The salaries were then delivered to the worker when the supervisor made the regular monthly field visit. This system worked well until a cash flow problem developed about a year and a half after the project began. For a period of two months, no salary payments were made either to the supervisors or to the workers. Understandably, morale dropped, enthusiasm waned, daily work patterns changed, and some family planning clients were not provided with services that they might otherwise have received. Equally important, the interruption of salary payments eroded the commitment of the fieldworkers, and the momentum of the project was lost during the last six months.

Project Evaluation

Three types of analyses were planned as part of the Gorkha and Dhanusha project evaluation. First, service statistics collected continuously during the project were to be used to compare the performance of panchayat workers and clinic workers. Second, the KAP survey data collected annually from 1975 through 1978 were to be used to compare the family planning knowledge, attitudes and practices of a panel of currently married women in panchayat worker areas and a similar panel of women in clinic worker areas. Third, the KAP data were again to be used to compare the family planning knowledge, attitudes, and practice of women interviewed in Gorkha and Dhanusha and all women interviewed in the matched control districts of Kaski and Parsa.

Given the disturbances to the original project design, it is not entirely surprising that the three analysis plans proved difficult to undertake and the results proved difficult to interpret. Each of the unanticipated events had one or more effects that represent threats to the validity of the evaluation. The most likely effects are presented in Table 1.

Discussion

Almost always, experimental field research projects face unanticipated events that present a dilemma for both the research evaluator and the program policymaker. The dilemma involves the extent to which field projects can maintain a high degree of internal validity without at the same time sacrificing external validity. Making causal inferences with some degree of statistical confidence (what Cook and Campbell term "statistical conclusion validity")[7] usually requires a randomized research design with rigid control over the introduction and measurement of the experimental variables. Yet the more rigid the design and the tighter the control, the less likely it is that the experimental project mirrors real field conditions and thus the less likely that the causal inferences can be generalized to other field settings.

Table 1. Probable effects of unanticipated events on project evaluation

Unanticipated events	Effects
Selection of project sites: Local committee selects some experimental panchayats that either are remote or do not coincide with KAP-sampled panchayats.	1. Remote panchayats difficult to service and supervise. Accuracy of worker performance statistics in these areas questionable. 2. Remote panchayats not initially equivalent on basis of many measures to more accessible comparison panchayats. 3. No baseline and subsequent survey measures in those selected experimental panchayats that did not coincide with KAP-sampled panchayats. Cases available for analysis reduced. Evaluation in non-KAP panchayats limited to consideration of service statistics or other data sources.
Project field staff: In Dhanusha, full field and supervisory staff lacking. In Gorkha, district family planning officer absent for 14 of 24 months.	1. Reduced field staff in Dhanusha limited geographic coverage of project. 2. Lack of full supervisory staff in Dhanusha probably affected worker performance and accuracy of field reports. 3. Project monitoring and supervision in Gorkha difficult without top administrative leadership. Worker morale, commitment, and performance probably reduced. Accuracy of field reports questionable.
Sterilization camps: Two large sterilization camps held in Dhanusha during project period.	1. Routine project health and family planning activities stopped for two months. 2. Intense publicity probably served to increase family planning knowledge and practice in district 3. Possible increase in method switching 4. Probably loss of confidence by people in field-workers and some client method discontinuation.
Experimental and comparison panchayats: Some panchayat workers begin to work in clinic worker areas.	1. Work effort in experimental areas reduced, effort in comparison panchayats increased. 2. Possible dual reporting of clients by panchayat and clinic workers resulting in inflated statistics.
Salary payments: Payments stopped for two months.	1. Morale and commitment of field staff declined. Momentum of project lost during last six months. 2. Some clients probably not provided services, resulting in some method discontinuation.

In the Gorkha and Dhanusha project, internal validity was repeatedly compromised by a series of unanticipated events. It might have been possible to lessen the effect of these events, or a least to account for them, by changing the field setting. The use of a local panchayat selection committee could have been avoided. A more-educated and better-paid field-worker could have been recruited and employed. More attention to project monitoring through a higher ratio of supervisors to field staff could have been instituted. While these and similar measures might have served to increase internal validity and allowed research hypotheses to be tested with a degree of statistical confidence, they would have created an atypical and somewhat artificial field setting that probably could not be duplicated elsewhere in Nepal.

Cook and Campbell ask the question, "What determines the extent to which one should assign higher priority to internal validity over other kinds of validity?" They answer by saying, "The interest of internal validity are paramount when the cost of being wrong about a causal inference is high—for example, when, because of experimental results, an ineffective policy could be implemented widescale or an effective one reduce in scope."[8]

The Nepal project began as an experimental research endeavor that required a high degree of internal validity in order to answer such questions as the extent to which panchayat workers could affect the family planning knowledge, attitudes, and practices of couples, and the degree to which their work performance would be significantly different from that of clinic workers. In retrospect, the "cost of being wrong" in answering these questions was far less than the "cost of being wrong" in answering a series of process questions related to external validity or to the extent to which project findings can be generalized to other settings. These questions, of primary importance to program policymakers, concerned such issues as: What type of problems would be encountered in organizing and conducting a training program at the district level? How should a local panchayat family planning committee be formed, what should be its functions, and how much authority should it have? Could local people be identified, recruited, and trained as health and family planning workers, and would they work in remote areas with minimal supervision? Would social or political opposition develop to panchayat workers? Would the workers be able to maintain forms, recruit cases, provide regular follow-up, and refer clients experiencing side effects from contraceptive use? Could a logistics system using porters be organized to provide supplies on a regular basis?

The Gorkha and Dhanusha project was able to provide answers for these questions. What began as a research endeavor with quantitative outcome evaluation, developed, through a series of unanticipated events, into a service delivery field demonstration with a process evaluation. The project had a number of important program implications, but three in particular stand out. First, it demonstrated that training programs could be organized and conducted in field settings on a mobile basis as needed. In part because of this demonstration and the experience and confidence it gave trainers, the panchayat worker training program in Nepal was decentralized and moved to three rural centers outside of Kathmandu. Training is now provided at these centers and it taken to districts when required. In addition, far greater emphasis is given to field training than to classroom training.

Second, the project demonstrated that locally recruited panchayat workers could and would work in remote areas without constant supervision. On the basis of services statistics from the project (admittedly often of poor quality) and subsequent evaluations in later year,[9] the workers have shown that they can cover a larger geographic area than their clinic counterparts and their work performance appears to be equal to or slightly better than the clinic workers in terms of monthly recruitment of new acceptors, pill user continuation rates, follow-up visits, and other indicators. In part because of this, the panchayat worker approach to service delivery was expanded to other districts of the country. Over 1,100 panchayat workers now operate in 13 of Nepal's 14 administrative zones.[10] Third, the project demonstrated that local leaders, if encouraged and given the opportunity, would become more involved in family planning activities. In part because of this experience with community involvement, local district and panchayat committees are now used in Nepal to help identify and recruit new panchayat workers.

The decisions to decentralize training, expand the panchayat approach to service delivery, and involve local committee in family planning program were made primarily on the basis of field experiences gained over the two-year period of the project. They certainly were not taken solely on the basis of the quantitative outcomsevaluation findings.

The Gorkha and Dhanusha project suggests several useful guidelines. First, the value of family planning field projects probably lies as much in the formative experience gained during the life of the project as it does in the summative evaluation of findings at the end of the project. Handling unexpected problems increases understanding and administrative skill. Second, and a corollary of the first point, it is important to devote as much time and attention to evaluating a project's process of development as it is to evaluating a project's final outcome. While there is an obvious need for concern with internal validity issues, particularly when the objective is to make causal inferences, there is an equal need for attention to external validity issues, particularly when the objective is to understand the operation of program processes in a natural setting.

References and Notes

1. R. Cuca and C.. S. Pierce, *Experiments in Family Planning* (Baltimore: Johns Hopkins University Press, 1977).

2. R. W. Osborn and W. A. Reinke (eds.), *Community Based Distribution of Contraception: A Review of Field Experience* (Baltimore: Johns Hopkins Population Center, Johns Hopkins University, January 1981).

3. B. R. Pande, A.A, Fisher, K. Vaidya and R. Carlaw, *The Gorkha and Dhanusha Experimental Service Delivery Project*, The Family P;anning and Maternal Child Health Project, Kathmandu, Nepal, August 1978. A complete report of the Nepal FP and MCH program can also be found in *Nepal FP/MCP Data Analysis Final Report*, His Majesty's Government, Ministry of Health, Nepal Family Planning and MCP Project, The Population Council, 1979.

4. A panchayat (community) is an administratvie unit in Nepal comprising, 1,000–6,000 people.

5. For an analysis of the four KAP annual surveys in Gorkha, Dhanusha, Kaski, and Parsa districts, see J. M. Tuladhar and John Stoeckel, "The Relative Impact of Vertial an Integrated FP/.MCH Programs in Rural Nepal," *Studies in Family Planning*, 13, no. 10 (1982): 275–286.

6. Donald T Campbell and Julian C. Stanley, *Experimental and Quasi-Ecperimental Designs for Research* (Chicago: Rand McNally, 1966).

7. Thomas D. Cook and Donald T. Campbell, *Quasi-Experimentation: Design and Analysis Issues for Field Settings* (Chicago: Rand McNally, 1979).

8. Cook an Campbell, cited in note 7, p. 385.

9. "Evaluation of th FP/MCH project's panchayat based health workers" prepared by NEW ERA, Kathmandu, Nepal, submitted to USAID, Kathmandu, Nepal, September 1981.

10. "Evaluation of the FP/MCH project's panchayat based health workers,: cited in note 9, p. 7.

Guidelines for Overcoming Design Problems in Family Planning Operations Research

Andrew A. Fisher, John Laing, and John Stoeckel

Since 1981, 14 research studies have been implemented in Thailand, the Philippines, Sri Lanka, and Nepal as part of an ongoing family planning operations research (OR) program in Asia. Eleven of these studies are small-scale, longitudinal field studies that test new approaches to service delivery. The other three seek to diagnose or explore particular problems affecting family planning programs. The 14 studies employ a variety of research designs and use different combinations of data collection techniques.

In this report, we are concerned with experimental designs for field intervention studies utilized in operations research in family planning. Because there are so many difficulties associated with using "true experimental" designs—such as the inability to meet random selection requirements and problems maintaining control over the study intervention—we propose the use of quasi-experimental studies, and describe guidelines for selecting and designing them. Focusing specifically on the use of multiple replications of the study intervention, these guidelines should help researchers and field-workers account for the possible effects of unexpected events during operations research field studies.

Operations Research Field Studies

Over the past decade, national health and family planning programs in Asia have expanded greatly in terms of expenditures, staff, geographic coverage, and activities. These programs have become large and complex undertakings that require detailed planning, close coordination of efforts, careful training and supervision, and continuous monitoring of program direction, process, and impact. For all of these areas, research and evaluation can play an essential supportive role as a source of information for program managers who are faced daily with vexing questions concerning the most efficient and cost-effective means of delivering services.

The numerous health and family planning surveys conducted in practically every country of Asia have been a valuable source of information for policymakers and others. Coupled with improved service statistics systems, large na-

Reprinted with the permission of the Population Council from *Studies in Family Planning* 1985. 16,2: 100–105.

tional surveys have been used to measure the impact of program activities on birth, death, and morbidity rates. On the other hand, because these surveys have not always focused on program problems and solutions, they have been somewhat less than useful to program managers.

Typically, managers are concerned on a day-to-day basis with such questions as: What type and length of training should field-workers receive? What is the most cost-effective means of providing accurate information to large numbers of rural people about the availability of services? Do incentives increase contraceptive prevalence and, if so, what type of incentives? How can informal community leaders be identified and used to promote health and family planning practices? What is the optimum price level to charge for contraceptives?

In general, these and similar questions cannot be answered satisfactorily on the basis of data from national cross-sectional surveys or from routinely collected service statistics. Many of the problems of primary concern to managers are not necessarily national in scope, but are limited to specific areas and can best be addressed through the design and implementation of operations research studies.

The term "operations research" causes confusion because it has several different meanings. As used here, it refers to research and evaluation studies concerned with the activities or "operations" of health and family planning programs. These studies tend to be small in scale, limited in time, and highly focused in objectives. They are intended to result in relatively rapid feedback of information for the purpose of program improvement. While they may draw on the data from large national surveys for problem identification, operations research studies can be categorized as either exploratory/diagnostic or experimental. Often they are both, beginning with an exploratory phase and followed by an experimental field intervention that tests a new approach to service delivery. The intervention to be tested might be the use of a new category of field personnel, a new training curriculum, a previously untried combination of communication channels, a new community organization strategy, or any number of other activities that might improve program efficiency and effectiveness.

Problems With Selecting a Research Design

Given the emphasis in operations research studies on testing the impact of a new service delivery approach, an experimental design would, ideally, be most desirable to use. Such designs, termed "true experimental" by Campbell and Stanley, include the pre-test–post-test control group design, the Solomon four group design, the post-test-only control group design, and variations on these.[1] As desirable as these may be, two features of true experimental designs often prove problematic for health and family planning field studies.

The first is the random selection of study units (individuals, households, villages, districts, etc.) from some larger grouping of these units, and then the subsequent random assignment of these units to experimental and control groups. Random selection helps assure, within known limits of sampling error, that the study units are representative of the universe from which they are drawn. Representativeness relates to external validity and the degree to which study findings can be generalized. Random assignment of study units to experimental and control groups relates to internal validity and is important if the objective of a study is to make causal inferences about the impact of a program intervention. The second feature of true experimental designs that is problematic in field settings is maintaining full control over the timing, intensity, and duration of the experimental intervention variables.

Random Selection and Assignment of Study Units

Usually, the initial selection of an operations research study area and population is purposive, not random. The selection tends to be based on considerations of availability of study resources, presence of the problem being addressed by the study, convenience for the investigators, and relative ease in implementing the experimental intervention, including access roads, communication and physical facilities, personnel in place, and the absence of civil disturbances. While purposive selection limits a study's ability to generalize findings, this may not be as important a concern for most operations research efforts as the ability to make valid causal inferences about the impact of a program intervention *within* a study area. Yet here too, operations research studies face difficulties.

Administrative, logistic, ethical, and political considerations often preclude the use of random procedures to assign study units to experimental and control groups. For example, health and family planning services cannot be delivered selectively to one household that is randomly assigned to an experimental group, and then denied to a neighboring household in the control group. Even in situations where it might be possible to deliver experimental services to larger units such as entire villages or districts, random procedures to assign these units cannot always be used. Village leaders sometimes fail to fully appreciate the logic of experimental design and become upset when their village is assigned to a control group while a neighboring and possibly rival village receives services as part of an experimental group. Program managers sometimes find that they simply cannot implement a particular experimental activity to a randomly selected district because roads, storage facilities, vehicles, trained personnel, or other prerequisites are absent.

In other cases, problems related to contamination and spillover effects occur when an experimental and control area are contiguous. For instance, directors of training centers that happen to be assigned to a control group have an uncanny way of obtaining a new curriculum used in experimental centers. Similarly, communications experiments directed at one province often affect neighboring control provinces. In part, to avoid these difficulties, operations research studies purposively select control areas that are similar yet geographically separated from the experimental area and population. This may result in the selection of nonequivalent comparison groups, which can complicate the task of making causal inferences.

Although random selection procedures offer a number of advantages over purposive selection, it should be recognized that they merely establish the initial conditions of equivalence between groups. They do not guarantee that subsequent experimental effects can be attributed with confidence to the intervention variables, or that these same effects can be expected from a similar intervention applied in another field setting. The initial equivalence established between groups through randomization cannot be assumed to continue indefinitely over time. Numerous factors extraneous to a research study may introduce a degree of nonequivalence between groups that can lead to spurious relationships and confound the study's results. While some of these factors may be evenly distributed between the experimental and control groups, and their effects cancelled out, this is not always the case.

Government program managers, for example, may decide to initiate special, intensive health and family planning campaigns in districts that service statistics indicate are low performance areas. These districts may consist primarily of control areas that are low in performance because they are being compared with experimental areas, where an operations research intervention is having an effect. Sometimes, two agencies may find that they are implementing similar service delivery activities in the same area and directed at the same population. In other situations, civil disturbances may affect out-migration from one district, but not from another that is being used as a control. Randomization, no matter how well implemented, cannot overcome the effect these situations may have on an operations research study.

Control Over the Study Intervention

A second aspect of experimental designs that is problematic in field settings is maintaining control over the timing, intensity, and duration of the experimental intervention. Although full control is probably never possible, in order to hypothesize expected relationships between independent and dependent variables and draw reasonable conclusions about these relationships, a research investigator needs to maintain control over when, where, to whom, in what amounts, and for how long an intervention is introduced. This degree of control, of course, is not always possible. Rarely do intervention studies begin, continue, or end according to schedule.[2] Equipment and personnel required to deliver a service may not be available in the amounts and kind originally planned. Activities may be implemented out of sequence or in greater or lesser intensity than expected. Some activities may not even be implemented. For example, the cold chain required for an immunization program may be broken in one area but not another. Newly trained multipurpose health workers may entirely avoid providing certain preventive services and concentrate instead on curative services. While the number of these problems can be reduced through careful planning and field supervision, it is unlikely that they can be eliminated altogether.

Selecting a Quasi-Experimental Design

The only reasonable alternative to true experimental designs is the use of quasi-experimental designs. Campbell and Stanley note that, while these designs do not allow an investigator to maintain full control over the "when and to whom of exposure and the ability to randomize exposures," they do at least allow control over the "when and to whom of measurements."[3] This will not assure equivalent groups, prevent the intrusion of extraneous factors, or guarantee control over the intervention. All it can do is help the investigator become aware of possible invalidating study factors and avoid making mistaken conclusions. A quasi-experimental design is "good" when it is able to measure whatever it is that happens in a field setting, whether a planned or unplanned event. Thus, the crucial factor to consider in selecting a "good" quasi-design is whether the timing and focus of measurement observations are adequate for the objectives of the study. In view of this, we propose as a guideline for selecting a field research design the *Principle of the Three Multiples:*

1 Seek multiple data sources to obtain information on the same variables.

2 Seek multiple measurements over time of the same variables.

3 Seek multiple replications of the study intervention in different field settings.[4]

The use of multiple data sources serves several purposes. First, each source can provide a reliability check on the other sources. Second, each source may provide additional insights about a particular event or relationship between events. Third, the use of multiple data sources provides the opportunity to obtain qualitative as well as the more usual quantitative information about a study intervention. Qualitative information on process can be particularly useful for determining how and why an intervention effect was obtained or not obtained.

Multiple measurements over time of the same variables can provide information on trends before, during, and after the introduction of an intervention. This type of information can be extremely valuable for field studies. Sudden and radical deviations from past trends can be the first indication that factors extraneous to a study intervention are affecting an experimental area or population.

Finally, multiple replications of a study intervention in different settings can provide information concerning the extent to which the intervention's effects are unique to a particular area and population, or can be generalized to other areas and populations. Ideally, the use of multiple replications means that one or more follow-up studies are conducted with the same objectives and research design, but are implemented in different areas. In practice, because of time and resource constraints, this is difficult to accomplish. An alternative, therefore, is to introduce the intervention into several types of field settings at the same time. This procedure not only provides an indication concerning the confidence with and degree to which the intervention's impact can be generalized, but also gives some guarantee that if one experimental area is affected by floods, riots, administrative delays, strikes, migration, or other happenings, at least the study may be able to continue in the other areas.

Obviously, there are many ways in which multiple data sources can be combined with multiple measurements over time and multiple replications to construct a quasi-experimental research design. While the particular mix of measurement observations and program interventions depends in large part on a study's objectives and available resources, our experience over the past three years with 14 family planning operations research field studies in Asia suggest that a "good" quasi-experimental design includes most, if not all, of the following procedures:

1 *Obtain background information from secondary sources.* Previous research data from national and local studies and from past and current service statistics should be obtained as a first step in designing an operations research field intervention. This information is helpful in identifying the parameters of a problem situation and defining the characteristics of a study area and population. It also can be used to match experimental and control groups on key variables or serve as a check on the degree to which these groups are equivalent if random procedures were used to select them.

2 *Select multiple sites for replication of the study intervention.* As far as time and resources permit, the study intervention should be introduced into as many different sites as possible—small clinics and large hospitals, farming communities and coastal fishing communities, highland and lowland areas, wet and dry areas, different religious and ethinic areas, and so on.

3 *Collect preliminary qualitative data.* Once the study sites have been selected, it is useful to collect qualitative data through such techniques as village meetings, focus group discussions, and informal meetings with village and community leaders, government officials, and private agencies. This type of information is particularly useful or constructing questionnaires and operational definitions of key study variables.

4 *Conduct a baseline survey.* In almost all operations research studies, it is essential to obtain initial quantitative measures on independent and dependent variables related to the study's objectives.

5 *Implement a study monitoring system.* Because of the many unanticipated events that usually occur during the life of a field study, it is important to establish a monitoring system that routinely collects both quantitative and qualitative data before, during, and well after the study intervention. Sources for this type of data include government and private agency service statistics, diaries maintained by field-workers, observational visits, group meetings, key informants, simple monthly record-keeping forms, financial records, and managers' opinions. It is useful to monitor data for an understanding of how and why an intervention was either successful or unsuccessful. In addition to continuous monitoring, it is often useful to conduct small-scale research activities during the study period in order to determine whether the intervention is being implemented as expected. Resarch methods designed to provide qualitative data, such as in-depth surveys of field personnel, focus group discussions with clients, or systematic observation of field operations, are particularly likely to be helpful. Project managers can use feedback from such research for identifying and responding to problems of implementation while the study is still underway.

6 *Conduct a follow-up survey.* An immediate post-intervention follow-up survey should be conducted along the lines of the baseline survey.

7 *Collect post-intervention qualitative data.* In order to obtain an in-depth understanding of study processes and client reactions to the intervention, a second round of village meetings, focus group discussions, and informal interviews with key informants should be conducted.

8 *Collect long-term follow-up data.* Sometimes there is either a delayed reaction to a field intervention or a decay in the initial reaction. In order to determine whether either of these possible situations exists, it is useful to collect long-term follow-up data. If study resources permit, this can be done through a second quantitative follow-up survey six months or a year after the first. Alternatively, all or part of the study monitoring system can be maintained so that monthly record-keeping forms and sources of data continue to be collected and maintained well after the intervention ends.

Some of these procedures may be inappropriate for a particular research effort. Others may be impossible to implement because financial resources are inadequate, trained research personnel are few in number, technical assistance is unavailable, data processing equipment is lacking, or other constraining factors exist. Nevertheless, and as a minimum, it is usually possible to include in the design of a field intervention study: (1) a comparison/control group, (2) pre- and post-intervention measurements, and (3) an ongoing study monitoring system. Indeed, without these three design features, it is unlikely that the impact of a study intervention can be determined with any degree of accuracy.

Case Example of an Operations Research Study

An ongoing operations research field study in Sri Lanka exemplifies many of the points discussed above. Started in 1982, the Sri Lankan study is being conducted by the Family Health Bureau of the Government and the Family Planning Association of Sri Lanka. The primary objective is to increase the number of new IUD acceptors in the country. The study interventions consist of providing initial training to public health nurses and retraining to medical officers in IUD insertion techniques; identifying satisfied IUD users and then training them to work on a part-time basis with government field-level midwives; and finally, upgrading rural clinics by providing equipment sterilizers, room partitions, cots, chairs, and other basic facilities required for insertions. The personnel training and upgrading of rural clinics are preliminary activities. The central focus of the study is an experimental test of the extent to which satisfied IUD users can be identified, trained, and encouraged to work on a part-time basis with government midwives, making home visits to recruit new IUD acceptors.

At the time the study was planned, there were 102 administrative health divisions in Sri Lanka. Twenty of these were purposively selected for the operations research study, and they included ten experimental divisions and ten control divisions. The selection was made with a view toward covering all major geographic regions of the island—north and south, east and west, highlands and lowlands, wet areas and dry areas. Experimental and control divisions were matched on the basis of similar topography, ethnic and religious composition, number of service delivery staff, and IUD insertion facilities.

Within each experimental division, half of the midwives were selected randomly and asked to find in their work areas four satisfied IUD users who would be willing to assist with IUD motivation, recruitment, and follow-up tasks. An initial two-day workshop was held in each experimental division and attended by all satisfied IUD users plus all midwives in the division. Subsequently, every six to eight weeks, one-day review meetings have been conducted in each experimental division. These meetings are attended by the medical officers, public health nurses, midwives, and satisfied IUD users.

The study was planned for an 18-month period, with the first three months devoted to data collection and training, the next 12 months for the intervention, and the final three months for follow-up data collection and analysis. Originally, it was expected that 196 midwives from all ten experimental divisions would be trained, and 98 of these would work alone while the remaining 98 would work with 392 satisfied IUD users.

The Sri Lankan IUD study is characterized by multiple replications of the intervention in ten geographically separate divisions, multiple sources of data, and multiple measurements over time. The basic design includes the following features:

1 *Background information.* An initial review of government service statistics and the findings from the Sri Lankan Fertility and the Contraceptive Prevalence Surveys was made to determine changes in the contraceptive method mix over the past decade (1972–1982), particularly the decline in new IUD acceptors.

2 *Multiple sites for replication.* Twenty of the country's 102 administrative health divisions were selected as study sites. The ten experimental divisions cover all major geographic, ethnic, and religious areas of the country.

3 *Preliminary qualitative data.* A profile of each of the study divisions was made by collecting information on staff and clinic facilities through group meetings with medical officers and informal interviews with key officials. In addition, research staff visited all divisions to collect basic service statistics.

4 *Baseline survey.* Midwives conducted a baseline survey in their areas to determine contraceptive prevalence.

5 *Monitoring system.* A variety of procedures are used to monitor the study. Satisfied IUD users, midwives, nurses, doctors, and IUD insertion centers maintain simple record-keeping forms that provide information on home visits, new IUD cases, withdrawals, reasons for withdrawals, and problems encountered. Regular research staff visits are made to all experimental divisions. Every six to eight weeks, each experimental division holds a one-day review meeting attended by doctors, nurses, midwives, and satisfied IUD acceptors. Government and private agency service statistics also are routinely collected each month.

6 *Follow-up survey.* A follow-up contraceptive prevalence survey will be conducted in each division at the study's completion. In addition, a more detailed survey of a randomly selected number of new IUD cases will be conducted in both the experimental and control divisions.

7 *Post-intervention qualitative data.* Focus group discussions will be conducted in selected areas with field and clinic staff and with village women in the reproductive ages.

8 *Long term follow-up.* Service statistics from each of the study's divisions will be collected for a period of approximately one year after the intervention ends.

Together, the multiple sources of data, multiple measurements, and multiple intervention replications have allowed the study to take into account and make adjustments for several unexpected events. Had the study relied exclusively on conventional pre- and post-intervention quantitative measurement, it is unlikely that all of these events would have been noticed. Even if they had been noticed, the additional information required to make adjustments would not have been available. For example, of the original 20 study divisions, four have been dropped entirely (two experimental and two control) because of civil disturbances that prevented the delivery of services. Multiple replications of the intervention have allowed the study to continue in the remaining eight experimental divisions. In some of these eight divisions, the initial training and subsequent delivery of services was delayed for about three months because staff did not attend offices and clinics, again because of civil disturbances. In one division, severe flooding prevented the delivery of supplies and the collection of data. These delays were first noticed on monthly record-keeping forms and subsequently verified through research staff site visits. Plans have now been made to extend the study intervention period to cover the unexpected delays that have occurred.

In one division, another service delivery agency is testing whether local agents can be used to sell cycles of pills door-to-door. These agents, who receive a small profit from each cycle sold, have viewed the IUD study as a rival and unwelcomed intrusion that is reducing the pool of potential new pill acceptors. In a number of cases, they have told women that the IUD is associated with severe and unacceptable side effects. Information about the activities of the agents was first obtained at a monthly meeting with the study's nurses, doctors, midwives, and satisfied IUD acceptors. Trends on new IUD acceptors (as well as pill acceptors) from this division can now be analyzed somewhat more meaningfully than might have been the case if only pre- and post-intervention measures had been taken, and the activities of the agents had not been noticed.

Finally, in some of the IUD insertion centers, nurses and doctors trained through the operations research study have been transferred and replaced by untrained staff. Besides the lack of training, the new staff are unfamiliar with the objectives and procedures of the OR study. There is every likelihood, therefore, that in divisions where staff transfers have occurred, the trends in new IUD acceptance will be affected. However, since the date when staff transfers occurred is known from monthly clinic records, trend changes can be analyzed with this knowledge in mind.

Summary and Conclusions

This paper has reviewed the difficulties of using "true experimental" designs for operations research field studies. The randomization requirement of these designs often cannot be met and, even if it is, it is almost impossible to maintain full control over the study intervention. Field-workers and researchers cannot prevent the intrusion of unexpected events. All they can hope to do is notice these events and account for their possible effects by using multiple sources of data, multiple measurements over time, and multiple replications of the study intervention. These procedures are being used in the Sri Lankan operations research study. This study has experienced numerous problems, but at least the research design will allow the investigators to isolate statistically the data from areas known to have been affected by nonstudy intervention variables.

References and Notes

The family planning operations research program in Asia referred to in this report is funded by the US Agency for International Development (AID).

1.   Donald T. Campbell and Julian C. Stanley, "Experimental and quasi-experimental designs for research on teaching," in N.L. Gage, (ed.), *Handbook of Research on Teaching* (Chicago: The American Educational Research Association, Rand McNally & Co., 1963), pp. 171–246.

2.   For a discussion of the difficulties often encountered in maintaining control over an experimental intervention, see Andrew A. Fisher and Raymond Carlaw, "Family planning field research projects: Balancing internal against external validity," *Studies in Family Planning* 14, no. 1 (January 1983): 3–8.

3.   Campbell and Stanley, cited in note 1.

4.   We should point out, of course, that these three multiples can lead to an unintended fourth, namely, multiple sources of error. This, however, is balanced by greater ability to detect error.

Introductory Small Cash Incentives to Promote Child Spacing in India

Janice R. Stevens and Carl M. Stevens

The Government of India plans to reduce the crude birth rate from the present level of approximately 33 births per 1,000 population to the low 20s by the year 2000. More than 80 percent of contraceptors in India have undergone sterilization and 88 percent have done so in Thanjavur District, Tamil Nadu, the original site of the program reported here. Sterilization (more than 90 percent of which is female) is now reported to cover around 30–45 percent of women in the rural areas of this district, and it surpasses 50 percent in some sections of Madras city. Sterilization rates appear to be reaching upper limits among those couples of age and parity that can be considered the natural market. Thus, it is recognized that if the fertility reduction goal is to be achieved, there will have to be a large-scale increase in the use of temporary methods of contraception in rural areas, from the present level of 3–5 percent to about 30 percent of eligible couples. The Indian government, which for many years has offered significant cash incentives to both acceptors and providers of male and female sterilization, has in the past several years increased its promotion of the pill, condoms, and intrauterine devices (IUDs). These supplies are provided free of charge, and, as with the sterilization program, targets have been set for distributing them. A small monetary incentive is also offered to women who accept the Copper-T IUD. Despite these measures and the widespread promotion of the small-family norm by radio, television, and billboards, realistic knowledge about and actual use of modern temporary methods of contraception remain very low; regular utilization rates were below 5 percent of eligible couples in rural areas of Tamil Nadu and Bihar when the program was implemented. The Ammanpettai Family Welfare Program, begun in 1985, attempts to address this critical problem by introducing incentives to advertise and promote knowledge and use of temporary methods.

There is a very considerable literature arguing the pros and cons of incentives, and concerning the advantages and disadvantages of immediate vs. delayed incentives; individual vs. group incentives; community vs. provider incentives; and money vs. food incentives, for the promotion of family planning (Repetto,

Reprinted with the permission of the Population Council from *Studies in Family Planning* 1992. 23,3: 171–186.

1968; Rogers, 1971; Perkin, 1971; Enke and Hickman, 1976; Cuca and Pierce, 1977; Veatch, 1977; David, 1982; Chomitz and Birdsall, 1990). The effectiveness of incentives for promoting sterilization is generally accepted, although the ethics of offering relatively large cash payments to very poor people for a permanent method causes concern (Cleland and Mauldin, 1991). In 1971, employers on three large tea estates in Tamil Nadu offered small monthly bonuses to women employees who did not become pregnant. These payments were deposited in a special account accessible only after the end of each woman's reproductive period. This program was reportedly associated with a clear decrease in fertility rates during its early period of operation, but nearly all the impact was due to sterilizations, because contraceptive supplies were not regularly provided. Since the employer kept the account books, few women knew how much money they had accumulated or were aware of the relation between no pregnancies and eventual expectation of a cash reward (Ridker, 1980).

The unique features of the Ammanpettai program are that it offers immediate, on-the-spot introductory small cash bonuses for a limited period to eligible women who elect to use a modern temporary contraceptive method of their choice—pills, condoms, and IUDs are the only methods provided by the Indian government—and it subsequently provides free contraceptive supplies through village contact women.

The design of the Ammanpettai program was based upon three hypotheses: (1) that a significant number of women who want to avoid pregnancy (but who reject sterilization) do not try modern temporary methods because of inertia, passivity, fear of ill effects, sociocultural constraints, or lack of accurate information about and access to such methods; (2) that small cash incentives, by overcoming such inertia or reluctance, would draw large numbers of women to a center where they could learn about and try a reversible method of their choice; and (3) that participation in this program, combined with subsequent easy access to supplies of contraceptives, would be a cost effective way to increase regular use of contraceptives.

To test these hypotheses, the program was publicized and implemented in selected villages. To follow the introductory incentive period, the program developed a village-based distribution system for condoms and pills, operating through village resident contact women.

The program may be compared to other marketing strategies that offer free small gifts for opening bank accounts, buying appliances, and so on. However, the Ammanpettai program is even less coercive, for nothing need be purchased; beneficiaries must only come to the center, hear about the methods and the reasons for using them, and understand the advantages and disadvantages of each available method. Potential beneficiaries are free to join or not to join as they see fit, to elect the temporary method of their choice if they do join, to use it or not to use it after joining, and to leave the program at any time. After they "graduate" from the introductory incentive program, they may continue to use or not to use any method. Women who have participated in the program are aware from that time forward what temporary methods of contraception are available, what they look like, how to use them, where to get them, and what the possible benefits and side effects are. At the same time, the staff at the clinic-based program has the opportunity to check the health of women who come to the clinic. All women are asked to bring their youngest child to the clinic; this child is weighed and immunized and particular attention is given to discussing appropriate weaning foods with mothers and offering health advice or treatment when necessary.

The first phase of the program began in 1985 in Stella Maris Clinic (SMC), a private charity clinic in the rural village of Ammanpettai, 10 km. north of Thanjavur in Tamil Nadu. At the outset, 75 percent of the women who joined the program stated that they wanted no more children, and more than 80 percent had previously been aware only of sterilization plus their own traditional methods as contraceptive strategies. Women were so afraid they might be tricked into undergoing sterilization that they would only come to the clinic in groups accompanied by their community creche teacher, a local woman whom they knew and trusted. As information about the program was publicized in other villages, the small cash incentives attracted very large numbers of women to the clinic.

A number of different formats for the promotional payments have been tried, including varying the number of paid monthly visits from one to 18 months and changing the amount of monthly incentive payments from 12 to 30 rupees.[1] Only married women under age 35, who have not been sterilized and whose husbands have not been vasectomized, and whose youngest child is six months to five years of age, are eligible to participate in the program. After participation in the introductory promotional payments component, women who have selected the pill or condoms are assigned to the contact person (CP) in their own village from whom they can continue to receive their contraceptive each month.

After a brief introductory training period, the CPs meet each month with clinic staff for further in-service training, to discuss any problems, to have their client registers checked by staff, and to receive new supplies and their monthly stipend, which was equivalent to US$7.00 in 1985 and US$6.85 in 1991. CPs also publicize the program and screen and supply new acceptors who have not been enrolled in the introductory incentive program.

Periodic surveys of acceptor knowledge and use by a team from Gandhigram University[2] not associated with program operation have guided and shaped program development. In 1988, the program was extended to selected areas in the city of Madras having a low rate of couple protection, and to two government primary health centers in rural Thanjavur District. In 1989, similar programs were developed in a semi-urban area and in several rural areas of Bihar. More then 6,000 women have participated in this program in the various areas.

Phase I: Pilot Study

Phase I of the project began in February 1985 by publicizing the program through creche teachers in five villages within eight km. of Stella Maris Charity Clinic in Ammanpettai and in one area of the town of Thanjavur. At the outset, 398 women—the upper limit constrained by funding—joined the program, most of whom were mothers of very young children who attended creches supervised by SMC teachers. This program offered 30 rupees per month for 6, 8, 12, or 18 months to program participants who remained nonpregnant. Pregnancy tests were performed monthly during the bonus periods: Fewer than 1 percent over the entire period were positive. (For this reason, in the following phase pregnancy tests were only performed in cases of suspected pregnancy; since nearly all tests were again negative, pregnancy testing was eventually eliminated altogether.)

Creche teachers in each village continue to distribute contraceptives monthly. As of June 1991, 284 women receive pills from these teachers. Of this number, approximately one-half are from the original 398 enrollees and the remainder have come to the teachers since bonuses were terminated in August 1986. Many of the "dropouts" have had tubal ligations or IUDs inserted, and others have moved away from the area.

Small cash incentives were very effective in promoting participation in the project. Moreover, the six-month period of participation appeared to be as effective as the longer periods of monthly payments in terms of postincentive continuation rates. This finding suggests that the incentives represented a "marketing" rather than a "conditioning" strategy. The first phase of the program achieved very high acceptor rates for temporary methods, compared with the rates achieved in a nearby control area (Nadakavery), which featured the regular, ongoing government family welfare program. Critics suggested that the better performance of the Phase I program might well be owing less to the incentives and more to the fact that women preferred to come to a high-quality private clinic where they were treated with concern and respect, rather than to regular government facilities where indifferent or coercive staff could be severe problems. In response to this critique, Phase II was designed as a controlled study specifically to test the power of small cash incentives to attract eligible women to the same clinic for family planning. Identical MCH and family planning services were offered to women in two separate clusters of villages, with only one cluster offering introductory incentives.

Phase II: Incentive and Control Villages

Two clusters of villages with socioeconomically matched populations of about 15,000 each were chosen; each cluster was located 5–6 km. from the SMC in Ammanpettai. In April 1987, a baseline survey of demographic characteristics and family planning knowledge, attitudes, and practice was conducted in both clusters by a research team from Gandhigram University Rural Development Institute. A sample from each cluster of 500 married women aged 18–45 was randomly selected from the government list of eligible couples. As Table 1

Table 1. Baseline survey of women in cluster A (control) villages and cluster B (incentive) villages, according to selected demographic, social, and economic characteristics, Tamil Nadu, 1987

Characteristic	Cluster A (N = 500)	Cluster B (N = 500)
Religion (%)		
Hindu	80	56*
Muslim	14	31*
Christian	6	13
Age group (%)		
15–19	3	3
20–24	14	20
25–29	28	25
30–34	24	22
35–39	21	19
40–44	9	11
Average age (years)	(30.7)	(30.4)
Type of house (%)		
Hut[a]	67	66
Pucca[a]	16	21
Kutcha[a]	18	13
Monthly income per household (rupees)	240	245

	Cluster A		Cluster B	
	Wife	Husband	Wife	Husband
Education (%)				
No schooling	42	20	35	14
1–3 years	10	5	9	10
4–6 years	26	25	35	33
7–10 years	17	24	17	27
10+ years	5	17	4	17
Occupation (%)				
Agricultural coolie	93	50	91	50
Farmer	—	17	—	14
Business	—	9	—	13
Other	—	23	—	23

*Population proportions are significantly different at 95% confidence limit.
[a] A hut is a small, usually windowless structure made of mud brick with a thatched roof; pucca means a well-built, permanent structure made of durable materials; and kutcha is a structure in between these standards.

shows, whereas education, income and other socioeconomic factors were very similar for the two clusters, compared with cluster B, cluster A had lower percentages of Muslims (14 percent vs. 31 percent) and Christians (6 percent vs. 13 percent). Cluster A also had higher rates of sterilization (35 percent vs. 25 percent) and use of temporary methods (3.6 percent vs. 3.2 percent) (not shown). Total contraceptive coverage was 33.1 percent for cluster A and 28.3 percent for B. In order not to give our program the benefit of cluster A's initial advantage in contraceptive coverage (and lower percentage of Muslims, who are generally less apt than others to accept family planning), women living in cluster B were selected as the experimental group and those living in cluster A were chosen as the control group for the introductory incentive study.

In May 1987, promotional announcements were made and notices (in Tamil) were distributed in both clusters of villages, inviting eligible women to come to the Stella Maris Clinic on specified days for free MCH services, contraceptive education, and supplies. For the villages in cluster B, the announcements offered women an incentive of 20 rupees (US$1.25) at their first visit and an additional 20 rupees per month for the next five months for coming to the clinic, continuing the temporary contraceptive method of their choice, and not becoming pregnant (see Figure 1).

Figure 1. Announcement distributed to women in cluster B (incentive) villages, translated from the Tamil

Stella Maris Family Welfare and Family Control Scheme
Ammanpettai
!!!!!!!
An Announcement for Married Women Between the Ages of 18 and 35

If you postpone pregnancy you can receive Rs. 20/- once in a month.

To be eligible you will have to be:
1. Married and between the ages of 18 and 35 years and not pregnant.
2. You should not be a widow or divorced or otherwise not living with your husband.
3. You or your husband should not have undergone tubectomy or vasectomy operations.
4. If you have children the last one should be more than 6 months old and not aged more than 5 years.
5. You must be a resident of Melathirruppanthuruthi or Kandiyur or Kellathiruppanthuruthi villages.

If you satisfy the conditions mentioned above please come every month to Stella Maris Hospital on any day except Sunday between 10 a.m. to 5 p.m.

If your last child is below 3 years please bring the child along with you.

This is not a scheme for permanent prevention of pregnancy. Family Welfare operations are not done here.

The first 500 women who are selected will alone be included in this scheme.

Similar announcements appeared in cluster A villages, but no incentive payments were offered (see Figure 2). Owing to budget constraints, enrollment from cluster B villages was limited to 1,000 women (estimated to be about two-thirds of the eligible women). Acceptors were enrolled in two groups of 500 each, spaced six months apart to accommodate the clinic's capacity to process the beneficiaries. No enrollment limits were set for cluster A, the control villages.

More than 1,000 women from cluster B villages came to the clinic on the first few appointed days of enrollment, overwhelming clinic resources and space. On the days appointed for women from cluster A villages, only 14 women came to the clinic for the same services. Of the 1,000 cluster B beneficiaries, 950 stayed with the program through the five months' introductory bonus period. Women who joined the program were younger, of lower parity, of lower income and caste, and were more likely to be illiterate than were those in the population-based survey of women in their catchment area.

When acceptors completed their initial and five subsequent monthly incentive-payment visits, they were referred for future supplies to the seven contact persons who were selected for their villages from among program participants. The CPs were literate, young, married women, most of whom had participated in the program themselves, had shown an interest in the program, were trusted by other women in their villages, and were able to maintain monthly rosters of the beneficiaries served by them. All of the CPs attended a brief course given by the clinic physician and staff on reproductive physiology, contraceptive methods and practice, indications and contraindications for specific methods, side effects, and

Figure 2. Announcement distributed to women in cluster A (control) villages, translated from the Tamil

Stella Maris Family Welfare and Family Control Scheme
Ammanpettai
!!!!!!!
An Announcement for Married Women Between the Ages of 18 and 35

Free supply of pills and nirodh for prevention of pregnancy.

Free offer of consultation and examination by qualified doctors.

To be eligible for the above you will have to be:
Married and between the ages of 18 and 35 and not pregnant.
You or your husband should not have been operated upon for tubectomy or vasectomy.

If you satisfy the above conditions kindly come to Stella Maris Hospital on any day except Sunday between 10 a.m. and 5 p.m.

This is not a scheme for permanent prevention of pregnancy. Family Welfare operations are not done here.

Note: Nirodh is the common term for condom.

register-keeping. The CPs were supplied with lists of acceptors' names. The CPs report monthly to the clinic as a group, for exchange of experiences, continuing education, resupply of contraceptives, checking of beneficiary rosters by the program administrator, and collection of their monthly stipend.

There were, of course, no incentive-program "graduates" to serve as clients for CPs in cluster A villages. Thus, the CPs appointed in cluster A were instructed to do some initial recruitment by publicizing the availability of their services in their villages. No targets were established for the CPs in either cluster. The intention was to test genuine continuation rates for the incentive-program beneficiaries by determining the extent to which they would come on their own initiative to the CPs for continuing supplies rather than having the CPs actively seek them out and carry supplies to them in their homes or elsewhere. (Subsequent surveys, however, showed that the CPs were much more active in taking supplies to the beneficiaries than had been intended.) By the time of the follow-up survey conducted by a team from Gandhigram Rural Institute during July–August 1989, more than a year after Phase II payments had ended, CPs in both clusters A and B reported about the same number of clients were obtaining contraceptive supplies from them—somewhat over 450 clients in each cluster.

This result was surprising. The large numerical difference in initial response to the program from the women in the cluster B villages and those in the cluster A villages (1,000 vs. 14, respectively) did not lead us to expect that the CPs in these clusters would develop the same apparent client load of acceptors. Subsequent surveillance by field monitors who visit a random sample of beneficiaries from CP lists has shown that two CPs in cluster A villages maintained large lists of acceptors, but many of the names were not valid. Ongoing surveillance of random samples of acceptors has resulted in the removal of dubious names from CP lists in all the villages covered by this project. This report classifies as "continuing acceptors" those beneficiaries reported by their CPs to be receiving supplies from them. The term "users" applies to pill acceptors who can show a partly used pill packet to field monitors (and exclude those who say they are taking pills but who present a full or empty packet, or no packet). Using this definition, users constitute about 60 percent of continuing acceptors.

Evaluation of the Phase II Program: The Follow-up Survey

In 1989, Gandhigram University conducted a follow-up population-based survey. As Table 2 shows, compared with women in cluster A villages, the random sample of women in cluster B villages showed a greater knowledge of all three available temporary methods and they experienced a greater increase in knowledge over the two years between the baseline and follow-up surveys. Table 3 shows that the percentage of nonsterilized respondents using a modern temporary method increased in cluster A from 3.6 percent to 13.0 percent. During the

Table 2. Percentage of women who know of specific contraceptive methods and percentage increase in knowledge of temporary methods between surveys (1987 and 1989), according to type of village [a]

Type of village	Female Sterilization	Male Sterilization	Pill	Condom	IUD
Ammanpettai program					
Cluster A					
Baseline	87	54	34	20	28
Follow-up	98	67	39	39	34
% increase	13	24	15	95	21
Cluster B					
Baseline	75	51	32	31	26
Follow-up	92	65	43	58	46
% increase	23	27	34	87	77
Government-only program [b]					
Varagoor					
Baseline	87	59	22	26	27
Vadukagudi					
Baseline	94	64	32	33	32

[a] In the Ammanpettai program, women in cluster A villages were not offered cash incentives for using temporary methods, but those in cluster B villages were offered such incentives. [b] Women in Varagoor and Vadukagudi received the regular government family planning services; thus, these two villages serve as controls. The baseline survey carried out in these villages was conducted in 1989, at the same time as the follow-up survey of cluster A and cluster B participants.

Table 3. Percentage of nonsterilized respondents currently using temporary contraceptive methods and percentage increase in use of such methods between surveys (1987 and 1989), according to type of village

Type of village	Baseline Survey	Follow-up Survey	% Point Increase
Ammanpettai program			
Cluster A	3.6	13.0	9.3
Cluster B	3.2	24.6	21.4
Government-only program			
Varagoor	na	6.0	na
Vadukagudi	na	5.0	na

Note: See notes to Table 2.
na = not available.

same two-year period, respondents in cluster B showed an increase in use from 3.2 percent at baseline to 24.6 percent at follow-up. Two control villages that were not touched by either program showed a utilization rate of 5 percent and 6 percent, respectively, at the time of the follow-up survey. Thus, while women in cluster A villages showed better knowledge and higher use rates of temporary contraceptives than did women in government program-only control areas, neither group did as well as women in cluster B villages.

For comparison and to check the validity of CP rosters, a separate survey was carried out at the same time by the Gandhigram team on two samples of 150 respondents randomly selected from CP rosters in cluster A and cluster B villages. This survey showed that only 4 percent of women in cluster A and 6 percent of those in cluster B had ever used any modern family planning method before participating in the program; 89 percent of cluster A and 85 percent of cluster B acceptors were still receiving supplies from their CP, and 4 percent of cluster A acceptors and 57 percent of cluster B acceptors had participated in the incentive program (indicating that 43 percent of acceptors on CP rosters for cluster B enrolled in the program after the incentive program was terminated). Thus, the actual continuation rate of bonus-program participants is only about 25 percent 15–22 months after the last bonus payment.

In answer to the question, "Explain exactly how you get or got your supplies from the CP," 136 (91 percent) of cluster A acceptors and 135 (90 percent) of cluster B acceptors reported that the supplies were brought to them by the CPs; only 10–11 percent of acceptors went to the CP's house for supplies. Further, there were no differences in the numbers of women in clusters A and B who could show a partly used pill packet (50 percent and 46 percent, respectively) or a full packet (8 percent of women in each group).

In June 1991, three and a half years after the last incentive payment, CPs from the incentive area (cluster B) reported that they were giving temporary methods to 324 women, and CPs from cluster A reported 447 women on their acceptor lists. As noted above, current field monitoring by Ammanpettai staff indicates that the latter figure is inflated.

In a further attempt to evaluate program performance, several focus groups of program graduates have been held by social workers not associated with operating the program. A most poignant comment at one such group was made by a young mother, who reported that use of the pill had brought "greater harmony" to her home. "I no longer have to refuse my husband. He no longer goes to prostitutes, thus five rupees are saved and home is more peaceful."

Although Muslim women made up 31 percent of the baseline survey population in cluster B villages, only 4.9 percent of acceptors were Muslim. When asked if using contraceptives conflicted with her religious beliefs, one Muslim acceptor replied, "Will religion feed my children?"

Phase III: Trials of Smaller Incentives, Fewer Visits, and CPs Only

Phase III of the program addressed two questions: (1) Could lower introductory incentive payments and fewer free visits attract and keep as many women as had the original offering? (2) Would appointing contact women alone in a cluster of villages be as effective as using incentives?

In July 1988, village leaders and pamphlets distributed in the villages advertised a payment of 12 rupees for a single, initial clinic visit to the first 250 women who enrolled in the program in Ammanpettai from the village of Mathur, population 4,500, located 10 km. from the Stella Maris Clinic. Unlike the response in Phase II, some three weeks and considerable promotion by program staff were required to enroll 250 women. One year later, at the time of the Gandhigram survey, the two CPs appointed for this area reported serving 242 continuing acceptors. In June 1991, three years after the incentive program ended, 113 women were reported by the CPs to be on their rosters. Current acceptors are not all "leftovers" from the original 250, as there is a continuous process of dropping out and replacement by new acceptors once the follow-up program is started in the community. In this case, incentives served for initial publicity and perhaps created a positive attitude toward the program.

Phase III further tested the impact on recruitment of acceptors and continuation rates of appointing just CPs without an antecedent incentive program. To prevent dissemination of the incentive concept from the Ammanpettai area, Vallum District—some 25 km. from Stella Maris Clinic—was chosen for this study. For a population of 6,000 in six hamlets, six CPs supervised by the two government multipurpose health workers (MPHWs) assigned to this area were appointed and trained to supply pills and condoms to eligible women. Within six months, these CPs reported 252 acceptors on their rosters. As of June 1991, 85 percent of the 245 acceptors were reportedly using the pill, and 15 percent were using condoms.

Evaluation of Program Performance

Phase II and Phase III: Follow-up Survey of Program Graduates and Other Users

Two years following the last incentive payment in cluster B and the single payment in Mathur, random samples were drawn from the CP rosters—150 each for Phase II clusters A and B, 100 each for Phase III Mathur and Vallum programs.

These surveys showed that the client relationships represented by the CP rosters were genuine, in the sense that the survey field enumerators were able to find nearly all of the individuals in their random samples drawn from the rosters and virtually all of these respondents testified that they had received contraceptive supplies from the CPs. This finding was important, because virtually all of the respondents testified that they had never used temporary methods before.

Nearly all of the respondents reported that they were in fact practicing temporary methods of contraception. One cannot, however, take such testimony at face value. Consequently, respondents were asked, "What does it (the method you are currently using) look like; how do you use it?" The percentages of respondents with fair or better knowledge of their method were: 87 percent of those surveyed in Phase II, cluster B (five-visit incentive program); 75 percent of those surveyed in Phase II, cluster A (CP-only); 44 percent of respondents in Phase III, Vallum (CP-only); and 57 percent of respondents in Phase III, Mathur (one-visit incentive program). As a further check on contraceptive practice, respondents who had said that they were using pills were asked, "Can you show us the packet you are now using?" Except for the Mathur respondents (at 28 percent), about 50 percent of the respondents in all of the other programs could show a partly used packet.

The evidence assembled here on contraceptive practice leaves a good bit to be desired. One of the big problems encountered when evaluating the performance of family planning programs is finding feasible ways to measure the true rate and quality of contraceptive practice—a problem for which, to our knowledge, there is as yet no entirely satisfactory answer (Potter et al., 1991). Surveys of fertility, measured by numbers pregnant and length of open birth interval, are in progress.

Phase IV: Implementing the Ammanpettai Program Through Government Facilities

The program appeared to operate well in the private-clinic setting provided by the Stella Maris Clinic. However, to be of significance in addressing India's need to rapidly increase the number of contraceptive acceptors, such a program must be able to operate with very large numbers of acceptors throughout the country. To do so, a much larger infrastructure (facilities/personnel) than can be offered by private clinics is required. Government health facilities provide the single largest and most dispersed system for implementing such a program. Consequently, in 1988, the incentive program was implemented in several government health posts in the city of Madras. At the same time, incentive-CP and CP-only programs were implemented in primary health centers in two rural areas of Thanjavur District (Kabisthalam and Mellatur).

The Madras program has been operated entirely by government family welfare staff, with support from the Ammanpettai program limited to consultations, the financing of incentives, and some transport and data collection. Trials in rural primary health centers have entailed finding ways in which one or both of the two central elements of the Ammanpettai program—the introductory incentives and the local contact persons as a distribution network—can be used to complement and improve the ongoing operation of the government's programs. Various division-of-labor patterns are, in principle, feasible for engendering collaboration between private and government clinics. To be successful, however, patterns of association cannot, at least initially, require major changes in the way the government programs operate—that is, they cannot require significant changes in the quantity or quality of government staff effort or performance. In the rural area, government facilities' assuring quality of service and regularity of supplies has proved to be a major problem.

City of Madras Program

Inaugurated in October 1988 at the invitation of Chandra Gariyali, Director of Family Welfare, Tamil Nadu, and Hyma Balachandran, District Family Welfare Officer, Corporation of Madras, the Madras program was the first effort to implement the incentive program through government facilities. The areas chosen for this study were "slums" (undeveloped areas), where women are particularly resistant to adopting any method of family planning. Following publicity by government health-post staff in two blocks, each with a population of about 5,000, and an official inaugural ceremony, women who joined the program received a promotional payment of 15 rupees for the first and two subsequent visits if they were new acceptors of temporary methods.

The Madras City program has been operated entirely by government family-welfare staff under the leadership of Sheila Sekar, Family Welfare Medical Officer. Female multipurpose health workers from the health post carried out a baseline demographic and KAP survey, publicized the program through pamphlets and door-to-door contacts, and provided all educational and delivery services, including payment of incentives and follow-up. Although the 168 new acceptors initially enrolled in this program was a small number by rural standards, it was considered to be a significant increase by health-post staff, because more women accepted IUDs and pills for the first time on the first day of the program than could usually be recruited over several months of door-to-door canvassing. Similar programs have since been initiated in 13 additional health posts, in each case selecting a block of 5,000 people that have been particularly resistant to accepting any contraceptive method. Incentive payments of 12 rupees for the first and two additional monthly visits are funded by a World Bank population grant to the city of Madras.

The strong performance of the Madras program was unexpected, as the program was originally designed for rural women, most of whom knew little or nothing about temporary methods. In contrast, the Madras baseline survey showed that all women respondents were "aware of" the existence of temporary methods, but few used them. Moreover, multipurpose health workers and nurses on staff at each health post frequently canvassed every household; considerable attention had already been given to promotion of any means of contraception for women with more than two children. In July 1991, 1–3 years after the last incentive payment reported by their health worker, 1,360 women out of an original 2,821 who received at least one incentive payment were continuing to receive the contraceptive of their choice.

A survey of acceptors and a control population in the Madras program, conducted by K. Srinivasan in June–July 1990 (22 months after the scheme began), indicated that the program had indeed effected a sharp increase in the number of new acceptors of temporary methods over the very short period of the incentive offer, with beneficiaries in the incentive group accepting these methods at a lower age and parity than controls (Srinivasan et al., 1990). Open birth intervals were longer for program "graduates" who, surprisingly, were also opting for sterilization at a younger age and parity than were controls. In 1991, these favorable results led the city of Madras to approve the requests of two health-post family welfare physicians to extend the program to their entire health-post catchment areas, each with a population of approximately 50,000, in addition to operating in specified blocks (each with population of 5,000) in 28 health-post catchment areas.

Kabisthalam Primary Health Center Program

In January 1989, following several planning meetings with Kabisthalam Primary Health Center staff, including a physician, multipurpose health workers, and computer and nursing supervisors, a program featuring an introductory incentive payment of 15 rupees for an initial and two subsequent visits was inaugurated in the Kabisthalam Primary Health Center. This health center is a government facility which, with eight subcenters, serves a population of approximately 26,000. The incentive-program catchment area was comprised of three villages within two km. of the health center. Another three villages were designated as control villages and were assigned CPs only. Ammanpettai staff conducted a baseline survey of 892 women that indicated that all the women were aware of sterilization, the pill, and condoms, and 60 percent reported knowing about the IUD. Of the women surveyed, 19 percent had been sterilized; 5 percent were current users of the pill; 12 percent used condoms; and 3 percent used an IUD. Eighty-seven percent of the women stated they wanted only two children. In January 1989, government multipurpose health workers publicized the bonus program through pamphlets and word-of-mouth; women were invited to join the program by coming to the primary health center on designated days for maternal and child health and family planning information and were offered 15 rupees for each of three monthly visits.

In working with the health-center staff a number of problems emerged, including conflicts with the Ammanpettai program which offered a choice of methods and did not maintain government targets for sterilization, and government rules for restricting pill use to women with one child. Government staff also refused to allow their female health workers or Ammanpettai staff to distribute condoms from the health center, because this job is reserved for male health workers who interact only with male acceptors. With very little help from the staff of the health center, the Ammanpettai staff registered and interviewed prospective beneficiaries who came to the center on the appointed days, measured blood pressure, weighed mothers and babies, advised clients about available methods, provided the chosen contraceptive, paid the 15 rupee bonus, and kept the records. For a number of reasons (including the health-center staff's brusqueness toward potential enrollees and the physician's lack of support for the pill and insistence on IUD or sterilization for women with more than two children), enrollee recruitment during the three-month incentive period fell below expectations: Only 173 women instead of the anticipated 250, or approximately 25 percent of eligible couples, enrolled. However, the program grew rapidly when it moved out of the health center and into the villages, where the CPs promoted it and provided contraceptive supplies. Two years later (in January 1991), the three CPs in the incentive-program villages reported 240 beneficiaries, and the three CPs in the control villages (no incentive, CP-only) reported 235 beneficiaries on their rosters, more than three-quarters of whom were reportedly taking the pill. This is a very considerable increase over the 49 women who reported taking the pill during the baseline study.

Surveys are in progress to check the reliability of these rosters. Even though strenuous efforts have been made to discourage CPs from inflating lists of their acceptors, this practice has been a serious problem with some CPs. Spot checks by supervisory staff of random acceptors on CP lists are difficult to carry out, as most acceptors work in the fields daily. Although all CPs receive the same monthly stipend regardless of the number of clients on their lists—a policy adopted to discourage false inflation of acceptors—it has proven necessary to maintain ongoing surveillance of CP lists through unscheduled visits by program staff who interview random samples of beneficiaries. As in other studies of compliance and usage from developing countries, we have found that misuse and nonuse of methods are common problems requiring continued surveillance and education of both providers and acceptors (Seaton, 1985; Potter et al., 1991).

Mellatur Primary Health Center

Because of the problems encountered working with the primary health center's physician in Kabisthalam, our next effort was preceded by discussions with the director of family welfare for Tamil Nadu, Chandra Gariyali. Through her good offices, the staff at Mellatur Primary Health Center was advised to interpret targets less rigidly during the implementation of the bonus program. It was also decided to operate through the subcenters rather than out of the health center headquarters, which is located at a considerable distance from most of the villages and hamlets to be served.

Mellatur is an expanded primary health center with 24 subcenters serving a population of 111,425. Each subcenter has a catchment area of about 5,000 persons. According to government statistics, when the program began there were 17,828 eligible couples in the Mellatur catchment area, 33 percent of whom were sterilized, 2 percent of whom were IUD users, 4 percent of whom used the pill, and 1 percent of whom received condoms through the health center's male multipurpose health workers.

The initial program in Mellatur was started in eight subcenters: Four of them offered an initial and two subsequent monthly incentive payments of 20 rupees and follow-up by CPs, and four featured only CPs. As in the Kabisthalam program, initial publicity was to be carried out by government multipurpose health workers in each subcenter catchment area. Initiated in October 1989, the program got off to a slow start due to poor publicity by the health workers and inadequate facilities at some subcenters. (Subcenters generally consisted of very small one- or two-room structures with, at most, a chair, a table, or a bench. Sometimes they were locked; and some were nonexistent, so the local nutrition center or creche was used instead.) As information about the program spread by word-of-mouth, larger and larger numbers of new acceptors (more than 100 per day at some subcenters) turned up on the appointed monthly enrollment day, so that the initially planned three-month enrollment period was extended for two additional months. The local health center was unable to keep up with the demand for the pill: During this period, 476 new pill acceptors were enrolled, 321 of whom were on CP rosters six months after the last payment. In CP-only villages, 165 women were receiving pills, and 150 were reportedly taking condoms. The very large turnout for the incentive program overwhelmed the small Ammanpettai staff. The multipurpose health worker who was scheduled to help with screening, education, and registration in each subcenter was generally kept too busy screening out sterilized women and giving immunizations to children brought by each mother to assist with the family planning work.

In March 1990 the program was extended to 14 additional subcenters, all offering three incentive payments of 20 rupees, with half of the acceptors to be followed by CPs and half to be followed by government multipurpose health workers. Again, the response was very large: A total of 3,068 beneficiaries were enrolled and received at least one incentive payment. This number of beneficiaries represented more than half of all of the nonsterilized eligible couples in these catchment areas. This substantial ratio of enrollment to eligible couples was achieved in catchment areas where the official temporary-methods prevalence rates were below 5 percent of eligible couples. Once again, to the considerable satisfaction of the multipurpose health workers, they were able to immunize many children at the time of beneficiary visits. This, however, left to the small Ammanpettai staff all of the screening, maternal and child health services, contraceptive education, and enrollment procedures.

The Mellatur program demonstrated the power of modest incentives to achieve one important objective of family planning programs—namely, bringing women to a center for family planning instruction and supplies and for health surveillance for themselves and their children. However, the response was too great for the small staff to provide adequate services on the designated enroll-ment days. Subsequent programs in government facilities have been designed to allow a longer enrollment period, so that only about 40–50 women maximum need to be seen on a single day. Follow-up surveys of the large Mellatur cohort have demonstrated that education in method use at the time of enrollment was inadequate, and that some CPs were poorly chosen. Particularly disappointing was the poor follow-up by government health workers who, although they were present at the incentive clinics, maintained no lists of acceptors, were often changed to other posts, or took leave from their posts without replacements being made. CPs have since been appointed to follow up in areas originally des-ignated for health workers who are no longer active. Given these difficulties, the combination of an introductory bonus with health worker follow-up has not been successful or easy to assess. Equally troublesome, government supplies of the pill (and occasionally of condoms) have often run out, leaving women without pills for months at a time. The much greater logistic success of the Madras pro-gram using government health workers may be attributed to the higher ratio of service personnel to population, their higher morale, far better supervision, and the considerable support for the program at the highest levels of the Family Welfare Service.

The Power of the Promotional-Payment Strategy

Knowledge of Use of Temporary Methods

For the purpose of evaluation, the promotional-payments program may be re-garded as essentially a marketing and educational strategy. It is a necessary (but not a sufficient) condition for the success of family planning programs that women who wish to reduce the number of their pregnancies know how to use contraceptive methods and have easy access to the method of their choice. An important result of this program is that the beneficiaries, through actual trials, have acquired realistic, hands-on knowledge of modern temporary methods of contraception. The program has demonstrated the impressive power of small cash incentives to rapidly attract large numbers of women—virtually all of whom testify that they have had no prior use of temporary methods—to participate in voluntary trials of these methods. In the Phase II program, in a catchment area where government figures reported prevalence rates of around 5 percent for temporary methods, promotional payments motivated about 70 percent of the nonsterilized and otherwise eligible women to take home either the pill or condoms. The experience has been similar in other settings. If supervised visits to a clinic to learn about temporary methods represent an effective strategy to teach women how to avert pregnancy, then promotional payments must be regarded as a very powerful means to accomplish one of the main objectives of family planning programs, namely, awareness of and knowledge about methods and where to obtain supplies. As was evident in Phase I, going to family planning clinics in village groups offers reassurance to women and may further stimulate interest and motivation to join the program.

The follow-up program, using village resident women who accept responsibility for supplying contraceptives to women in their village for a small stipend of about US$5–$7 per month, was developed to assure continued availability of supplies, because these were not easily obtainable from health workers at the time the program was started. Five years later, even though the number of MPHWs was supposed to have doubled in Tamil Nadu and targets have been established for pill acceptors, multipurpose health workers (now called village health nurses) with their mandatory sterilization targets have great difficulty in attracting a large roster of acceptors of temporary methods. The CPs, who reside in the village they serve and therefore gain the trust of potential acceptors more readily, provide education and advice to program graduates and are also a major source of knowledge about and supply of temporary methods. Through the use of a screening questionnaire, they recruit new acceptors who choose methods in the absence of incentive payments.

Theoretically, the MPHWs, who visit each of these villages at least once a month, should be able to take over the CP functions once a woman has been established as an acceptor either through the incentive program or CP recruitment. To test this possibility, which would make sense economically and logistically, we have attempted to transfer the acceptor lists from the CP to the MPHW serving her village, while assuring the CP that her stipend will continue and she will thereafter be asked only to check up on whether her acceptors are being served. This effort has been entirely unsuccessful. CPs insist that their clients have little confidence in the MPHWs and are therefore unwilling to rely on them for the pill and to subject themselves to the pressure for permanent methods so integrally associated with MPHWs and all government family planning functions.

The CPs also provide vital feedback to program developers by reporting the problems in the field—whether these be side effects of drugs, fears of cancer, or attitudes of acceptors—and their suggestions for improving the program. The 58 Thanjavur District CPs form a new professional cadre; they are well-known in their community and are active in district family planning meetings. Their suggestions have been valuable to the development of the program. Continuation rates of about 25–30 percent were documented on rural CP rosters 15 months into Phase II, a figure comparable to that from other nonincentive temporary-method programs (Loza et al., 1990). The addition of new clients means that approximately 50 percent of those on current CP rosters "graduated" from the incentive program and 50 percent are new users who did not receive introductory incentives but were recruited by CPs in the villages after the incentive program ended.

CP-only vs. Incentive Formats

Although CP rosters indicate nearly equal numbers of acceptors in nonincentive and incentive villages, other factors need to be taken into account when comparing the relative effectiveness of the CP-only and promotional-payment programs. Surveys of Phase II incentive-program acceptors indicate that supervised visits in a clinic setting result in beneficiaries acquiring higher quality knowledge about temporary methods than is derived from learning about methods only from CPs. Promotional payments for family planning also have the advantage of bringing women to the health center for maternal and child health services. Malnutrition, anemia, and parasitosis were endemic among the Thanjavur rural enrollees, where the average hemoglobin level of mothers was 7–8 gms. (compared with a normal range of 12–13 gms.) and their average weights were under 40 kg. Important aspects of the program include teaching women about the importance of child spacing, adequate diet, and available weaning foods; dispensing iron to severely anemic women; weighing mothers and infants; and immunizing children and giving them vitamin A. Although the women rarely had elevated blood pressure or other contraindications to pill use, the clinic-based program has the advantage of being able to measure blood pressure and offer physical checkups by a physician. It has not been possible to systematically implement these services in the CP-only program or in the government pill-distribution program.

Cost Effectiveness and Sustainability

The Ammanpettai program, as it has operated to date in each of its settings, may be considered an evolving experimental program format. An important yield of this trial has been testing the hypotheses—set out at the beginning of this discussion—that informed the design of the program. The program performance has generally supported the validity of these hypotheses, findings which are of significance for the design of family planning programs in general. Beyond this, the Ammanpettai program will be of greater interest if it is sustainable and cost effective.

However satisfactory the performance of the Ammanpettai program, if the same results (outputs) could have been secured by an alternative program using fewer resources (inputs), then the Ammanpettai program would not be cost effective.

The program is now supported by two American foundations, the Hewlett Foundation and the Buffett Foundation. The question of *financial sustainability* is whether the Government of India could support such a program on a wide scale without help from donor funding. The question of *operational sustainability* is whether organizations exist or could be put in place to implement a program of the Ammanpettai type on a wider scale. At issue here is the capacity and willingness of such organizations to manage and administer an Ammanpettai-type program (assuming funding were available).

An adequate evaluation of the Ammanpettai program would include analyses of the cost effectiveness and financial and operational sustainability of each of the program components—incentive payments and CP distribution—in each of the settings in which it has operated. Space considerations preclude such analysis here. It is, however, important to consider whether the novel promotional-payments component is practical in the sense of being sustainable financially: Could it potentially be extended to cover wide areas of India insofar as budget constraints are concerned?

Financial Sustainability of Phase IV
Promotional-Payments Component in Rural Areas

To ascertain whether promotional payments are financially sustainable in rural areas, we begin by determining the budget size for this program were it to be extended to the population of Tamil Nadu as a whole. In March 1987, there were about 9 million eligible couples in Tamil Nadu, about 40 percent of whom are said to be effectively protected by sterilization. (The unprotected rate is officially reported at about 46 percent of eligible couples, but, owing to likely inflated figures of acceptors, is probably somewhat lower.) This leaves about 5 million unprotected eligible couples as potential candidates for a Phase IV-type promotional-payments program. We assume a promotional-payment program that enrolls 80 percent, or 4 million of these women.

The yearly budget of a generalized Phase IV promotional-payments component would depend upon the scale of the program adopted—that is, upon the number of participants to be carried in the program each year. The fewer the number, the smaller the budget, but the longer it would require to give all eligible unprotected couples an opportunity to participate in the program. For example, a program that enrolls one-eighth of the 4 million eligible couples each year would enroll about 500,000 women per year. With an additional (marginal) budget cost estimated at 63 rupees a year per benefiiciary (60 rupees for the incentive payment plus 3 rupees for administrative costs at 1987 prices), the total budget cost per year would come to 31.5 million rupees. This figure is about 4.3

percent of the Revised Estimate 1987–88 for public health and family welfare of 736 million rupees.[3] The fiscal burden implied by the budget necessary for generalizing the Phase IV promotional-payment component might thus be regarded as relatively modest.

Program Scale: The Early Years vs. the Steady-State Maintenance Scale

During the early years, the program would be operated at a scale to process the backlog of eligible couples at a rate acceptable in terms of fiscal burden. For example, at a scale covering one-eighth of the eligible couples with a Phase IV promotional-payments schedule, and processing, say, two such groups each year, the backlog would be processed in about four years at an annual *gross* additional budget cost of about 10.8 percent of the current rate of budgeting for public health and family welfare in Tamil Nadu. The *net* budget cost may be significantly less than the gross budget cost.[4]

At this point, by analogue to an immunization program, the promotional-payments component would go into a maintenance phase, adopting the smaller scale appropriate to processing the new additions to the cohort of eligible couples each year. This point is central to evaluating the fiscal burden implied by this type of program over the longer run.

With these longer-run considerations taken into account, the very modest relative size of the additional fiscal burden implied by generalizing the promotional-payments component would suggest that the question of financial sustainability per se should not be regarded as a serious problem. This discussion has directed attention to the power of promotional payments as a strategy to accomplish information, education, and communication (IEC) functions. In this domain, this program economizes on scarce resources committed to these functions by focusing them on the target population most likely to benefit from education in contraceptive use and for whom such information is most likely to effect behavioral changes.

The CP Component: Budget Cost and Financial Sustainability

The burden on fiscal capacity entailed by the CP program depends upon the scale of the program and upon the productivity of the CPs. We assume a program that enrolls as clients 2.5 million eligible couples (this is about one-half of those reported as uncovered in 1987). We assume that each CP serves 60 clients on average. The cost of the CP component includes CP stipends of 105 (1987) rupees per month and additional costs for field staff, who monitor the performance of the program on a continuing basis. Each field worker currently monitors the performance of 58 CPs. Salary (2,000 rupees per month) and transportation costs (1,000 rupees per month) for each field worker add up to about 10 rupees per client per year. CP stipend costs are about 21 rupees per client per year, or a total of 77.5 million rupees for the 2.5 million enrollees; this comes to about 10.5 percent of the 1987–88 government budget for public health and family welfare in Tamil Nadu.

From Pilot Program to State-wide Program

The significance of a pilot program depends in large part on the feasibility of increasing its scale, say, to state-wide dimensions (in this case, to cover the state of Tamil Nadu). In evaluating the prospects for doing so, it is necessary to distinguish the promotional-payments component and the CP component.

In the immediately preceding sections of this paper, the conclusion was reached that, particularly with longer-run considerations taken into account, the very modest relative size of the additional fiscal burden implied by generalizing the promotional-payments component statewide suggests that the question of financial sustainability per se should not be regarded as a serious problem. That is, financial sustainability should not be regarded as a barrier to increasing the scale of the program from pilot to statewide dimensions.

The question of operational sustainability—whether organizations exist or could be put in place to implement an Ammanpettai-type promotional-payments component—is another matter. It was, of course, with an eye to increasing the scale of the program to state-wide dimensions that we began in Phase IV an attempt to implement the program in government facility settings.

The first point to be made in this context is that the Madras City promotional-payments program, which began on a pilot basis in October 1988 in a block of about 5,000 inhabitants in each of two health posts (Villivakkam and Kolathur), is already being rapidly scaled up. Promotional payments for the initial pilot program in Madras were funded by the Ammanpettai Program. Shortly thereafter, the promotional-payments program was adopted and became the "Innovative Spacing Scheme" of India Population Project V, funded by the World Bank. This funding source is now used for most of the promotional payments in Madras. The program is entirely executed by the staff of those health posts where it operates (there being no need for CPs, since the health workers attached to the health posts discharge these functions effectively). As of October 1991, the promotional-payments program was operating in one block in each of 14 health posts. The program coordinator has requested authorization to expand to all of the catchment areas of these health posts, an expansion which would add about 13,000 eligible beneficiaries. Four additional health posts were added to those in the program, and a request has been made to authorize the inclusion of 12 more, bringing the total number of participating health posts to 30. These new additions will begin on the one block per health post catchment area pattern and then, if the small-scale initiatives are successful, may expand to include all of the catchment areas of these health posts. The population in the catchment areas served would be about 370,000 (about one-tenth of the total population of Madras). Assuming there is no funding constraint, there would seem to be no reason why continuing expansion of the program in Madras City could not take place.

As the Madras experience testifies, increasing the scale of the promotional-payments program operating in government facilities is clearly feasible when the program is implemented and executed by the staffs of these facilities. Madras affords a peculiarly favorable environment for this approach. It is, at this point, far from clear that this approach is feasible for operating the program in government facilities in rural areas. Insofar as family planning activities are concerned, in the rural areas the staff of government facilities focuses almost exclusively on meeting sterilization targets and the hard-sell approach to clients thought to be necessary for doing so. There seems to be little genuine interest in an Ammanpettai-type program, which emphasizes a couple's right to freely choose any temporary method, if they so desire. This may change in the future, if policymakers are convinced that significant increases in temporary-method prevalence rates will be necessary for India to achieve its population goals.

In rural government facilities in Thanjavur District, the pattern that evolved for fielding the promotional-payments component entailed cooperation between our program staff and the government staff, but only minimal contributions from the government side were required: MPHWs were only required to publicize the program and to go to their regularly assigned subcenters one or two days a month for a few consecutive months to open the facility and assist with screening and crowd control. Ammanpettai program staff visited the subcenters on these dates, educated potential acceptors about temporary methods, and made the promotional payments to acceptors. Health workers used the opportunity to immunize the the infants and children brought by their mothers. Some problems with this format did arise, but were of a kind that could be readily managed by scheduling more visits and using group educational activities for the large numbers of women attracted by the introductory bonus. Cooperative arrangements of this kind, between a private agency and a public program, may get increasing attention in the coming years in India, where plans are now being developed to rely more upon private voluntary or nongovernmental organizations for implementation of the family welfare program.

In principle, this format could be scaled up. In fielding the promotional-payments component in government facilities in Thanjavur District, a three-person team from the Ammanpettai program made site visits. To scale up would require increasing the number of teams cooperating with government facilities. How many such teams would be needed would depend upon the desired pace for processing eligible couples. We have suggested a program scale that would process about 1 million eligible couples a year (for four years) as a financially feasible pattern. A very rough estimate is that such a program would require about 100 teams of three persons each, or a total of about 300 field workers. Just in terms of numbers, the training of only 300 workers should surely be feasible. We do recognize, however, that some overarching organization would be needed to coordinate, manage the logistics of, and supervise the field workers' activities.

Turning to the CP component, the enterprise of scaling up from pilot to state-wide dimensions would run into a number of problems. Fielding the promotional-payments component under the cooperative pattern necessitates intermittent, short-term visits by project staff to the various program sites. The CP component would entail ongoing training, supervision, and resupply through monthly meetings that could, in principle, be managed by the current medical, nursing, and block education staff of each primary health center. Pilot experiments are now in progress using this format. Success depends heavily on the interest and dedication of the chief medical officer and his or her ability to motivate staff. If this program were to be extended, a private-agency staff could provide some technical assistance, visiting government facility sites on a rotating basis from time to time. But major responsibility for implementing and administering the CP component—selection of CPs, training of CPs, field supervision of CPs, and the like—would have to be assumed by the government staff itself. It is not clear to us that government personnel in the primary health centers have a genuine interest in fielding the CP component to the extent that they would be prepared to commit the necessary time, attention, and effort to it. Part of the problem, as with the promotional-payments component, is the government family planning program's almost exclusive focus on sterilization targets, with very little interest and confidence in the ability of their generally poor and illiterate clients to voluntarily choose and use a temporary method. Another problem is that, on paper, the CPs are not needed, since the existing multipurpose health workers are supposed to distribute temporary methods (although their target of 30 pill acceptors for a catchment area of 5,000 population exemplifies how little importance is attached to this effort).

Conclusions

Each of the four phases of the Ammanpettai program have yielded important information for developing and testing the introductory incentive concept to encourage use of temporary methods of contraception. Measures of program performance to date support the validity of the hypotheses that led to the program development. Preliminary cost effectiveness and financial sustainability data appear favorable. In Phase I, small monthly cash incentives brought large numbers of rural, predominantly illiterate women to a clinic where they learned about and procured supplies of condoms or pills for the first time. Follow-up of this program revealed that continuation rates were independent of the duration of monthly payments, which varied from 6–18 months, suggesting that introductory incentives were serving a promotional or marketing rather than a conditioning function.

In Phase II, a carefully controlled study showed that small monthly incentives of 20 rupees per acceptor for five months drew more than 70 percent of eligible women to a clinic for maternal and child health care and family planning information and supplies, whereas an offer of exactly the same services from the same clinic without incentive payments to a matched control population drew almost no women. However, subsequent delivery of condoms and pills by village resident contact women to both populations was successful in maintaining approximately equal numbers of clients in both incentive and nonincentive villages. Follow-up population-based surveys indicated that the quality of knowledge was better and the number of users was greater in the incentive villages.

In Phase III, trials of a single introductory payment or appointment of village resident contact women without antecedent client payment were successful in recruiting acceptors, but knowledge of contraceptives and evidence of use of condoms or pills were not equal to those of Phase II introductory-incentive graduates.

Finally, in Phase IV, the attempt to introduce the introductory incentive program in urban and rural government clinics has yielded mixed results. In the urban setting provided by Madras City, the program has been adopted by the government and is rapidly being scaled up, implemented entirely by the staff of government facilities. Operating in rural clinics in Thanjavur, with the support of our program staff, the program has enrolled large numbers of acceptors of temporary methods. However, unlike the situation in Madras, the staff of these rural government facilities does not entirely implement the program; our staff continues to play a major role in implementation. This raises some problems for scaling up the coverage of the program.

It is evident that introductory promotional incentives do overcome disinterest, inertia, and passivity, drawing large numbers of poor and illiterate women to a clinic where they hear about available contraceptive methods and can obtain a temporary method. Approximately half of those who accept the pill packet and introductory payment do not continue or may not even start to use the method they take home, but all clients have learned about the method, held a packet of pills or condoms in their hands, and know where they can be obtained and how they are used. During this visit to the clinic, the new acceptor is surrounded by a crowd of her own neighbors—her peer group—who, by their very presence, give sanction to an activity she might otherwise be reluctant to undertake alone. Finally, in the rural areas, the great majority of acceptors work in the fields whenever work is available: The introductory incentive of 15 rupees compensates for the loss of a day's wage, which most of these women would otherwise be unwilling to forgo. In the village, a local contact person who does not implicitly or explicitly "out-rank" the acceptors or pressure them to undergo sterilization is ready to supply their needs, clear their doubts, and answer their questions.

Introductory incentives may be particularly suited to communities where young married women's activities are severely restricted by husbands and in-laws; this is especially true where there is a strong tradition of female submission or subordination to the husband and his family, and also where, as in India, poor rural women of "backward" castes often feel intimidated by government workers. Thus, many women distrust government primary health centers and outreach workers who frequently deal rudely and harshly with them. To some extent, the small introductory incentive serves to diminish the timidity these women must overcome in order to challenge powerful traditional restrictions on their mobility and choices. In that sense, introductory incentives must be seen as much less coercive than the conditions under which poor rural women already live.

Notes

1. In 1985, 1 rupee = US$.07; presently, 1 rupee = US$.04.

2. These surveys and their analysis were carried out under the supervision of R. Subramanian, Director, and C. Sivapragasm, Lecturer, Department of Research, Centre for Research, Extension and Integrated Rural Development, The Gandhigram Rural Institute (deemed University), Gandhigram 624 302 Tamil Nadu, India. Findings are reported in Srinivasan et al. (1990).

3. Ideally, to compare this cost with the current expenditures in this domain the comparison would be with prevailing rates of budgeted expenditures for family welfare in Tamil Nadu. As the medical, public health, and family welfare budgets in India are functionally comingled although separately titled, it is not possible to separate these budgets into resource commitments to health or family welfare services. Taking as the budget for comparison the sum of Account 2211 Family Welfare and Account 2210 Medical and Public Health, the Revised Estimate for 1987–88 comes to about 736 million rupees. For readers interested in consulting the budget documents, see *Detailed Demands for Grants 1988–89*, 18 Medical, 19 Public Health, 49 Water Supply, budget Publication of the Government of Tamil Nadu. The Revised Estimate under Demand 18 Medical is about 610 million rupees, none of which has been included in the 736 million rupees reported in the text, although some part of Demand 18 Medical also should be allocated to family welfare.

4. By counting only the additional (marginal) budget costs, we make the assumption that the primary health center staff can implement the promotional-payments program without decreasing their provision of other services (that is, that in this sense, some excess capacity exists). To the extent that this is not true, these budget costs are understated. On the other hand, they may be overstated if the promotional payments should prove a much more powerful strategy for discharging various functions now budgeted for existing program activities, such as mass media, field staff motivators, and so on. The economic cost of the promotional payments component is much less than the budget cost, because the amounts budgeted for promotional

payments do not represent an economic cost. These payments do not represent a claim by the program on real resources (such as labor and materials), which might alternatively have been utilized by some other economic activity. Thus, these payments do not represent an "opportunity cost" in the form of forgone outputs from other economic activities. Rather, these payments are what is known as "transfer" payments—from whoever would pay for the program if it were ongoing (e.g. taxpayers), to the participating beneficiaries who receive the promotional payments. The economic cost of the program is particularly relevant for cost-benefit analysis, or cost-effectiveness variants on such analysis.

References

Chomitz, Kenneth M. and Nancy Birdsall. 1990. "Incentives for small families: Concepts and issues." *Proceedings of the World Bank Annual Conference on Development Economics, 1990*. Washington, DC: World Bank.

Cleland, John and W. Parker Mauldin. 1991. "The promotion of family planning by financial payments: The case of Bangladesh." *Studies in Family Planning* 22, 1: 1–18.

Cuca, Roberto and Catherine S. Pierce. 1978. *Experimental Efforts in Family Planning: Lessons from the Developing World*. Baltimore: Johns Hopkins University Press.

David, Henry P. 1982. "Incentives, reproductive behavior, and integrated community development in Asia." *Studies in Family Planning* 13, 5: 159–173.

Enke, Stephen and Bert D. Hickman. 1976. "Offering bonuses to reduce fertility." In *Population Public Policy and Economic Development*. Ed. M.C. Kelley. New York: Praeger. Pp. 191–210.

Hande, H.V. 1984. "Seven Years of Progress of Health and Family Welfare Services in Tamil Nadu." Report to the 10th Joint Conference of the Central Council of Health and the Central Family Welfare Council, New Delhi, July 1984.

Loza, S.F., H.A. Sayed, and L.S. Potter. 1990. "Oral contraceptive compliance and continuation in Egypt: Complementary findings of DHS and focus group research." Report to USAID and the National Population Council, Cairo, Egypt.

Perkin, G.W. 1971. "Non-monetary commodity incentives in family planning programs: A preliminary trial." *Studies in Family Planning* 1 (57) 12–15.

Potter, Linda, Malcolm Potts, Gary Grubb, and Mark Steiner. 1991. "What do we know about how women take the pill?" (Unpublished).

Repetto, Robert. 1968. "India: A case study of the Madras vasectomy program." *Studies in Family Planning* 31: 8–16.

Ridker, Ronald G. 1980. "The no-birth bonus scheme: The use of savings accounts for family planning in South India." *Population and Development Review* 6, 1: 31–47.

Rogers, E.M. "Incentives in the diffusion of family planning innovations." *Studies in Family Planning* 2: 241–259.

Seaton, Brian. 1985. "Noncompliance among oral contraceptive adopters in rural Bangladesh." *Studies in Family Planning* 16, 1: 52–58.

Srinivasan, K. D.A. Pandey, V. Ramamurthy, and A. Krishnamurthy. 1990. "Experimental Bonus Scheme for Promoting Spacing Methods in Slums of Madras City." Deonar Bombay: International Institute for Population Sciences.

Srinivasan, K., P.C. Saxena, T.K. Roy, and R.K. Verma. 1991. "Effect of family planning program components on contraceptive acceptance in four Indian states." *International Family Planning Perspectives* 17, 1: 14–24.

Veatch, Robert M. 1977. "Governmental population incentives: Ethical issues at stake." *Studies in Family Planning* 4: 100–108.

Acknowledgments

The authors gratefully acknowledge the collaboration of Lakshmi Alber, Albert Charles, Laura Mahendran, Umayal Das, and all members of the Stella Maris Clinic staff in Ammanpettai; Sheila Sekar, Hyma Balachandran, and Chandra Gariyali in Madras; and R. Subramanian and C. Sivapragasm of Gandhigram Rural Institute, without whose ideas, cooperation, and assistance this project could not have been carried forward.

Operations Research on Promoting Vasectomy in Three Latin American Countries

Ricardo Vernon

Vasectomy is one of the least known and least used family planning methods in Latin America and the Caribbean: Even though vasectomy is simpler and usually less expensive than female sterilization, as of 1991, just 0.7% of Latin American married couples of reproductive age were protected by vasectomy, and the proportion reached at least 1% in only three countries (Brazil, Guatemala and Mexico).[1]

The recent success of some programs in promoting vasectomy, however, suggests that the procedure's low prevalence results more from an inadequate supply of services than from a lack of demand. In Colombia, for example, the number of vasectomies performed by Profamilia, the country's primary family planning organization, increased from 92 procedures in 1970 (when the method was first introduced) to 1,064 in 1973; however, after Profamilia began offering female sterilization, the annual number of male operations decreased steadily, falling to 480 procedures in 1981. This number did not increase appreciably until 1985, when Profamilia opened its first two clinics for men; in that year, a total of 1,241 vasectomies were performed. The number of vasectomies continued to increase through 1992, when the annual number stood at 5,872.[2]

The situation in Mexico followed a similar pattern. From 1980 to 1988, the Mexican Social Security Institute (the Instituto Mexicano de Seguro Social, or IMSS) performed fewer than 5,000 vasectomies per year. In 1989, the IMSS launched a program to open at least one no-scalpel vasectomy training center in each state. By September 1994, 44 centers had been established, 116 physicians had been trained in the technique and 93 outpatient clinics offered no-scalpel vasectomy. Consequently, the number of vasectomies performed by the IMSS increased from 6,283 in 1989 to 16,882 in 1993. At the same time, the ratio of female to male procedures decreased from 21:1 in 1989 to 10:1 in 1993.[3] Thus, the experiences in Colombia and Mexico suggest that men respond when vasectomy services are made accessible.

Reproduced with the permission of The Alan Guttmacher Institute from *International Family Planning Perspectives* 1996. 22,1:26–31.

This article presents information collected in six operations research projects in Brazil, Colombia and Mexico:

- The Brazilian agency Promocão de Paternidade Responsável (PROPATER) evaluated a mass media vasectomy promotion campaign by one of its São Paulo clinics in 1985.[4]
- The Colombian agency Profamilia evaluated male-oriented clinics and promotion campaigns at six clinics in medium-sized cities in 1988–1989.[5]
- The Mexican fertility research organization Centro de Investigación Sobre Fertilidad y Esterilidad (CIFE) assessed the effects of worksite talks and brochure distribution on clients of a Mexico City clinic in 1988–1989.[6]
- The IMSS, which provides medical services to employees and their families, examined the effectiveness of informational videos and of male promoters at six of its clinics (four in Mexico City and two in provincial cities) in 1994.[7]
- The International Planned Parenthood Federation affiliate in Mexico, MEXFAM, conducted a small follow-up survey of vasectomy acceptors in a Mexico City clinic in 1988.[8]
- The Mexican social marketing research organization Mercadotecnica Social Aplicada (MSA) evaluated the impact of a vasectomy promotion campaign at a Mexico City clinic in 1988.[9]

The main characteristics of the projects are presented in Table 1. These projects tested various vasectomy promotion strategies, collected service statistics and conducted quantitative and qualitative follow-up studies of acceptors. The data collected may prove useful in the design and marketing of vasectomy services in these and other Latin American countries, specifically by identifying the market segment of potential vasectomy clients, describing the vasectomy decision-making process, and assessing the effectiveness of several service delivery and promotion strategies.

Characteristics of Acceptors

Identifying the characteristics of potential vasectomy clients is an indispensable first step in targeting promotional campaigns and designing appropriate service delivery strategies. To uncover who potential acceptors might be, we have only to look at current users. The service statistics and follow-up studies in the six operations research projects show that acceptors average 32–35 years of age, with over 70% aged 28–40. Men who choose vasectomy have relatively high levels of education (at least some secondary schooling) and relatively small families of fewer than three children, with their youngest child aged 2–5 (i.e., beyond the peak ages of child mortality). They tend to live in large cities. Almost all vasec-

Table 1. Selected characteristics of six operations research projects on vasectomy in Brazil, Colombia and Mexico

Country and agency	Interventions tested	Service delivery sites	Data sources
Brazil PROPATER (see reference 4)	4 ads ran in monthly news magazines with an estimated target readership of 4.4 million men >30 years of age. A precampaign promotion (using news reports and interviews on radio, TV, daily newspapers and advertising weeklies) was conducted to coincide with international conference on sterilization counseling.	1 São Paulo clinic	Clinic admission forms for 10,266 clients; clinic records of 7,403 vasectomy acceptors and records of 4,393 telephone calls and 386 letters.
Colombia PROFAMILIA (see reference 5)	Male services (urology, vasectomy, sexually transmitted disease treatment, ambulatory surgery) were offered by specialized personnel in two settings—an exclusively male context (1 male clinic and 1 clinic that followed a male-only, segregated schedule) and a traditional, female-oriented context (2 clinics). Each conducted a media campaign with radio and newspapers, and a promoter conducted information, education and communication activities. Two clinics were designated as controls.	1 clinic each in 6 mid-sized cities—Manizales, Ibague, Pasto, Pereira, Neiva and Bucaramanga	Clinic histories of 628 vasectomy acceptors; follow-up survey of vasectomy acceptors (N=306); 3 focus groups (1 group each in 3 clinics); service satisfaction survey with clients at all six clinics (N=736); clinic accounting records.

(continued on next page)

Table 1 (continued). Selected characteristics of six operations research projects on vasectomy in Brazil, Colombia and Mexico

Country and agency	Interventions tested	Service delivery sites	Data sources
Mexico			
CIFE (see reference 6)	Worksite talks and brochures given by 8 promoters to publicize vasectomy services offered by a private physician.	1 Mexico City clinic	Survey of persons who attended talks or received brochure (N=3,589); follow-up survey of vasectomy acceptors (N=50).
IMSS (see reference 7)	In 2 clinics, vasectomy information video shown in waiting rooms; in 2 clinics, acceptors were trained to promote vasectomy and refer friends for information and services; delivery personnel of these 2 clinics and nearby ones also received a talk and survey manual on vasectomy, and were asked to refer potential clients. 2 clinics served as controls. (All six used promotional posters and brochures.)	4 Mexico City clinics, 1 clinic in Pachuca and 1 clinic in Ciudad Juárez	Follow-up survey of vasectomy acceptors (N=444); survey of married male clients aged 18–55 at all 6 clinics (N=421); survey of married survey women clients aged 18–49 at all 6 clinics (N=524).
MEXFAM (see reference 8)	None.	1 Mexico City clinic	Follow-up survey of vasectomy acceptors (N=37).
MSA (see reference 9)	Advertising on billboards and in community newspapers; male promoter for clinic's services for men, and for vasectomy in particular.	1 Mexico City clinic	Clinic records of 259 vasectomy acceptors; 3 focus-group sessions conducted with middle-class couples not protected by sterilization; surveys of men who had requested vasectomy information (N=25) and of acceptors one hour before their operation (N=25); a follow-up survey of men who had had a vasectomy 1 month to 1 year earlier (N=50).

tomized men are married or in a union and their spouses are, on average, five years younger than they are.

A high proportion of vasectomy clients or their wives (ranging from 56% to 98%) were practicing contraception at the time they decided to have the operation, with 18–39% using methods that require male participation—i.e., the condom, withdrawal or periodic abstinence. Moreover, these men appear to feel comfortable talking with their wives about contraception and display a high sense of family responsibility and concern for their wives' health and well-being.

According to this profile of vasectomy acceptors, men who elect vasectomy do so at a younger age and have fewer children, on average, than men who chose vasectomy a decade ago.[10] Moreover, early acceptors of vasectomy tended to be of comparatively high socioeconomic and educational status, and proportionately more were protected by a contraceptive method at the time of the operation. It thus appears that as vasectomy has become more widely known and used among Latin American men, the characteristics of acceptors have moved closer to the average.

The Decision-making Process

The vasectomy decision-making process, as revealed in the surveys, follow-up studies and focus groups conducted in conjunction with the six projects, follows the four stages that accompany the adoption of any innovation in general*—awareness, information-seeking, evaluation and adoption.[11]

Early events in the awareness stage include realizing that one has reached or exceeded the desired number of children and that continued use of temporary methods is inconvenient. Another key event is finding out about vasectomy. Most vasectomy acceptors in the six operations research projects first became acquainted with the procedure through friends and other relatives, their wives, health personnel, and radio and TV.

During the information-seeking and evaluation stages, the men most often consulted their wives (74–88% of men in four projects), followed by health personnel (more than 40% of men in two projects) and relatives and friends (more than 20% in four projects). In addition, at least 11% of acceptors in four projects mentioned that they had talked with a vasectomized friend at this stage, and 26–66% of men in four projects said they knew other vasectomized men. This relatively high proportion, given the overall low prevalence of vasectomy in these countries, confirms the importance that information provided by other vasectomized men plays in the decision-making process. In fact, some focus-group participants in Colombia mentioned that the information given by vasectomized friends had been the deciding factor in their contraceptive choice.

Although vasectomy candidates also seek information from the media during the decision-making process, it is not easy to predict when the media will provide information on vasectomy. Thus, materials produced by vasectomy providers themselves are important sources of information during this stage. In the IMSS project in Mexico, for example, 62% of acceptors read the brochures they were given by their provider before they made their final decision, more than double the proportion who were exposed to information in the mass media. Finally, 44–51% of respondents in all six projects said their wife influenced their decision most, followed by the service delivery staff. Other sources seem to have had little influence in the final decision-making process.

In the Profamilia, MSA and CIFE projects, clients were asked how long they had thought about having a vasectomy before making their final decision. One-third of men in the MSA study and two-thirds of those in the Profamilia project decided within four months; fewer than 20% in both studies said the decision had taken more than one year. Thus, the length of the decision-making process seems to have been relatively short, especially compared with the mean duration revealed in a U.S. study (approximately 20 months).[12]

Since the projects used a variety of techniques and questions to explore men's reasons for having a vasectomy, their results are not strictly comparable. The data, however, suggest several important reasons. When asked to state the advantages of vasectomy, 40–90% of acceptors in the CIFE, MSA and MEXFAM projects mentioned the method's permanence and effectiveness, since they had had all of the children they wanted. The method's permanence, in fact, was the main reason for obtaining a vasectomy among just under half of the respondents in these three projects; their wife's health was cited as the main reason among 21–57% of acceptors.

In four projects, the proportions who said they had considered female sterilization ranged from 51% (in the Profamilia project) to 81% (in the IMSS project). Thus, for a majority of these men, vasectomy was the more attractive alternative. The reasons given most often for choosing vasectomy over tubal ligation were that vasectomy was simpler, easier, quicker and more comfortable (cited by 39–60% of those who had considered female sterilization). In addition, 39% of IMSS acceptors mentioned the greater safety of vasectomy compared to female sterilization as most important.

The next most commonly cited reason for preferring vasectomy over female sterilization was concern over the wife's health, mentioned by proportions ranging from 20% (CIFE) to 44% (MSA). Finally, about 10% of the respondents also mentioned a desire to collaborate with their wife and to take responsibility in planning their family. Focus-group participants talked about their wife's health, their love for their wife and the convenience of vasectomy over female sterilization and over temporary methods as reasons for preferring vasectomy.

Another influential factor in the decision was the specific surgical technique used. Thirty-nine percent of IMSS vasectomy acceptors said the no-scalpel technique made their decision easier because they feared surgery in general. Focus-group sessions conducted with nonsterilized couples by the MSA and with vasectomized males by MEXFAM also revealed fears of surgery; the no-scalpel technique could thus be an important promotional feature.

Although 10–20% of respondents in all six projects reported side effects, such as swelling and pain, almost all of the men were satisfied with the services and with the method itself. In the three projects that asked about the quality of sexual relations after the procedure, 35–52% of respondents said sex had improved. Conversely, only a negligible proportion said that the quality of their sexual activity had worsened, a finding confirmed in focus-group discussions conducted by Profamilia and MEXFAM.

Only 1% of men in the Profamilia project and 2% of acceptors in the MSA project regretted having had a vasectomy. About 75% of participants in five projects talked about vasectomy with other men or recommended it to others, and 82–96% indicated they would do so in the future. This suggests that vasectomy acceptors could be actively recruited and encouraged to be promoters for the method.

In the United States, vasectomized men are the key component of the vasectomy information diffusion network;[13] in the three Latin American countries studied here, however, family members seem to have a greater influence. In most countries, reaching the desired family size, financial reasons and dislike for other methods are the most common reasons men give for choosing vasectomy.[14] Concern for the wife's health, love for the wife and the desire to take more responsibility in family planning seem to be of particular relevance in the three Latin American countries studied. Finally, previous studies conducted in developing countries (Bangladesh, Colombia, Guatemala, India, Korea and Malaysia) and developed countries (Australia, United Kingdom and the United States, including Puerto Rico) have reported the same positive or neutral effects on libido and on the quality of sexual relations after vasectomy, and the same low proportions of men who said they regretted the procedure.[15]

Effectiveness of Strategies
The results of the promotion strategies tested in the operations research projects are not strictly comparable, for several reasons. First, the projects tested a different mix of promotional strategies, and some did not try to assess the relative contribution of each or did not employ a strong experimental design that would have enabled them to do so. Second, although most projects that used an experimental design asked acceptors how they learned about the operation, each project used different data-collection instruments, which did not systematically list the same information sources, so some men may have been offered a more limited choice than others. Thus, the proportions of men who relied on such

nonlisted sources may be underestimated. For these reasons, the results presented in this section should be considered suggestive only.

The projects that used at least a quasi-experimental design to evaluate the effects of promotional strategies found the campaigns to be effective. PROPATER, in São Paulo, Brazil, conducted a 10-week advertising campaign in weekly and monthly magazines for men, using four different ads. In the year before the campaign, PROPATER performed a mean number of 11 vasectomies per day; during the campaign, that mean rose by 76%, to nearly 20 procedures per day. In the year that followed, this number stabilized at about 17 daily, a level 54% higher than that in effect before the campaign.

Examining men's sources of information about vasectomy showed that during the 10-week campaign, 18% of new clients had seen a magazine ad about vasectomy, compared with 4% in the year following the campaign. In contrast, during the campaign, 74% of new clients said they had spoken to a clinic patient, compared with 88% in the postcampaign period, and a smaller proportion of new clients had spoken with the traditional sources of information (relatives and friends) during the campaign than afterwards.

In the Colombia project, Profamilia conducted a five-month radio and newspaper campaign to promote men's services (including vasectomy), which were offered by four clinics in four cities; each clinic had also hired a promoter to give talks in the clinics and in the communities. For comparison purposes, two clinics that used routine interpersonal promotion only were designated as controls. The average number of vasectomies performed in the four experimental clinics increased by 120% from the previous year (means of 57 and 125 procedures, respectively), while the number of procedures performed in the two control clinics increased by just 59% (from 40 to 63 per clinic).

Patient records showed that while a much larger proportion of men at the experimental clinics than at the control clinics mentioned radio as their information source (22% vs. 5%), the situation was reversed for other sources of information: clinic staff (23% vs. 27%), newspapers (3% vs. 9%) and the clinic sign (3% vs. 5%). There was virtually no difference, however, in the proportions who cited relatives and friends as their referral source (39% vs. 40%).

In the IMSS project, two clinics tested a one-year intervention using vasectomized men as volunteer promoters and an interclinic referral system from within the wider IMSS network. This intervention increased the number of vasectomies by 25% (from 375 to 470 procedures), while a comparison technique used by two clinics of making an informational video available in the waiting room increased vasectomies by 8% (from 495 to 534 procedures). Moreover, the number of vasectomies increased by 6% in two control clinics over the same period (from 694 to 738 procedures).

Other promotional campaigns in Latin America have also increased the demand for vasectomy services. For example, the family planning organization in Guatemala, APROFAM, compared three promotional approaches in 1983–1984—radio only, radio and promoter, and promoter only. In all three interventions, almost three times more vasectomies were performed than would have been expected in the absence of such a promotion.[16] Furthermore, an evaluation of a six-week multimedia campaign conducted by PROPATER found that the number of vasectomies performed increased by 80% over the course of the campaign period, and remained 55% higher than precampaign levels in the six months following the end of the campaign.[17]

Most of the experience accumulated in Latin America shows that traditional sources (relatives, friends and provider staff) usually account for the largest proportion of referrals. One way to gauge the effectiveness of promotional campaigns, especially when clinics open, is to examine the proportion of vasectomy clients who cite the campaign as their referral source. In the MSA project, a Mexico City clinic was launched with a promotional campaign that included advertisements in community newspapers and on billboards, as well as the services of a male promoter. More vasectomy acceptors reported having learned about the clinic through the billboards (44%) than by means of the clinic sign (22%), the newspaper ads (21%), the promoter and other clinic staff (15%) or relatives and friends (15%).

What makes for successful vasectomy promotional campaigns and programs? Experience in the region shows that strong program leadership is essential for success. This leadership is often achieved by setting up a team to expand vasectomy or male services. The team conducts activities that effectively show the importance the institution places on vasectomy as a method, such as establishing clinics or schedules exclusively for men, starting a strong vasectomy training program, expanding services for men, and conducting information, education and communication campaigns. In large programs, the effect that a single enthusiastic person can have on the number of vasectomies performed is often noticeable.

The experiences documented in these six operations research projects suggest that increases in the numbers of vasectomies often reflect a campaign's ability to reach large numbers of individuals who may be interested in vasectomy. Both the PROPATER and Profamilia projects showed that the social and demographic characteristics of men who responded to the campaigns did not differ substantially from those of men who came to the clinics prior to the campaign. Men who heard about vasectomy through the campaign were also very similar to those who learned about it through a traditional source. This suggests that, at least in the initial stages of the diffusion of vasectomy, promotional campaigns tend more to reach clients who are similar to previous clients, rather than to attract a new, different population of men.

The importance of targeting the appropriate audience is perhaps best illustrated by projects that have failed to do so. Unfortunately, few experiences of promotional failure have been adequately documented, and even fewer have attempted to explain the reasons for the failure. The CIFE project is an exception, however. Eight promoters were hired for one year to publicize vasectomy services offered by a private physician. The promoters gave talks and handed out brochures to mixed audiences at factories and offices. Only 55 men received vasectomies over the course of the project, and of these, only two mentioned the promoters as their referral source.

In testing the hypothesis that the campaign failed because of an inadequate targeting strategy, researchers compared the social and demographic characteristics of the target audience with those of vasectomy acceptors in the MEXFAM, Profamilia, PROPATER and MSA projects; according to the researchers' definition, men who had at least one characteristic that was not shared by 80% of the acceptors in the four other projects should not have been considered a target of the promoters' messages.

More than two-thirds (69%) of the 3,589 individuals who attended the promoters' talks or received brochures had at least one characteristic that disqualified them from the composite audience and should not have been targeted for the campaign in the first place—i.e., they were younger than age 24 or older than 52, they had not yet had at least two children, their youngest child was older than age 19, they had fewer than four years of schooling, they were unmarried or not in a consensual union, or they were already protected by sterilization (male or female).

Thus, the ineffectiveness of this interpersonal promotion strategy seems to have resulted largely from poor audience segmentation and targeting. This conclusion is strengthened when one considers that Mexican law requires all employees to be affiliated with the IMSS, which provides vasectomy at no cost to subscribers of social security insurance. This audience of factory and office workers would seem to be an inappropriate target for the services of a private physician.

The cost-effectiveness of promotional strategies is usually estimated as a ratio of vasectomies, or couple-years of protection (given that each vasectomy confers an average of 12.5 couple-years of protection), to program costs. In analyzing the cost-effectiveness of the PROPATER project, for example, researchers first assumed that the number of vasectomies would have remained at the same level in the absence of the promotional campaign; they then attributed the 54% increase to the campaign. They divided the total campaign costs by the additional number of vasectomies performed and estimated the cost per each additional vasectomy acceptor recruited by the magazine ad campaign to be US $39 (or $3.12 per couple-year of protection).

The Profamilia project provides another example. Using the same method-ology, the authors estimated the cost-effectiveness of the campaign, which used radio, newspapers and promoters, to be US $7.50 per each additional couple-year of protection. These are both just one-year returns, however. The researchers point out that cost-effectiveness needs to be estimated for longer periods of time, given the cumulative effects of referrals made by satisfied vasectomy ac-ceptors and of staff training over the following years.

Potential Demand

What is the potential future demand for vasectomy in these areas of Latin America? The IMSS project attempted to answer this question by surveying 421 male and 624 female clinic patients in the waiting areas of six of its clinics. All respondents were either married or in union; the women were aged 15–49 and the men, 20–59. Only 15% of the men and 19% of the women had fewer than six years of schooling; about 50% and 61%, respectively, had two or fewer children. Overall, more than 80% of respondents knew about vasectomy, and around 20% knew about the no-scalpel method.

Regarding contraceptive use among the women, 31% were protected by female sterilization, 2% by their husband's vasectomy and 42% by a temporary method; 25% were using no method at all. Among the men, 33% were protected by their wife's sterilization, 4% by their own vasectomy and 37% by temporary methods; 26% used no method. Among respondents protected by female sterilization, more than 11% said they had considered vasectomy during the decision-making process.

To assess the potential demand for vasectomy, respondents not protected by a permanent method were asked if they thought that they or their spouse would be sterilized in the future. A larger proportion of women than men (73% vs. 52%, respectively) replied affirmatively. When asked if they would likely choose vasectomy over female sterilization, 31% of the men said they would, but only 22% of the women said their spouse would likely do so. However, just 30% of the men and 55% of the women reported having actually discussed vasectomy with their spouse, and 21% overall said they knew a vasectomized man.

Further analysis showed that men were more likely to say they would adopt vasectomy in the future than women were to say their husband would do so. The potential demand for vasectomy is higher among men who are compara-tively young, who are more educated and who have fewer children, and it is also slightly higher among current users of temporary methods than among nonusers.

Conclusions

The data collected in these six operations research projects suggest some of the following conclusions and implications for promoting vasectomy in Latin Ameri-can cities.

- *Potential clients are a well-defined segment of the population.* These men tend to be relatively young and comparatively well-educated and have small families, steady jobs and a stable family life. Most are already using a contraceptive method, and a large proportion use methods that require their active participation, such as the condom and natural family planning. Thus, vasectomy programs should design service delivery and promotion strategies that reach and meet the needs of this specific population.

- *Informal interpersonal sources, especially wives and vasectomized men, are very influential during the decision-making process.* Vasectomy promotion efforts thus need to involve wives and vasectomized men more effectively. For example, vasectomy might be presented to women as an alternative to female sterilization—especially when they would be most receptive to such information, such as in the postpartum period. In turn, all vasectomy acceptors should be invited to collaborate in promotional efforts, taught to identify friends who may be interested in vasectomy and provided with promotional materials to distribute to friends as needed. Mechanisms for maintaining contact with these acceptor-promoters and for handling their referrals need to be developed.

- *Health care personnel are among the most consulted sources during the evaluation stage of the adoption process.* Staff thus need to be well-trained in counseling techniques and more involved in promoting vasectomy and referring potential clients. Providing minimal training to all clinic staff appears to be more effective than offering training only to those who provide vasectomy services; some clinics also tend to be much more effective in referral networks than others.[18]

- *Mass media promotional strategies tend to be effective, particularly in large cities where there are high-quality clinic services.* Because vasectomy is still in the early stages of diffusion in Latin America, mass media that reach the largest possible number of potential acceptors should be emphasized. Media that have been most effective include men's magazines, evening TV shows that cater to a male audience and radio newscasts; media with a smaller market share and those aimed at a more diversified audience, such as newspaper ads, appear to be less effective. The failure of promotional strategies seems to be more often a consequence of poor media selection rather than a lack of response among men. Efforts to identify and test other efficient media and formats should be made.

- *The reasons men give for adopting vasectomy suggest a well-defined set of vasectomy campaign themes.* These themes include: that vasectomy—and no-scalpel vasectomy especially—has many advantages over female sterilization and over temporary methods; that men elect vasectomy out of love for their wife and concern for her health, as well as out of a desire to take responsibility for and collaborate in planning their family; and that vasectomy confers peace of mind and greater sexual enjoyment by eliminating worries about unwanted pregnancy.

- *Some couples who currently do not rely on sterilization will consider vasectomy when they achieve their desired family size.* Although this conclusion is based on a relatively small IMSS study in six clinics in three cities, the strong potential demand for vasectomy in Latin America is suggested by the rapid increase in services in the few institutions in the region that have made a strong effort to popularize the method, including the IMSS and Ministry of Health in Mexico, Profamilia in Colombia and PROPATER in Brazil. Although these three countries have moderate-to-high contraceptive prevalence rates and relatively high socioeconomic indicators, the fact that the countries differ so much culturally suggests that similar demand may exist in cities of over 100,000 throughout this highly diverse region. Further studies need to be conducted to assess this potential demand.

References

1. L. Liskin, E. Benoit and R. Blackburn, "Vasectomy: New Opportunities," *Population Reports*, Series D, No. 5, 1992.

2. Profamilia, "Informe de Actividades de Servicio, Año 1993," *Boletín de Evaluación y Estadística*, No. 72, Bogotá, Colombia, 1994.

3. C. Juárez and F. Alarcón, "Prestación de Servicios de Planificación Familiar a Varones en el IMSS," paper presented at the Second Latin American Operations Research Conference, Ixtapa, Mexico, Sept. 19–22, 1994.

4. M.P.P. de Castro, B.M. de Castro and K.G. Foreit, "Measuring the Effectiveness and Cost-Effectiveness of Mass Media Promotion of Vasectomy Services," Promoção de Paternidade Responsável (PROPATER) and The Population Council, São Paulo, Brazil, 1987; and K.G. Foreit, M.P.P. de Castro and E.F. Duarte Franco, "The Impact of Mass Media Advertising on a Voluntary Sterilization Program in Brazil," *Studies in Family Planning*, 20:107–116, 1989.

5. R. Vernon, G. Ojeda and A. Vega, "Operations Research on Different Approaches for Vasectomy Service Provision in Colombia," final technical report, Asociación Pro-Bienestar de la Familia Colombiana (Profamilia) and The Population Council, Bogotá, Colombia, 1989; and —, "Making Vasectomy Services More Acceptable to Men," *International Family Planning Perspectives*, 17:55–60, 1991.

6. L. Nuñez et al., "The Effectiveness of the Private Physician and Male Promoter in the Implementation of a Male-Only Clinic," final report, Centro de Investigación Sobre Fertilidad y Esterilidad (CIFE) and The Population Council, Mexico City, Mexico, 1989.

7. C. Juárez et al., "A Strategy to Increase the Acceptance of No-Scalpel Vasectomy in Out-Patient Clinics of the Mexican Social Security System," final technical report, Academia Mexicana de Investigación en Demografía Médica (AMIDEM) and The Population Council, Mexico City, Mexico, 1994.

8. A. López Juárez et al., "A Follow-up Survey of Men Undergoing Vasectomy," final technical report, Fundación Mexicana para la Planeación Familiar (MEXFAM) and The Population Council, Mexico City, Mexico, 1988.

9. L. de la Macorra, R. Sánchez and L. Varela, "The Effectiveness of Social Marketing Strategies in the Implementation of Male-Only Clinics," final technical report, Mercadotecnia Social Aplicada (MSA) and The Population Council, Querétaro, Mexico, 1989.

10. R. Santiso, J.T. Bertrand and M.A. Pineda, "Voluntary Sterilization in Guatemala: A Comparison of Men and Women," *Studies in Family Planning*, 14:73–82, 1983; S.G. Philliber and W.W. Philliber, "Social and Psychological Perspectives on Voluntary Sterilization: A Review," *Studies in Family Planning*, 16:1–29, 1985; and M.P.P. de Castro et al., "An Innovative Vasectomy Program in São Paulo, Brazil," *International Family Planning Perspectives*, 10:125–130, 1984.

11. J.M. Bohlen, "Research Needed on Adoption Models," in W. Schramm and D.F. Roberts, eds., *The Process and Effects of Mass Communication*, revised edition, University of Illinois Press, Urbana, Ill., 1977.

12. S.D. Mumford, "The Vasectomy Decision-Making Process," *Studies in Family Planning*, 14:73–82, 1983.

13. Ibid.

14. S.G. Philliber and W.W. Philliber, 1985, op. cit. (see reference 10).

15. R. Santiso, J.T. Bertrand and M.A. Pineda, 1983, op. cit. (see reference 10); S.D. Mumford, 1983, op. cit. (see reference 12); S.G. Philliber and W.W. Philliber, 1985, op. cit. (see reference 10); M.P.P. de Castro et al., 1984, op. cit. (see reference 10); and K. Ringheim, "Factors that Determine Prevalence of Use of Contraceptive Methods for Men," *Studies in Family Planning*, 24:87–99, 1983.

16. J.T. Bertrand et al., "Evaluation of a Communications Program to Increase Adoption of Vasectomy in Guatemala," *Studies in Family Planning*, 18:361–370, 1987.

17. L. Liskin, E. Benoit and R. Blackburn, 1992, op. cit. (see reference 1).

18. A. Estrada, senior medical advisor for the Association for Voluntary Surgical Contraception, personal communication, June 1994.

Note

*According to one U.S. researcher, almost all vasectomy acceptors experience six significant events in the decision-making process—becoming aware of vasectomy, talking with a man who has had a vasectomy, deciding to have no more children, seriously considering vasectomy, deciding that temporary methods are no longer acceptable and considering vasectomy to be the best method. In addition, more than half of the men who elect vasectomy do so after a pregnancy scare (see reference 12).